The Patients

Also by Jürgen Thorwald

The Century of the Surgeon

The Triumph of Surgery

Science and Secrets of Early Medicine

The Century of the Detective

Crime and Science

The Patients

Jürgen Thorwald

Translated by Richard and Clara Winston

A Helen and Kurt Wolff Book

Harcourt Brace Jovanovich, Inc.

New York

ISBN 0-15-171300-6
Library of Congress Catalog Card Number: 72-78461
Printed in the United States of America
First published in Switzerland under the title *Die Patienten*
B C D E

With this experimental work as a background it was decided to attempt to apply the data to a patient suffering from coronary sclerosis. To select a satisfactory case was not without difficulty, and then to have the selected patient give his consent to have an operation performed on his heart (an operation that had never been done before on a human being) required something of the heroic spirit. For this reason I wish to mention the name of the patient, Joseph Krebmar of Chardon, Ohio. I believe he has made a contribution to surgery. —Claude S. Beck, M.D.

Annals of Surgery, November 1935

Despair stalked before us. . . . I remember saying to my team that we could do only one of two things—give up or go on. . . . The great pressure to aid the development of mitral valve surgery came not from the doctors, but from the patients who, in their frustrated desires to obtain help in their disability, brooked no interference.

—Sir Russell Brock of London in a symposium
at Henry Ford Hospital, Detroit, 1955

Contents

Illustrations

Esperanza del Valle Vásquez, 1966
Associated Press

Esperanza del Valle Vásquez with her son, Pepe, 1970
Martha Low

Editorial Note

This book is based on a variety of source material, collected and selected over a number of years. Articles in the medical and general press, reports at medical conferences, letters of physicians to the press or to colleagues, to which the author was given access, have been used and quoted from. Whenever the source is not fully identified, this conforms to the wish of the person quoted.

The main material, however, is drawn from personal interviews with patients, their families, friends, and physicians, undertaken for the author by highly qualified researchers in Europe and America.

A number of deletions, corrections, and additions prepared by the author for German revised editions have been incorporated into the English translation.

Mended Hearts

To operate on a "blue baby" and to give to it a whole new life has become an everyday occurrence, and the name of the inventor of the operation, Dr. Alfred Blalock, is famed the world over. He and the surgeons who followed him know, however, that they owe their success to the small beings on which they tested the operation which, at the time, was considered a bold experiment. As these children stayed alive and grew into adults, they furnished the doctors with the knowledge from which we profit today.

—Dr. Marcus Schneider, in an address of 1966

1 / Marvin Mason
Eileen Saxon
Barbara Rosenthal

Marvin

When Marvin Mason was born in ancient St. John's Hospital in Brooklyn on July 15, 1938, he looked like a healthy baby. He weighed six and a half pounds, was neither premature nor late, had dark hair like his father and beautiful eyes like his mother, and cried as vigorously as a baby should. His father, Lewis M. Mason, had just lost his post-office job and was pounding the pavements of New York day after day, like thousands of other victims of the Depression, looking for work. He did not know how he was going to pay the rent, the doctor, and the hospital bills. But he was young, tough, and healthy, for all that he was a slight fellow. And he felt that things could only look up.

He had been hoping for a son. As soon as the call from the hospital came, he took the subway to St. John's. He embraced Ruth, his young wife, whom he had met and married in Atlanta only a year ago, and looked contentedly at his son. Ten days later he brought Ruth and Marvin home to their apartment.

Lewis Mason proved to be a devoted father, who never left in the morning without saying good-bye to Marvin and never failed to go straight to Marvin's crib the moment he came home. He was sure the baby was going to be a remarkable boy. Then one evening his wife greeted him with the news that the baby's lips and fingers had suddenly turned blue while she was bathing him. Lewis thought Ruth must have done something wrong. But he soon realized that it was not her fault, for Marvin's lips, fingers, and feet became blue when he himself took care of the bath or fed the infant.

At first the two of them attributed the trouble to the muggy summer heat. But then they began to worry and decided to take Marvin to a doctor. Ruth appealed to an uncle who lived in Manhattan and had a pediatrician friend who might not ask too much for a consultation.

3

In August they took Marvin to the doctor's office and looked on anxiously while he examined the crying baby. When he finally laid his stethoscope aside, he told them: "I'm sorry, but the child was born with a heart defect. . . . I'm afraid you must adjust to the idea that he isn't going to live long—at most another six months."

"That's impossible!" Lewis burst out. "There's nobody in our whole family ever had a weak heart. Examine him again. Please."

The doctor shook his head. "The result would be just the same," he said. "And there's nothing I can do about it. There's nothing to be done about this kind of defect. It's just one of those bitter things we have to accept."

Lewis's shock at learning that their baby had something fatally wrong with him turned to anger at this doctor who would let Marvin die without trying to do anything. He swooped up the baby and, followed by his wife, hurried out of the office.

The two of them did not calm down until they were back home. Then they thought of going to another doctor. But they were both afraid that a second doctor might only confirm the terrible verdict they had just heard. And so they decided simply not to believe it and to give the baby the best possible care. They checked Marvin's weight every day, and when at last, in December, the child for the first time was able to hold up his small dark head without support, they felt they had cause to celebrate.

But when the stormy and wet New York winter of 1938–39 began, Marvin's whole body took on a bluish color. The strange tint remained even when he lay quietly in his bed. As soon as he cried, he turned dark blue. Around this time Lewis learned that Ruth's father had suffered from a heart murmur all his life. And two of Ruth's siblings had been born with their hearts on the right instead of the left side of their bodies. But neither had ever been sick and their hands or bodies had never turned blue. So whatever was wrong with Marvin must be something different.

In the spring Lewis came upon a magazine article entitled "Blue Babies." It dealt with a highly complicated disease, and Lewis found the article rather hard to understand, even though the writer tried his best to explain how the human heart functioned. He described the heart as a carefully constructed pump that forces the blood through a system of pipes. The "pipes" that lead from the heart into the body are called arteries; those that return the blood to the pumping heart are the veins. On its way through the arteries the blood carries oxygen to all parts of the body, from the brain to the toes. The oxygen keeps the body alive. At the same time the blood takes up carbon dioxide from the cells of the body. When it streams through the body rich in oxygen, it is glowing red; when it is loaded with carbon dioxide and without oxygen, it is purple to dark blue in color. After returning to the heart, the article explained, the blood is pumped through the lungs, where it gives up its carbon dioxide and obtains fresh oxygen. When the lungs inhale, they suck in fresh oxygen for the blood, and in exhaling get rid of the carbon dioxide.

Next, the article described the auricles and ventricles of the heart. The author began with the first of the two auricles, or atria, the one in the upper right quadrant of the organ. Two large veins carry the blue, carbon-dioxide-laden blood from the body into this auricle. From here the blood flows through a flap valve that has three points, or cusps—for which reason it is called the tricuspid valve—into the right ventricle. The contractible walls of the ventricle can squeeze the blood out again. The right ventricle pumps the blood through a second valve, the pulmonary valve, into an artery leading to the lung. Thus the blue blood reaches the lung and flows from it newly charged with oxygen and bright red once more, through the two pulmonary veins back into the pumping heart. These veins now lead to the left auricle, and from this through the mitral valve to the left ventricle. The walls of this chamber are the strongest of all, for its task is to pump the oxygen-rich blood through the body. To do so it forces the blood through a fourth valve—the aortic valve—into the thickest artery of the body, the aorta, whence many main and subsidiary arteries branch off to various parts of the body.

The man who had written this article obviously knew a good deal. But when he tried to explain what blue babies were, he got into difficulties. He had to describe a considerable number of malformations affecting the heart of a blue baby from birth. One of these defects consists of holes in the septum, or dividing wall, between the left and right ventricles. According to the author, nobody knew what caused these holes in certain babies. In any case, the blue, oxygen-poor venous blood flows or seeps through the holes from the right ventricle into the left, which is supposed to contain only red blood full of fresh oxygen from the lungs. Red and blue blood mingle, and, instead of pure oxygenated blood, the heart of a blue baby pumps this mixture through its body, which therefore never receives as much oxygen as it needs.

There is another possible defect. If the valve through which the blue blood from the right ventricle is pumped into the pulmonary artery and on into the lung is too narrow, too little blood reaches the lung. Thus the left ventricle receives too little red blood from the lungs.

The article admitted that doctors were only beginning to investigate all the varieties of "blue-baby disease." But the description of these two principal defects gave Lewis some notion of what Marvin's trouble was. Obviously, the baby's blood was not receiving enough oxygen, and this was why he did not look as pink as other babies. The article ended by stating that many blue babies died within a few months. Others lived longer, but as children every exertion was difficult for them and caused their lips, hands, and feet, or their whole bodies, to turn blue. All ultimately died of heart failure or cardiac infections. A very few attained the age of fifteen or twenty—a particular tragedy, the article concluded, because so many of them were handsome and intelligent children.

The whole tone of the article was gloomy. But for a man of Lewis Mason's fighting temperament, the article seemed encouraging. If blue babies could reach the age of fifteen or twenty, why should Marvin not be one of those destined to live at least that long? And by then science might have found some way to repair the defects. Lewis managed to inject this confidence into Ruth, and both agreed that their Marvin was one of those handsome and intelligent children the article mentioned. They must do their best to care for him, and must also be careful not to miss any story about some new possibility for saving Marvin.

In March 1939—by then Marvin weighed thirteen pounds and had learned to sit up—Ruth received a piece of news from her mother, who lived in Baltimore. There was a woman physician at the Harriet Lane Home for Children at Johns Hopkins University, her mother wrote, a Dr. Taussig, who was said to be one of the foremost specialists on blue babies in the country.

Lewis and Ruth seized on the chance. Since Lewis had just found a job in New York and dared not take time off from work, Ruth wrapped her baby in a warm blanket and took a Greyhound bus for Baltimore.

From the recollections of a former nurse at the Harriet Lane Home for Children in Baltimore:

"It was at the end of March or the beginning of April 1939 that I first saw Marvin Mason and his mother at the clinic. I was struck by the boy at once because of his marvelous dark eyes and because I had the feeling that his mother was a woman prepared to go through hell for her son.

"The Harriet Lane Home, one of the children's clinics of the Johns Hopkins Medical School, has 113 beds, and its outpatient clinic was then, as it is now, always filled with a great many parents and children—it treats as many as 60,000 children a year. The building was an old one, dating from 1912, and we called the outpatient clinic, which was open from early in the morning until midnight, 'the Pit.' The Depression was still not over. Mothers and fathers who had brought their children often sat waiting all day long before their turn came. Most of them could pay little or nothing.

"Dr. Helen Taussig had taken over the heart clinic in 1930, and around 1937 word went around that she was particularly interested in children born with cardiac defects. At that time she was about thirty-nine and some of her fellow doctors thought of her as a suffragette. Her father was a professor of economics at Harvard, and she had studied medicine in the days before Harvard admitted women medical students. For that reason she had taken her anatomy courses at Boston University. There Dr. Begg, the anatomist, had once tossed the heart of an ox to her with the remark that it would do her no harm to study it. That was the beginning of her career as a heart specialist. She had come to Johns Hopkins because women were allowed to work there.

"Compared with our present knowledge, precious little was known about heart diseases in those days. Aside from the stethoscope, X rays, and a rather primitive electrocardiograph, there were virtually no instruments in a cardiac laboratory. Nevertheless, Dr. Taussig had profited from her wide experience at the clinic. In examining a great many children, she had repeatedly encountered the same pattern of symptoms. Ultimately, the blue babies attracted her special attention. A Frenchman—Fallot, I think his name was—had described the blue-baby syndrome earlier. But on the whole not much was known about it. From around 1938 on, more and more blue babies were brought to the clinic.

"I think Dr. Taussig must already have had some idea of how the poor infants could be helped. It was obvious that medicines would not do; somehow, the heart defect would have to be repaired. Yet if anyone had declared at the time that twenty years later surgeons would be cutting open living hearts and operating on them, he would have been called a dangerous fool. And not even Dr. Taussig had the imagination to indulge in such visionary dreams. But from observation of blue babies she had made a remarkable discovery.

"In addition to blue-baby disease, there are quite a number of other heart defects in children. One of these is called the open ductus arteriosus, or open ductus Botalli. It is not until birth that the child begins lung breathing. For this reason, the lungs are not supplied with blood so long as it is in the womb. It is the task of the ductus arteriosus to prevent the supplying of blood to the lungs by diverting the blood stream, before it reaches the lungs, directly from the pulmonary artery to the aorta. In some children the ductus does not close, as nature intends, after birth. It remains open. This also occasionally happens to blue babies—in addition to the other heart defects they have. In such a case the condition of the babies ought to be even worse. But in practice the opposite happens. They are better off than others, and Dr. Taussig grasped the reason for this contradictory situation.

"The open connection permits part of the oxygen-poor mixed blood, which the left ventricle of blue babies pumps into the aorta, to return to the lungs. There it has a second chance to take up oxygen. Dr. Taussig's conclusion was simple. She assumed that blue babies could be considerably helped if an artificial connection could be established between the aorta and the pulmonary artery. At the time she had no idea of how such a connection could be made. For the present it was just an idea, and for the time being Dr. Taussig and her assistants and students merely continued observing as many blue babies as they could, and noting their findings.

"The mothers who brought their children to us did not realize, of course, that we had no cure to offer and that their babies were merely guinea pigs who might teach us how to arrive at some solution in the future."

On March 25, Ruth Mason carried Marvin up the six steps at the entrance to the rather depressing Harriet Lane Home for Children. She was sent to a large room with beds and examining tables separated by curtains. There were also chairs and benches on which mothers and fathers sat waiting with their children until a nurse behind a desk called them.

Ruth undressed Marvin so that he would be ready for the examination. She wrapped him in his blanket, and then she waited patiently hour after hour until her name was called. She carried Marvin behind one of the curtains, but she saw nothing of the woman doctor her mother had spoken of. Instead, a young male doctor applied his stethoscope to Marvin. He was followed by other young doctors, who likewise listened to the baby's breathing, until Marvin began screaming in fear and turned blue. Finally Ruth was told to come back at the beginning of April. The young doctors did not say what they had learned or whether they could help Marvin.

From then on, the way between 3314 Garrison Road, where Ruth's mother lived, and the blocklike buildings of the Johns Hopkins Hospital became all too familiar to Ruth. The trip back and forth plunged her repeatedly from hope to disappointment. It was April 24 before a nurse at last told Ruth that Dr. Taussig in person would examine the baby.

Dr. Helen Taussig was a trim, athletic-looking woman. She wore rimless glasses and her hair was parted in the middle. She knew how to deal with children, and understood that mothers were fearful about their little ones and hated to leave them alone for examination. Ruth was allowed to hold her baby and comfort him when he cried or gasped for breath. The doctor's manner gave her great confidence. She began to feel she had found the place where something would be done for Marvin.

But soon afterward all hope vanished.

Ruth Mason's recollections:

"She told me, 'I want you to have another baby right away,' and what she meant was she didn't think the child would live a year and that if I had another one right away the loss wouldn't be so hard. Well, the first doctor said six months and the second doctor said a year, maybe, and I was determined that I would do something—we weren't going to let him die. You know, when you are young like that your shoulders are a lot wider and you can carry a lot."

Ruth was supposed to bring the baby to the Harriet Lane for observation once a month. After a few weeks, Lewis, who had again lost his job in New York, also came to Baltimore. Now the couple waited together at the Harriet Lane.

Lewis M. Mason's recollections:

"There's nothing so infuriating as the way we waited and waited, hour after hour, to be called in. . . . Once when they kept the child in the hospital my wife had to be over there every day, and she brought bottles of milk to the baby, and she waited and waited and waited and never found out anything. But one particular day, we had been waiting a long time—hours—and there, up in front at that desk, there were several interns sitting around with a nurse, smoking cigarettes, talking and giggling as though they had all the time in the world. I told my wife: 'Dress the baby, we're leaving,' and we started out. Well, the head nurse came running after us and asked what was wrong. I blew my top and told her, and she said: 'You're absolutely right and I'm going to report it.' We went back the next time and it was a lot better—actually, yes, the nurse came out to the house and told us to come back."

By the autumn of 1939 they had lost their last hope that anything could be done for Marvin at the Harriet Lane. The child had grown somewhat. But he would be struggling for breath as he tried to crawl or to stand up. Lewis Mason got a job at a Navy Department office in New York; men were suddenly needed because war was brewing. The Masons therefore decided to return to New York. During the winter months they took turns sleeping, so that one or the other was always watching Marvin to make sure he did not throw off his blankets. They were afraid his heart would not hold up if he caught a cold. On one occasion they were forced to call a doctor, who said that Marvin would surely die in New York, but they might be able to keep him for a while if they moved to sunny California. Lewis Mason promptly gave up his job at the Navy Department and bought a bus ticket. After days and nights of riding, he arrived in Los Angeles and at once set about looking for a job. Ruth packed up and followed with the baby. Her mother was afraid that Marvin might not survive the long journey; but all Ruth could think of was the possibility that sunlight might help Marvin. She refused to be deterred.

Ruth Mason's recollections:

"When we first got to California, some of our relatives there insisted that it was best for the child to be put into an institution where he could be visited once a week without so much strain on us. Well, we actually did go to one to see what it would be like, but we were both against it and we hardly ever left there, so we took the baby home with us again after several days. We never liked the idea in the first place. I swore I'd never allow it, but the relatives really tried to pressure us. . . . He was such a wonderful child. Of course, he would turn blue so easily; his lips were blue all the time. I had to take him everywhere with me, and it was so hard for him to walk. He would try, bless his heart, but he'd just go a few steps and then squat down because he was all worn out. What I did—particularly so that nobody would notice that he wasn't normal—was to get him a little red wagon, and I pulled him with me everywhere I went. But he didn't live just one year, like Dr. Taussig said. We had him 1941, 1942, 1943, and 1944—all the years we stayed in California."

In the fall of 1944, Lewis Mason entered the army. Ruth decided to go back to stay with her mother in Baltimore. Once there she took the boy—now six years old—to see Dr. Taussig again. She had no inkling of what had been happening at the Johns Hopkins Hospital in the meantime.

Notes of a former intern at Johns Hopkins Hospital:

"I think the decisive moment came at the end of November 1942. The chief of the surgical division was Dr. Alfred Blalock, who at that time was relatively little known. When he was invited to Baltimore in 1941, he encountered a good deal of opposition because some people thought he was not important enough for the great medical tradition at Johns Hopkins. He was a slim, unimpressive man of forty-two who had been through a whole series of illnesses. His left kidney had been removed; he had had a bout of tuberculosis; and as recently as 1938 his gall bladder and a quantity of gallstones had been removed. This record of illnesses prompted a good many people at Hopkins to feel that he was physically not up to the demands of such an important position. Hardly anyone expected that within a few years he would make Johns Hopkins more famous than had many of his predecessors.

"By November 1942, however, his opponents had learned that they had to take him seriously. His method of treating shock with blood plasma had meanwhile saved the lives of thousands of American soldiers. Moreover, in spite of his physical ailments, he was a sometimes impatient, sometimes rough, but always sure-handed and coolheaded surgeon. And whenever he ran into difficulties there was his assistant, Vivien Thomas, a kind of alter ego, whom he had brought with him from his previous post at Vanderbilt University in Nashville. Thomas was a young black whom Blalock had discovered at a Negro high school in Nashville. Although Thomas had never studied medicine, he was one of the most gifted surgical experimenters in the country. He carried out most of the experiments on animals in Blalock's laboratories, and in addition always stood at his chief's side during operations. Blalock had not the slightest hesitation about asking him: 'Do you think that's right, Vivien?'

"In Nashville, Blalock had specialized in chest surgery, or what went by that name at the time. In 1938, Dr. Robert Edward Gross in Boston made the first successful attempt to close surgically an open ductus arteriosus, in a seven-and-a-half-year-old girl. Blalock promptly took up the operation. By the time he came to Baltimore he was among the few surgeons in the country who had carried out this operation with success several times. In other words, he had worked in the immediate vicinity of the heart.

"At the end of November 1942 he performed the first closing of an open ductus arteriosus in Johns Hopkins. Practically every doctor of any consequence gathered in the operating room, including Helen Taussig from the Harriet Lane. At the time we did not know how long she had been considering the idea of establishing an artificial connection between the aorta and the pulmonary artery, in order to provide her blue babies with more oxygen.

"Now, after Blalock had brilliantly performed his ductus operation, Helen Taussig went straight up to him and in her usual blunt manner said: 'That was magnificent work and this is a great day. But it would be an even greater day if instead of closing a duct you would implant a new one in one of my children.'

"On the whole Blalock did not usually react amiably to such approaches. He was a southern gentleman, to be sure, but he also had the very devil of a temperament. But this time, instead of getting angry, he just stared for a moment. Then he said: 'Well, if the day ever does come, what I've just done will really seem like child's play.' That seemed to close the subject. But Blalock did not forget his brief exchange with Dr. Taussig.

"Among the many experiments he and Vivien Thomas had carried out during their studies of shock at Nashville, they had tried, for one thing, to create artificially excessive pressure in the pulmonary circulation of animals. For that purpose Thomas had severed either the left or right arteria subclavia in animals and sewed the ends of the cut into the left or right branch of the pulmonary artery. I suppose I ought to explain this procedure in more detail. After leaving the left ventricle, the aorta turns in a great arch. Along this arch arise several arteries which supply blood to the left arm, the head, and the right arm. From right to left, first there is the arteria innominata, or 'nameless artery,' which splits somewhat higher up into two branches. One of these branches, called the right arteria subclavia, or collarbone artery, leads to the right shoulder and arm. The other branch, the right arteria carotis, or head artery, supplies blood to the head and brain. The next artery leading from the arch of the aorta, called the left arteria carotis, also serves to supply blood to the head. Finally there comes the left arteria subclavia, which extends into the region of the left arm.

"In their attempts to pump more blood to the lungs and so produce excessive pressure, Blalock and Thomas had never dared to establish a direct connection between the aorta and the two branches of the pulmonary artery which lead to the right and left lobes of the lungs. The aorta and pulmonary artery are quite close to each other. But the idea of opening the aorta seemed to them at the time far too bold. They had hoped to attain the same end by connecting one of the branches of the aorta with the pulmonary artery. When Vivien Thomas demonstrated that, for example, the subclavian artery could be severed without interrupting the blood supply to the arm, the way for such experiments was opened. For many small subsidiary arteries took over the task of supplying blood. Thomas had therefore severed the left or right subclavian artery in dogs and bent the stump of the artery downward until the cut surface touched the right or left pulmonary artery. Then he cut an opening in the pulmonary artery and sewed the subclavian artery into this opening. The blood stream to the lungs had promptly been increased.

"Now, after that brief conversation with Helen Taussig, Blalock recalled the experiments in Nashville. He discussed the matter with Thomas, who made the guess that it might not be necessary to establish a dangerous direct link between the aorta and the pulmonary artery, such as Taussig had in mind. Thomas became convinced that the same effect could be achieved if an artery branching off from the arch of the aorta were connected to the pulmonary artery, as he had done in Nashville. In December 1942 he began a new series of experiments on dogs. By 1943 he had performed two hundred such canine operations, by 1944 another hundred more. At first he produced in the animals the same cardiac defects that belonged to the blue-baby syndrome—in other words, he had blue-baby dogs. After he had succeeded in this end of the experiment, he shifted to connecting the pulmonary and subclavian arteries. By the beginning of 1944 he felt sure enough of his results to let me see his work occasionally. It was really incredible—as soon as the new arterial connection was established in a blue-baby dog, the animal's condition changed radically. The miserable creature suddenly came to life and began to run and play. There could be no clearer proof that its oxygen supply, though not normal, had been enormously improved. The actual heart defects, such as the holes in the septum or the narrowness of the entrance to the pulmonary artery, had not been removed. The heart was not touched. Who would have dared such an operation then! But the 'rerouting' proved enough to permit the experimental animals to lead virtually a normal life.

"But Blalock was cautious by nature. He was afraid that blue babies, with their innate handicaps, might not even be able to survive the anesthesia essential for an operation. There was another difficulty. In order to join the subclavian artery to the pulmonary artery, it would be necessary to clamp off both and thus interrupt the blood stream. He had no idea whether blue babies could endure checking of the blood stream in a pulmonary artery. During the summer and autumn of 1944, therefore, Thomas began a new series of experiments on animals. He anesthetized them and stopped the flow of blood in the pulmonary artery for varying lengths of time. And in the autumn of 1944 he assured Blalock that the risk could be taken.

"The pair then tried out the details of the operative technique on child cadavers. In the course of this work they realized how thin the blood vessels are in a child and how difficult it would be to find them. Making the sutures to connect the arteries was in itself a feat—Blalock had to work with what we now think of as primitive needles. But in the end Blalock decided to risk the operation on a child.

"I don't know when he informed Helen Taussig that he thought he had solved her problem and that the 'great day' was near if she could provide him with a small patient. On November 29, at any rate, Helen Taussig picked out a blue baby on whom Blalock agreed to try out the new procedure. As always in such initial experiments, the baby was one who had no other chance. It was a girl, fifteen months old, who had been in an oxygen tent for weeks. The tiny thing weighed only nine pounds and kept dropping from one blue fit into another and from one coma to the next."

Eileen

Almost every day, that autumn of 1944, Dorothy Saxon walked through Patterson Park in Baltimore. She was a pretty young woman of twenty-two who lived with her husband, Francis, in one of the uniform row houses on South Milton Avenue. She no longer remembered how many times in the last eleven months she had walked the distance to the park and then along the mile or more of path that ended at Johns Hopkins Hospital.

Dorothy and Francis had married in November 1941, but had not had much of each other's company since. Francis was a sheet-metal worker at the Glenn Martin aircraft plant, where bombers for the air force were being built. The honeymoon they once dreamed of had shrunk, because of the war, to a weekend in New York. Francis rarely came home from the factory before nine in the evening. And things had turned out rather badly with the child they had longed for. It was born at last, after nearly two years of marriage, but seven weeks premature. It was a girl; they named her Eileen.

Ever since, Dorothy had often thought that it was unwise to wish for anything too intensely, or to be happy about anything too soon. Every time she walked through the park she passed other mothers with their laughing or crying, crowing or screaming babies; but those children were healthy, pink-skinned or dark-skinned. Every such encounter forced Dorothy involuntarily to compare the other children with Eileen, who had been born so tiny that for four months her mother had been able to look at her only through the glass window of an incubator.

Some eight months had now passed since she had first learned, at the Harriet Lane Home, that Eileen would never be a healthy girl and would never reach the age to wear a white bridal gown—an event Dorothy sometimes dreamed of in her romantic moments.

After four months she had been allowed to take Eileen home, although the doctors recommended that she bring the baby in regularly for check-ups. Francis had noticed before Dorothy did that Eileen changed color when she was given her bottle. He had also noticed that she scarcely grew and moved with difficulty. One day, the baby lost consciousness and turned such a dark blue color that Dorothy rushed her in a cab to the Harriet Lane Home.

Dorothy Saxon's recollections, 1970:

"I heard the truth there by accident. One doctor said to another while they were examining Eileen: 'Blue baby.' I wasn't supposed to hear it. But now it was said, and I insisted that the doctor tell me the truth and explain what a blue baby was. He explained it. But at the time I understood no more than something about twenty-four hours when the heart of a newborn baby closes—that it's open before and has to close, and that this hadn't happened inside Eileen. It was a terrible shock to me. I told Francis about it that night, and from then on we brooded about Eileen's future night after night. But I couldn't give up hoping."

Eileen had spent most of June and July 1944 under an oxygen tent in the Harriet Lane Home. She would turn completely blue as soon as she was taken out of it. She weighed only nine pounds and in many weeks had gained only six and a half ounces. In July she was sent home again because all treatment seemed useless. But since October she had been placed under the oxygen tent again, because at home she would have died in a few hours or days. Her whole body was swollen. She was too weak to drink. Syringes were being used to remove blood and fluid from her cranium. There seemed little doubt that the baby was going to die.

Every day, on that long walk to Johns Hopkins, Dorothy feared that she would not find Eileen in her bed. Sometimes, early in November particularly, she thought that death might be the best thing for the poor little one.

And Francis, after learning that he was about to be drafted, had volunteered for the navy, because he wanted to pick his service, and had been sent to Norfolk, Virginia. Now Dorothy was left alone, and all her thoughts fastened upon Eileen—although only the grip of one of her tiny blue hands around a rattle revealed that there was a little life left in her. Each day Dorothy felt relieved when she approached the bed, covered with the oxygen tent, and saw that the baby's hand still held the rattle.

Dorothy Saxon's recollections, 1970:

"One afternoon in November, when I arrived at the Harriet Lane, they told me that Dr. Taussig herself wanted to talk to me. I knew she was the head of the heart section and I'd often seen her from a distance. I was frightened. In my experience, you seldom find out anything from the doctors, and if she herself wanted to talk to me it must be something important. Maybe she wanted to tell me that Eileen was dying. There were some other doctors with her. They told me what I knew myself, that all their efforts to help Eileen had been useless. But now they thought they had found a way to help her by an operation. But this was the kind of operation that had never been done before and they could only undertake it if they had my and Francis's permission. . . . Then they took a piece of paper and drew a kind of tree with lots of branches and explained that this was the heart and these were the arteries coming from the heart. They showed me how they hoped to correct the defects so that the blue blood would go away. . . . They tried their best, but how could a young woman understand all that when it was hard enough for the doctors themselves? I said I'd have to get in touch with Francis and ask him. They agreed, but told me not to wait too long and that there wasn't any other hope for Eileen."

Torn between hope and fear, Dorothy went to the Red Cross office and explained that Francis had to be given a leave because she needed him to make a decision. She did not make herself very clear, but after the Red Cross had telephoned the Harriet Lane Home the arrangements were made. A few days later Francis arrived in Baltimore, in a state of intense anxiety. He and his wife went immediately to the Harriet Lane Home for Children. They were shown in to Dr. Taussig. With her they found a diminutive doctor with a kindly face.

Dorothy Saxon's recollections, 1970:

"Dr. Taussig said she wanted to introduce us to Dr. Blalock, who would perform the operation on Eileen if we consented. Dr. Blalock had soft but big hands, so that I asked myself how he could operate on a little baby like Eileen with such big hands. But he was very patient and said it was a great risk and he didn't want to talk us into it. At the same time he said it was Eileen's only chance. We thought about it and thought about it. But, after all, we had no choice, so at last we said yes. They decided to operate on November 29. By then Francis had to be back in Norfolk. I went to the hospital very early in the morning, so I could at least see Eileen once more if it went wrong. She was so tiny. They let me walk beside her bed as far as the entrance to the operating room; then they sent me to a little room one or two floors down—with iron bars on the window and a bench. I waited there for hours and hours—I don't remember how long it was. Not a soul came in to see me—it was hard on me, because sitting all alone like that I began to realize for the first time that they were trying something absolutely new. Dr. Blalock was something like that doctor in South Africa, the one who transplanted the heart, I mean. He was trying something new, and Eileen was the first patient he had for it."

. . .

Blalock's operation began at eight o'clock. With him, aside from his assistant, Dr. Longmire, were the anesthetist, Dr. Harmel, and Vivien Thomas. Helen Taussig stood to one side of the operating table to watch this operation she had so long hoped for. Longmire afterward remarked that at the sight of the baby, so small and emaciated, weighing little more than nine pounds, with her bluish skin and glassy eyes, he had the strong conviction that the operation would fail. Harmel, too, feared surprises. How could this tiny creature with her feeble heart withstand anesthesia and an arterial operation? He had no apparatus small enough to use on the child and therefore had to work with open ether anesthesia. Blalock seemed the calmest person in the room.

Blalock began with an incision over the left breast all the way to the armpit, and then he opened the chest—no bigger than his fist—between the third and fourth ribs. When the first blood vessels were exposed, they were filled with such alarmingly viscous blood that Longmire felt all his doubts return. But Blalock only beckoned to Vivien Thomas to come a little closer. He now began a more or less blind search for the left pulmonary artery. After some difficulties, he managed to expose it. Without touching the heart, he then searched for the aortal arch and the arteria innominata branching off from it. Once more he thrust his fingers into the mediastinum, parted several tissues, and either by luck or by trancelike certainty brought the subclavian artery into the light.

Up to this point the baby's circulation had stood the shock of anesthesia and operation. But the sight of the subclavian artery gave Blalock an unpleasant surprise: the artery was unusually delicate and thin. Moreover, he had to clamp and sever several smaller arteries that were in his way before he could expose enough of it to work with. Only then did he clamp off the subclavian artery, sever it, and draw the lower end of the cut up to the pulmonary artery. The operation had already taken between forty and forty-five minutes before he was ready for the next decisive stage, dual clamping of the left pulmonary artery above and below the spot where he wished to suture the subclavian artery to it.

Blalock applied the clamps and paused to note, with obvious tension, the child's color. Even though Vivien Thomas had established that his animals survived for a long time after the flow in one branch of the pulmonary artery was checked, the appearance of the child boded ill. But to Blalock's surprise the blue coloration had scarcely deepened. Swiftly, he made an incision into the clamped-off part of the artery, introduced the end of the subclavian artery, and began the suturing. Ten minutes passed. He asked Thomas: "Are the stitches close enough together?" Thomas nodded. Twenty-five minutes more had passed before Blalock was close to finishing. It seemed incredible that there was still no deepening of the blueness. Everyone sighed with relief when the last stitch was in place after exactly thirty minutes. Blalock removed the clamps and no blood trickled through the suture. The crucial part of the operation was over—and the baby was alive.

A few seconds later, however, Blalock was assailed with fresh doubts. He had counted on additional blood pouring from the subclavian artery into the pulmonary artery to produce a tangible increase in the blood stream. But when he laid a probing finger on the pulmonary artery, he could feel nothing of the sort. Perhaps the subclavian artery, whose weakness had surprised him, was too thin to carry into the lung the increased stream of blood on which the success of the operation depended.

Blalock could not understand the absence of a reaction in the pulmonary artery. He had no choice but to wait and see. If the cyanosis—the shortage of oxygen—diminished or disappeared in the next few days, he would know his procedures had worked. If it persisted, that would be proof that the tiny diameter of the subclavian artery had not sufficed to allow enough blood to flow through. If this was so, he had two options. He could try to repeat the operation on the right side, hoping that the child's right subclavian artery would be stronger and wider. Or he would have to give up the idea of operating successfully on babies as small as Eileen and make another attempt with a bigger child.

Shortly before 9:30 A.M. Blalock sewed up the thoracic wall.

Dorothy Saxon was still waiting in the dismal small room with the barred windows. It was nearly ten o'clock when a nurse opened the door and told her: "It's over. They're bringing her down." Dorothy rushed to the door. Then she heard the baby crying—and realized that Eileen had survived the operation. "If she's crying that loud she wants to live," she told herself. "And she will live, she will."

Dorothy knew nothing of Blalock's doubts. An intern assured her that everything had gone well. They would let her know when she could come to see her baby.

Dorothy returned home at last. But she could not bear to wait patiently. Every day she came to the hospital, hoping to get news. Once she managed to reach the room where Eileen lay, separated from other babies by curtains. But she saw so many doctors there that she did not dare go in. She was not told that for two weeks Eileen had been passing from one crisis to another, and that Blalock, Helen Taussig, and several other doctors—Dr. Kay, Dr. Whitemore, Dr. Gilger—were taking turns keeping her alive.

The child had begun to have unexpected violent attacks of pneumothorax—air entering the thoracic cavity and exerting pressure on the tiny lungs. Yet her blue color seemed to be diminishing. Her left arm, which had lost an important blood vessel because of the diversion of the subclavian artery, felt somewhat cooler than the right arm, but its mobility was unimpaired. This seemed to suggest that the operation itself had been a success. But the pneumothorax attacks were followed by infections and fever.

Day after day passed, while Dorothy waited in growing anxiety. Then, about two weeks after the operation, the pneumothorax abruptly stopped. Infection and fever vanished. Eileen remained for a while longer under the oxygen tent. But within a few days she was removed from it, and did not turn nearly so blue as had been the case before the operation. Blalock and Helen Taussig continued to look in on her several times a day, because the sudden turn seemed almost too good to be true—so good that they kept fearing they might be deceiving themselves. Soon, however, Eileen showed an interest in her surroundings for the first time. She tried to raise her head, and moved the arm with the rattle, which she was still clutching tightly.

Dorothy Saxon's recollections, 1970:

"When I was allowed to see Eileen for the first time, it was like a miracle. . . . I'd never seen her with such a pink color, just like other children. She still turned blue when she kicked her feet hard. But otherwise she looked like a normal child. I was beside myself with happiness. Dr. Taussig or one of the other doctors told me it would be best from now on if I came every day, because she would recover soonest if she had her mother with her. They let me go everywhere around the hospital and gave me a white smock just like the doctors. I was able to feed Eileen and play with her. Every day it seemed to me she was making progress. She really wanted to eat for the first time, and started gaining weight. She couldn't talk yet, but she babbled as happily as other children. Her eyes, which had been dull for such a long time, were shining now. It was like she was wearing make-up. And the blue color went away from her hands. She turned back and forth, as if she wanted to show herself that she'd changed and wanted to be admired. The doctors and nurses treated her like a little princess because she proved that the new operation was a success.

"On January 25, 1945, I was allowed to take Eileen home. For the first time I felt confident that she would be a normal, healthy child and grow up to be a big girl. And I became certain of it when Eileen later pulled herself up and stood in her playpen for the first time, and when she said her first words."

Notes of a former intern at Johns Hopkins Hospital:

"Those last weeks of December 1944, when Blalock's first patient turned the corner from being on the verge of death to obvious new life, really were crucially important. They proved to Blalock that he was on the right track—although he still had certain doubts. He had held the child's subclavian artery in his hand, and he could not forget how fragile it was. He kept fearing a relapse and was emotionally preparing himself for the possible need to perform the same operation on the girl on the other side.

"Blalock decided to choose older children with stronger arteries for his next patients, so that he would be able to provide a conclusive demonstration of the value of the operation. He also considered the possibility, if he nevertheless encountered such a thin subclavian artery again, of using the arteria innominata in its place. The problem was that the innominata was the source not only of the right subclavian artery, but also of the right carotid artery. He did not know whether interrupting the carotid artery would be as harmless to the circulation of the brain as temporarily shutting off the subclavian artery had been to the supply of blood for the arm. But early in 1945 further experiments on animals convinced him and Vivien Thomas that this was the case. In other words, if necessary the innominata could be used.

"In January, after these preparations, Blalock and Taussig chose their next two patients. They were an eleven-year-old girl, B.R., and a six-and-a-half-year-old boy, M.M. They had known the boy over a long period of time. Because the parents had moved to California, he had vanished from sight for a while and they had thought him dead. When the parents returned Dr. Taussig learned that by devotion or a miracle they had kept the child alive—and brought him back to Baltimore just at the right moment."

But for the time being their attention was fixed on the girl, who had been under Dr. Taussig's care for about a year.

Barbara

When Shirley and Leonard Rosenthal set out from Buffalo to Baltimore on January 5, 1945, it was not their first trip to the Harriet Lane Home for Children and Dr. Helen Taussig.

Leonard Rosenthal was highly regarded in the jewelry trade and was considered a wealthy man. But only a few of his friends and neighbors knew that he and his wife, Shirley, carried a heavy burden of grief that wealth could not dispel. Their daughter, Barbara, born in 1933, had suffered from shortage of oxygen since babyhood. Barbara was an unusually intelligent and sensitive girl. She had suffered intensely from never being able to move freely, never being able to live and play like other children.

Two years earlier, the family physician, Dr. Dexter Levy, had recommended to Shirley and Leonard Rosenthal that they consult Dr. Helen Taussig. They had taken Barbara all the way to Baltimore. At the time the child could scarcely walk twenty yards without having to crouch down and struggle for breath. Her arms and legs, her lips, even the conjunctiva of her eyes were colored blue. Her slender fingers were so distorted by lack of oxygen that they resembled small drumsticks.

In February 1943, Barbara was admitted to the hospital for observation. Familiar as Dr. Taussig was with so many unfortunate children, Barbara made an even more piteous impression. When the child had to go up the few steps to the hallway on which her room was situated, she would start gasping for breath and rush the last few feet down the corridor, her body pitched steeply forward, to fall on her bed with knees drawn up close to her body. There she would struggle for air for half an hour before she was able to say a word. Examination had suggested that Barbara's pulmonary artery was virtually closed, and that only auxiliary arteries which had formed in the course of years served to carry some blood into her lungs. In her organism's desperate efforts to secure more oxygen, her body had produced nearly double the usual number of red blood corpuscles.

Like so many other parents, the Rosenthals had gone home to Buffalo with, for the moment, nothing more than an accurate diagnosis. Ever since, Barbara's condition had slowly but inexorably worsened. At the end of December 1944 she was no longer able to move from her wheel chair to her bed without severe shortness of breath. At this point Dr. Levy had advised another visit to Baltimore. When the parents agreed, Dr. Levy telephoned Helen Taussig and learned about the operation on Eileen Saxon. Helen Taussig proposed that Barbara's parents bring the child so that they could determine whether Dr. Blalock thought an operation possible.

The Rosenthals arrived at the Harriet Lane on January 6, 1945. They pushed Barbara in a wheel chair down the halls to Helen Taussig's office. During the subsequent tests, Barbara proved unable even to get up on the examining table without agonizedly gasping for breath. Her mouth was as blue as ink by now.

Dr. Taussig showed the parents a drawing outlining the nature of the operation and explained to them the risks and the possibilities. The Rosenthals did not need convincing. They knew that there was no other hope. Even if Barbara lived a few months more, it would be a time of torment. But before they finally made up their minds, they wanted to talk with Barbara herself.

They returned to tell Dr. Taussig that Barbara understood the risk and wanted the operation. First she would like to visit New York once more. Perhaps, the parents thought, it would be a good idea to give her this pleasure. Since Blalock intended to leave on a trip on February 7, February 3 was set as the day for the operation. The Rosenthals promised to return to Baltimore on January 29.

They arrived punctually. One of the first bits of cheerful news they heard was that Eileen Saxon had been discharged and gone home to her mother.

Blalock began his second operation at 8:45 A.M. Barbara submitted quietly to the anesthesia, with the composure of children familiar with suffering. At 9:10 A.M. Blalock made his first arc-shaped incision. Helen Taussig had warned him that he would find a tangle of morbidly altered blood vessels inside Barbara's chest. Nevertheless, he was surprised by the actual extent of the changes. The intercostal artery was unusually thick. Bronchial arteries blocked his way. Blalock encountered all kinds of difficulties before he finally located the arteria innominata. Blalock decided not to lose time exposing the subclavian artery; instead, he would connect the innominata to the pulmonary artery. In Barbara's case, it was at least one-half inch in diameter. This time, as soon as he had finished the suture and opened the clamps, his probing fingers immediately found what they had sought in vain in the case of Eileen Saxon: the pulmonary artery was expanding. Blalock distinctly felt the intensified blood stream pulsing in it.

Fifteen minutes later his second operation was over. This time he had taken two hours and forty minutes. Barbara Rosenthal awoke almost immediately. She talked, moved her limbs. There was no sign of any disturbance in the blood supply to her brain. Blalock wrote into his record: "Postoperative condition of the patient: very good."

This was no exaggeration. Barbara was kept under an oxygen tent for a few days. But within three days after the operation the morbidly high red blood corpuscle count diminished. This was the surest sign that the oxygen supply was improving. In the following days the bluish coloration of her lips, hands, and feet receded dramatically.

On March 13, Blalock, Helen Taussig, and all the nurses at the Harriet Lane accompanied Barbara to the entrance, where her parents were waiting for her. They promised to bring Barbara back for a checkup within a year at the latest. Then they went home.

As good as their word, all three came to Baltimore on February 12, 1946. Dr. Taussig noted: "Barbara R. came in today for a checkup. She looks like a million dollars. Her lips have a lovely red flush, and the color persisted even when she . . . cried during the arterial puncture. . . . She is extremely active; I was overwhelmed by her condition."

Marvin

Ruth Mason had been through several difficult months after returning to Baltimore in October 1944.

She had become so used to having her husband at her side, sharing in the care of Marvin, that she found it hard to manage without him. She had moved in with her mother on Garrison Road again. But Mother was no substitute for Lewis. Ruth's anxiety increased when the authorities in Baltimore ruled that Marvin would have to go to school, since he was now six years old. At the same time she realized how small the dependency benefits for a soldier's wife were; she would have to try to earn a few additional dollars.

Faced with so many problems, the courage she had displayed for years temporarily deserted her. The fear that she would be unable to attend to Marvin day and night made her forget the vow she had taken never to let Marvin be sent to an institution. She was so discouraged that she took a cab and for the first time in four years brought Marvin to the Harriet Lane Home for Children. She no longer believed that anyone there could restore Marvin to health. But she hoped that perhaps the people there would help her place him in some home like the Happy Hills Hospital, where he would be well cared for while she worked.

As in the past, she waited for hours before she was seen by a welfare worker and later by an intern. When the doctor looked up the name in the file, he was surprised that Marvin was still alive and noted him as an interesting case for Dr. Taussig. But he told Ruth that there was no prospect of a place in the Happy Hills Hospital. Because of the war and the fact that so many mothers were now working, all such institutions were overcrowded. Wearily, Ruth took Marvin home again. During the following weeks she found a solution on her own. She took Marvin to the William S. Baer School for physically handicapped children in the morning and fetched him in the afternoon.

Marvin was by now so weak that he could not take a step without having to rest for a long time afterward. His lips were bluish violet. He learned to read and write, but his drumsticklike fingers made all schoolwork doubly hard for him.

In December 1944, Ruth again took Marvin to the Harriet Lane, but this time, too, she did not see Dr. Taussig. A young doctor who examined Marvin sent him to the dental clinic for removal of several teeth. And there, while Ruth was waiting as usual, some of the other mothers told her about a mysterious operation on a blue baby. They had met the baby's mother and heard that the child was now much improved. Ruth could scarcely believe it, but when she at last obtained an appointment with Dr. Taussig, she decided to ask about it.

Helen Taussig was also surprised to find Marvin still living. She at once told Ruth about Dr. Blalock's operation and said there now might be a chance to help Marvin.

Lewis M. Mason's recollections:

"I was in Camp Roberts in California when I heard the news from Ruth. I felt terribly alarmed that the doctors might be rushing things, and I insisted that nothing be done until I came to Baltimore. They gave me a long leave from the camp when they heard what it was about. In Baltimore, Ruth and I went to see Dr. Taussig right away and we discussed the whole thing. But it was strange. We'd been praying for years that the doctors would find some way to correct Marvin's condition, but now that there was something, we were scared. . . . But finally we were convinced and said yes. The operation was set for February 10; we were supposed to bring Marvin to the hospital on February 7. Of course, we had to explain to Marvin why he was going to the hospital and that he would have an operation so he could be well. But he was much too little to understand it all. He told Ruth he'd go to the hospital if she'd give him something."

Ruth Mason's recollections:

"I said I'll give you anything you want for a gift, and he said, then I want a baby sister so I can play with her. Well, because of his condition I had been afraid to have another child, but I promised him, you are going to have a baby sister."

Lewis M. Mason's recollections:

"Then came the day before the operation. At the last moment we had new doubts. I remember walking the streets of the city, and we decided once and for all, no, we weren't going to do it. Let someone else be the experimental one, we decided. We've held out for years and it's best to wait a little more. We went to Dr. Taussig and told her of our decision. She said she understood our feelings, but would we first let her introduce us to Dr. Blalock. Well, she introduced us. Now, here was such a gentle, soft-spoken man. After talking to him we had such confidence and hope that we decided to go ahead. He gave us some pills and told us to get some sleep and be at the hospital at eight o'clock the next day for the operation. We arrived at seven and they had been operating since six."

Before Blalock began his third operation, on the morning of February 10, he had already decided to proceed on the right side this time, in order to explore the surgical possibilities there. After his excellent results with Barbara Rosenthal, moreover, he had determined to connect the innominata with the pulmonary artery once more.

There was one moment when human feeling broke into the coolness of the surgical world. As Dr. Harmel was giving the abnormally slight little boy on the table a last injection, Marvin whispered: "My mother's going to have a baby."

The operation began in routine fashion. But it quickly turned out that it was more difficult to expose the pulmonary artery on the right side than on the left. It seemed as if the task were taking forever. Afterward, however, everything went smoothly until it came time to clamp off the pulmonary artery. There was a hemorrhage. When this was checked, the operation proceeded without further hitch until the suturing of the innominata and pulmonary artery was complete. But when Blalock opened the clamps, blood spurted through the suture. Before Blalock succeeded in clamping the artery again, Marvin had lost a pint of blood, and he fell into shock. Hurriedly, blood plasma and glucose were administered while Blalock closed the leak with an additional suture. After some nerve-racking moments, Marvin's blood pressure became measurable again. After three hours of operating Blalock closed the opening in the thoracic wall.

In spite of the shock, Marvin awoke from the anesthesia twenty minutes after the operation in a surprisingly vigorous state. He moved his arms and legs on command, and asked in a clear voice: "Can I get up now?" It was as if he had decided in his unconscious that after the operation he would immediately be well. He fell asleep once more while he was being taken to a glass-enclosed nursery. As the stretcher rolled past Lewis Mason, who had been waiting in the corridor hour after hour, Marvin awoke for the second time.

Lewis M. Mason's recollections:

"He saw me and started calling, and do you know what the first thing he said to me was? 'Daddy, I want some water.' Well, I couldn't move, I was so happy. All I could do was look at him. He was pink, the blue was gone; his lips, his cheeks were pink."

. . .

The change in Marvin Mason was truly dramatic. On the fourth day after the operation the oxygen tent was removed. The oxygen saturation of his blood, which had been 23.4 per cent before the operation, shot up nine days later to approximately 80 per cent. The sole complication was a slight rise in temperature, for which reason Blalock and Helen Taussig kept Marvin in bed. But from the fifth day on he insisted more and more urgently on getting up.

Lewis M. Mason's recollections:

"He kept wanting to get up but the doctors wouldn't let him. . . . I remember one day in March, Dr. Taussig came in and Marvin said: 'Dr. Taussig, don't you remember you promised me I could walk today?' But Dr. Taussig said: 'Don't you want to wait for Dr. Blalock to watch?' But Marvin said: 'Well, why don't I do it first, then we'll know what he'll see?' So they opened up the drapes and put on a bathrobe and he walked off, beautiful. Dr. Taussig asked: 'Don't you feel a little weak?' and he just kept on going. They couldn't keep him down after that."

At the same time the onsets of fever stopped. On March 20, forty-one days after he had entered the hospital, Marvin was so far recovered that Blalock and Helen Taussig permitted him to go home.

Lewis M. Mason's recollections:

"By the time we took him home he had become almost like a son or a grandson to Dr. Blalock and Dr. Taussig. He was a kind of symbol of the success of their operation. We had to promise to bring Marvin in for a checkup every year. But I didn't have the heart to leave Ruth and the boy in Baltimore, and so we decided to buy a car and drive to California together. On the way we wanted to visit my parents in Atlanta and show them how well Marvin was. When we told Dr. Blalock about that, he asked us to visit his mother in Jonesboro, a few miles from Atlanta, and show her Marvin, because Marvin was the biggest success of his new operation. We were glad to do it. We bought the car and packed our things on the back seat so Marvin would be able to lie on them. Then we drove to Atlanta and Jonesboro. Mrs. Blalock lived in a white house on Main Street. We were bragging about Dr. Blalock so much, we almost considered him like a god, and you know, his parents weren't so enthusiastic as we were. Their attitude was, sure, he's great, but our other children are just as good.

"Then we drove on to California. It took us eight days. That was the happiest time in our lives. Marvin came into every restaurant with us just like a normal boy, and he kept getting stronger every day. Finally we reached Long Beach and—and then we kept the promise Ruth had made to Marvin. . . . From the start we never had any doubt it would be a girl, the way Marvin wanted. We picked out only one name, Jocelyn. She was born in 1946. The nurses at St. Mary's in Long Beach said she was pretty as a song, so we made it Jocelyn Melody, and that's what we call her, Melody."

Baltimore Sun, *May 12, 1945:*

"Hopkins doctors' new surgical method aids blue baby for the first time."

New York Sun, *December 10, 1945:*

"Their genius gave blue babies sole chance."

New York Herald Tribune, *February 15, 1946:*

"How two doctors give new life to blue babies."

From an unpublished interview with a German cardiologist on the sixth anniversary of the first three blue-baby operations (February 20, 1951):

QUESTION: Six years ago, in November 1944 and February 1945, Dr. Alfred Blalock operated on three blue babies for the first time. In spite of the Second World War his method of operation became the greatest medical sensation of these two years. How do you explain that?

ANSWER: Blalock's report on his operation was first published May 19, 1945, in the *Journal of the American Medical Association.* The fighting in Europe had just come to an end. But if the war did have any effect upon the tremendous public interest in the operation, it was because it created the proper psychological mood. There was, as it were, something like a psychological reorientation from mass killing to a desire to heal. Probably millions of people were unconsciously waiting for news of the kind that came out of Baltimore. But all this doesn't really touch the heart of the matter. Blalock was the first to treat successfully by surgical methods a hitherto incurable heart ailment and—this was what most people actually thought at the time—to cure it. Besides, children were involved, which naturally touched people on their sentimental side.

QUESTION: You were one of the witnesses to the world-wide rush to get into the act that the operation produced, weren't you?

ANSWER: Well, it certainly surprised Helen Taussig, Blalock, and especially the Johns Hopkins Hospital, which so far had always avoided publicity. Doctors came to Baltimore from virtually every country in the world. The gallery in the operating room was crammed with them whenever Blalock undertook another of his operations. When he began spraying his arterial sutures with a novel gelatin foam, dozens of Frenchmen, Englishmen, Turks, Swedes, Australians, and Chinese could be seen leaving the hospital with packages of gelatin foam and Blalock's or Helen Taussig's publications under their arms. But the storm of patients and the press was even more turbulent. Parents with sick children came to Baltimore from everywhere. The impecunious were arriving at the hospital entrance after riding in busses for days. Many of the children were not suitable for operation because they were not blue babies, but patients with simple aortic, pulmonary, or mitral valve defects. At the same time Baltimore swarmed with reporters. It became fashionable to have children sent to Blalock from all over the world at the expense of local newspapers —so that the papers could publish more or less sensational stories on the operations. Amid all this crazy publicity the fact wasn't even noticed that Blalock's first little patient had to be brought back to Johns Hopkins at the end of July 1945, after a few months of apparent improvement, because she was suffering from renewed attacks of cyanosis. And shortly afterward she died.

QUESTION: You mean Eileen Saxon?

ANSWER: Yes. I seem to recall that a few newspapers dealt with the child at the start and published some touching stories. There were mentions of every gain in weight, and stuff about how Eileen and her dog, Chin-Chin, sat on the steps of her house waiting for her father to come home—I suppose he was in service at the time and coming on leave. But when the child was brought back to Blalock and died, there was no publicity, because a failure didn't fit into that hectic atmosphere of triumph, not as far as the journalists were concerned. From the medical point of view, the result only proved what Blalock had feared during the operation. The child's left subclavian artery was too weak, and on August 1, Blalock performed a second operation, on the right side this time, because he hoped he would find a stronger artery there. But the condition of the arteries on the right side was the same as on the left—and the child died five days later.*

QUESTION: To return now to the international repercussions . . .

* After Eileen's death Dorothy and Francis Saxon had two healthy children, Patricia Adette, born on February 25, 1947, and Francis, Jr., born on July 28, 1952.

ANSWER: During 1945, Blalock remained the only surgeon to risk the operation. That year he operated on 247 children. Twenty-three per cent, approximately 60 of them, died. That ratio of mortality nowadays seems terrifying—today we have a death rate from the operation of only 5 or 6 per cent. In addition, there were many cases that showed no improvement after the operation. But since all the children were hopeless cases, saving some two-thirds of them was a sensational achievement. In 1946, surgeons outside the United States began their first operations. In 1947, Blalock and Taussig (who, incidentally, did not get on particularly well, because they had such divergent personalities) went on a veritable triumphal tour. They traveled to London, Stockholm, and Paris to introduce the operation into Europe. At Guy's Hospital in London, Blalock operated on ten blue babies without a single death. At a lecture in the auditorium of the British Medical Association, at which movies were shown in the darkened room, the scene would have done credit to a public-relations firm. A spotlight suddenly illuminated a nurse holding on her lap a blonde girl with rosy cheeks—Blalock had performed a successful operation on the child a week before. The applause was thunderous. Later, he and Dr. Taussig returned to a rousing welcome in Baltimore.

QUESTION: To come to the present, what is the state of medical opinion on the operation now, six years later? Does it provide a lasting cure and give the patients the life expectancy of a normal person?

ANSWER: It cannot lead to a normal life expectancy because the actual heart defect remains. In fact, in order to improve the oxygen supply to the body it introduces a new anomaly, the artificial connection between two arteries. But this operation does mean restoration of an almost normal life and a considerable prolongation of life expectancy for children who previously, in the best of cases, reached an average age of fifteen years. Naturally, we cannot yet say how great a prolongation of life expectancy we can count on. Only observation over a period of years can teach us that. In any case, a wholly new medical development in the past two years has opened up new prospects.

QUESTION: What do you mean by that?

ANSWER: I am referring to a revolutionary development in heart surgery prompted partly by Blalock's work, although it also goes back to other sources. Since the war a new generation of surgeons has come home, surgeons who no longer regard the heart with the same timid respect as did the previous generation—including Blalock. A man such as the young American surgeon Dwight Harken, now working in Boston, who during his military service removed 134 bullets or shell fragments from the hearts of wounded men, including 13 directly from the beating ventricles of the heart. He learned that the heart is much more resilient than was previously assumed. His experiences were shared by many doctors of his generation. They have reminded us of several forgotten surgeons who decades ago made occasional attempts to correct defects in the cardiac valves. The Parisian surgeon Tuffier tried it in 1912, the Englishman Souttar in 1925, the American Curler around the same time. All of them dealt with specific valvular defects, called stenoses, which are adhesions and other hindrances to the flow of blood that occur after rheumatic attacks. They opened the chest cavity and made a small incision in the wall of the heart. Then they swiftly thrust one finger into the opening. The finger acted like a cork, preventing the blood from spurting out. Inside the beating heart and in the midst of the swirling blood, the finger groped its way forward to the faulty valve. Then they pushed a knife along the finger and tried to sever the adhesions and thus open the valve.

QUESTION: Were they successful?

ANSWER: Partly so. In 1925, Souttar operated on a ten-year-old girl, Lily Hime, in London's East End. She was suffering from mitral valve stenosis and was on the point of death. A hemorrhage prevented Souttar from introducing his scalpel. But he discovered that it sufficed to break open the adhesions on the valve with his finger alone. The patient survived for seven years after the operation. Nevertheless, the widespread fear among physicians of any operation on the heart was so great that Souttar's experiment was rejected and forgotten until the views of the younger generation began affecting medical practice, as I've just mentioned.

About three years ago, early in 1948, the British surgeon Russell Brock at Guy's Hospital operated on a number of patients, introducing a specially constructed instrument through the right ventricle as far as the scarified pulmonary valve and trying to break the adhesion. His first patients died on the operating table. But then he succeeded in three cases in a row—the patients are still living. That same year two American surgeons, Horace Smithy in Charleston and Charles Bailey in Philadelphia, operated on the mitral valve by a similar method. Smithy succeeded four times in eliminating a cicatrix before he himself died of a defect in the aortic valve for which no operative method has as yet been discovered. Bailey, after three failures in which his patients died during or after the operation, succeeded, on June 10, 1948, in repairing the stenotic mitral valve of a twenty-four-year-old woman. His patient, Claire Ward, was able to accompany him, shortly after the operation, to the Fourteenth Congress of Thoracic Surgeons in Chicago as living proof of his success. Bailey has meanwhile experimented in repairing holes in the walls of the ventricles, those same defects that have such fateful effects upon blue babies. He has tried folding part of the auricular septa over the holes and suturing them there.

QUESTION: What are you implying by this statement? Are you suggesting there are forms of heart surgery that in the near future will replace the present blue-baby operation because they will directly eliminate the basic heart defects of the children?

ANSWER: Within limits, yes. So far all the operations have been "blind operations" in the closed, beating heart. Their possibilities are limited. In the case of large ventricles, it will never be possible to close the holes in the septa in this way, not with any real prospect of success. To do that it will be necessary to open the heart and operate directly on the septa. Brock's or Bailey's valve operations also can work only where there is a cicatrization or stenosis of the valves. With many valve defects the opposite is the case: parts of the valves have been destroyed and the valves are therefore not too narrow, but too wide, so that they no longer close. Here there is scarcely any prospect of carrying out blind repairs from outside or (though this is conceivable) of replacing parts of valves with plastics. For this purpose, too, one would have to open the heart and operate undisturbed by the heartbeat or the flow of blood. But such possibilities are actually within sight. The idea of constructing a pump that will take over the work of the heart for the duration of the operation has been under discussion for some time, and experiments are in progress in Philadelphia. If such a pump becomes a reality, it is conceivable that the heart can be by-passed by the circulating blood, briefly opened, and the deformations of blue babies repaired.

QUESTION: Aren't those dreams that will probably never come true?

ANSWER: No, I think they can come true. They contain the ultimate answer to your question about the life expectancy of blue babies as a result of Blalock's operation. We have reason to assume that their life expectancy after the operation amounts to twenty-five years, rather than the ten or fifteen years we previously counted on. That may mean that they'll live until a way is found to eliminate their heart defects directly. Blalock has thus done something that means more than merely a postponement of death—he's opened a bridge to real life for them. But only the future fate of his patients can give us any final answers.

Marvin

At Hamilton High School in Los Angeles, situated between the busy Pico and Venice boulevards, an unusually slender but lively boy with a shock of dark hair participated in the life of the school in 1952. Lewis Mason had made his way in business. He or Ruth took Marvin to Baltimore to have Helen Taussig examine him, and year after year they came back feeling more optimistic. Marvin still occasionally suffered from shortness of breath, but he climbed three stories without having to stop. He was determined to prove that he was no different from the other boys at Hamilton High. It was a keen disappointment to him when, on Helen Taussig's orders, he was not allowed to take part in the school athletic programs. Secretly he practiced in a friend's swimming pool. His mother was quite horrified one day when she saw how long he swam under water. But his skill at swimming filled him with fierce pride. He was a member of the school orchestra and played the drums in the band. He would protest energetically whenever his friends tried to carry his instruments because they thought him frail. In 1954 he learned that he would receive a scholarship to the Pacific College of Music after he finished high school. His future looked very bright.

On April 25, 1955, while going barefoot, Marvin stepped on a splinter of wood that pierced deep into his flesh. A doctor removed the splinter, and the incident had almost been forgotten when, a month later, Marvin suddenly returned home on May 17 with a high fever. He had been on a school outing, and since he said he had drunk water from a brook, several doctors thought he had contracted an intestinal infection. The attacks of fever returned at regular intervals, and when Marvin's hands, feet, and lips once more turned blue, his parents became so anxious that on June 6 they flew with him to Baltimore. The Douglas prop plane took almost ten hours for the trip. Marvin was deathly ill by the time they arrived at the Harriet Lane Home for Children.

Helen Taussig could not conceal her alarm. The fever was very high; a bacteriological examination showed that Marvin's blood was swarming with streptococci. It turned out that in April only part of the splinter had been removed; the rest had caused septicemia, and Helen Taussig knew only too well how easily such blood poisoning could affect the heart and its valves. Undoubtedly inflammation of the inner lining of the heart—endocarditis—was developing. The only hope consisted in shock treatment with massive doses of penicillin. Perhaps that would check further deterioration. For several days Lewis and Ruth Mason did not sleep. They felt as if they had been transported back to those years during which they took turns watching over their imperiled little boy.

On the third day the temperature dropped. But Helen Taussig feared the infection might turn chronic, and she decided to keep Marvin under observation for several weeks and to continue the penicillin treatment. The injections became a torment to the boy, because there was soon not a muscle left in his body that had not been injured by the needle. Ultimately it became impossible to give him further injections without local Novocaine anesthesia.

Lewis Mason had to fly back to Los Angeles, so Ruth stayed with

Marvin, who recovered slowly. By the end of July, after six weeks of treatment, he was well enough to return to California. But new bouts of endocarditis were a distinct possibility, Dr. Taussig said, and Marvin would have to take penicillin capsules constantly. The doctor also suggested that Marvin come back to Baltimore for checkups at more frequent intervals, and made an appointment for the following November 5.

The Masons went home in a depressed mood. Marvin had changed. Some of his optimism and determination seemed to have been shattered. The following year he passed his final examinations at Hamilton High School, and he had continued to play in the orchestra and band, but he discovered that he could complete a drum roll only while sitting down. His lips were gradually turning bluer, and his fingers tended to assume the shape of the drumsticks he worked with. He did not attend the College of Music, but remained at home—feeling that at eighteen he was an invalid, a hopeless invalid. During 1956 he read an article on heart diseases and found out what defects in his own heart had remained after Dr. Blalock's operation. This information deepened his depression, but it also made him want to read more medical material, and to find out why he was so sick and why nothing could be done about it.

It happened that in the summer of 1957 he came across a newspaper account about "open-heart surgery." In England and America, he read, doctors had begun opening hearts in an incredible way and operating directly on them. He found similar stories in *Time* and in *Reader's Digest*, as well as other magazines. They explained it all so clearly that Marvin could follow the operations without difficulty.

Toward the end of the year he came upon the story of an eighteen-year-old girl, Cecilia Bavolek, who from birth had had one of those abnormal openings in the septum of the heart that—with other defects—were characteristic of the blue-baby syndrome. In April 1953, Dr. Stanley Rienkiewics, the family doctor, had sent the girl to Dr. John H. Gibbon, a surgeon at Jefferson Medical College in Philadelphia. Gibbon had been working for the past twenty years on a pumping machine that could temporarily assume the functions of the heart. His hope was that with the aid of this machine he could suspend the heartbeat long enough to operate on the heart without interference. The idea seemed so wild that he was considered something of a nut. Undeterred, he had gone on tinkering with his machine.

He had early realized that the machine must take over the work not only of the heart but also of the lungs. Otherwise he would have to make two pumps, one to drive the blood through the body and the other to force the returning blood through the lungs. It would have been difficult indeed to connect two such pumps to the complex network of arteries and veins involved. Gibbon constructed an apparatus he called a heart-lung machine. Using cats as laboratory animals, he placed catheters in the two great veins that transport the blood from the body to the heart. He connected these catheters by tubing to his machine and thus diverted the blood. As the blood flowed into the machine, it was guided over metal surfaces that were exposed to a constant stream of oxygen. In this way the blood became enriched with the oxygen it would normally absorb by circulating through the lungs. It was then pumped back into the animal's body through a second piece of tubing connected to a catheter that entered the artery of the thigh or one of the subclavian arteries. Thus oxygen-rich blood reached the arterial system directly, and thence all parts of the body. In order to prevent any blood from flowing into the heart, Dr. Gibbon clamped off the aorta close to the heart. The blood, after flowing through the animal's body and discharging its oxygen, again reached the two great veins leading to the heart. There it was once again diverted, led through the machine, charged with oxygen, and pumped back through the body. Although the heart was almost empty of blood during this procedure, it continued to beat slowly. When Dr. Gibbon opened the clamps, restoring normal circulation, the heart began once more to work vigorously.

By 1951, Dr. Gibbon was convinced that his machine worked, and would keep his animals alive while he opened their beating hearts, performed his experimental operations, and sewed up the hearts again. He had encountered skepticism and rejection from almost all the doctors in Philadelphia, and this attitude grew worse in 1952 when he employed the machine to operate on a child who suffered, he thought, from an opening in the septum of the heart. He succeeded in opening the heart, but did not find the hole—because there was none. He had been mistaken in his diagnosis, and the baby died.

Either Dr. Rienkiewics had not heard of this disaster or he did not consider it conclusive. At any rate, a year later he sent Cecilia Bavolek to Philadelphia and persuaded her parents that Gibbon should be allowed to repeat his experiment. And this time Gibbon succeeded. As soon as the machine began running, he opened the heart and sutured the hole in the septum. The article concluded with an enthusiastic description of the healthy new life that had started for Cecilia after the operation.

When Marvin first mentioned his reading to his parents, they were alarmed. It was clear that he was applying everything he read to himself and hoping to be healed permanently, like Cecilia Bavolek. But they no longer had that naïve trustfulness that had helped them struggle through so many years. The fateful blow of the spring of 1955 had sapped their confidence. They, too, read Marvin's articles, but what struck them was less the successes than the failures and the deaths, the implications of experiment upon human beings. Twelve years ago they themselves had decided for such an experiment. Now they were no longer so young and hopeful as they had been then; and they told themselves that, although Marvin was sickly, his life, at least, was not immediately threatened. Everything described in the articles seemed to them terribly hazardous.

Marvin read more and more, and finally he learned from an article in *Time* that a Dr. Clarence Walton Lillehei in Minneapolis, Minnesota, had also attempted to work with a machine. His heart-lung machine differed from Gibbon's in not conducting the blood over plates, but letting it run through a tube into which bubbles of oxygen had been forced. The blood absorbed the oxygen, and at the end of the tube superfluous bubbles were removed, so that they did not enter the patient's circulation, with the risk of creating a deadly embolism. Since 1955, Dr. Lillehei had opened many hearts and repaired damages to the septa. He had also undertaken experiments in narrowing leaky valves or reinforcing them with small bits of plastic, and in widening the entrances to the pulmonary artery—one of the troubles with Marvin's heart. When Dr. Lillehei had to cut away pieces of the heart wall, he tried to replace them by the plastic Teflon. *Time, Newsweek, Scientific American,* and *Reader's Digest* described the work of other American and British surgeons who were following Dr. Lillehei's lead and employing heart-lung machines to perform open-heart surgery. As the year 1958 advanced, Marvin's hopes waxed.

On his next trip to Baltimore he asked whether Dr. Blalock would not be willing to operate on him, using a heart-lung machine. But he was told that Blalock was not attempting open-heart surgery and did not intend to try it. The doctor no longer felt young enough for such bold experiments. When Marvin persisted, he learned that Dr. Jerome Harold Kay, one of Blalock's former colleagues, had moved to Los Angeles, was working at St. Vincent's Hospital, and had already done several operations with a heart-lung machine. Marvin was now twenty years old; on the flight back to California he made up his mind either to regain complete health or to die. He went to see Dr. Kay, who confirmed the story: yes, he had operated on defects of the septa and stenoses of the pulmonary valve, using the heart-lung machine. But the work was still in its initial stages.

When, in the summer of 1958, Marvin suffered unbearable attacks of a wildly racing heart, he decided to take the gamble.

Ruth Mason's recollections:

"It was his own decision. He insisted he wanted to live a normal life. He had to sign for it himself; I wouldn't sign. I was afraid."

. . .

The operation was scheduled for January 28, 1959. At eight o'clock in the morning Marvin lay on the table in St. Vincent's, and Dr. Kay, Dr. Anderson, Dr. Meihaus, and several assisting doctors began the operation. It was the sixth open-heart operation Kay was undertaking.

It took six hours, until early afternoon. Dr. Kay noted in his operation record: "Reasons for the operation: a subacute bacterial endocarditis which appeared three years ago, and auricular tachycardia in the past year." He wrote to Helen Taussig that he had had to suture into the heart an "outflow patch," and another patch to close the defect in the septum. By patch Kay meant pieces of Teflon. Along with all this he undid the operation that Dr. Blalock had performed fourteen years before, severing the connection Blalock had made between the innominate artery and the pulmonary artery. The cool, clinical report made the operation sound almost routine. To Lewis and Ruth Mason the memory of it was quite different.

Lewis and Ruth Mason:

"They were finished with the operation and were about to close him up when he started to hemorrhage. Dr. Kay had come downstairs and was talking to us; he was putting on his jacket and said he was going to a coffee shop for a moment and would be back. Then we heard the emergency call for Dr. Kay and saw him go running back. We believed Marvin was dying, and after a while they told us he was. We waited outside his room for six hours. His body was black, and there were many doctors in and out. The mother superior told us they were praying for Marvin. Finally the crisis passed, but more followed. One day, for some inexplicable reason, a nurse coming on duty varied her routine. She would always arrive, check her charts, and then hang her coat in a locker at some distance. Somehow, on this night, she felt she had to check on Marvin immediately. He was in a private room and was strangling on his saliva. She pressed the panic button. Dr. Kay performed a tracheotomy to save him. Two days later a lung collapsed and he needed a great deal of blood to pull him through that, but there were a thousand volunteers. How could he live through all that?"

No one knew. But Marvin himself thought it was his absolute determination to be well. Kay's assurance that he had removed the cardiac defect sounded to him like the announcement of a new life—and in this conviction he left St. Vincent's Hospital. He got a job as assistant film editor at the Film Fair Company in Studio City. His confidence in his new life and his future was now so rooted that he began dreaming the dream shared by almost everyone in his new environment—the dream of becoming an actor, perhaps a star. His dream had no more prospect of fulfillment than the dreams of thousands of others. But now that his new life had begun, he had the firmest faith in his luck.

From a second interview with a German cardiologist
(April 18, 1959):

QUESTION: For several months there have been more and more reports of blue babies operated on by Dr. Blalock years ago who have now been undergoing a second operation, with the aid of the heart-lung machine, to correct their basic heart defects. In January of this year, Marvin Mason, one of the early patients on whom Blalock tried out his method in 1945, underwent such an operation and has been in good health since. For this reason we would like to take up the theme we discussed with you in our interview of 1951 on the future prospects for Blalock's operation. At the time you predicted the development of open-heart surgery. Our present question is: Is the Blalock operation, after barely fifteen years, outmoded? Is the same Marvin Mason who in 1945 was a prime example of the validity of Blalock's procedure now a prime example of the fact that this procedure will have to give way to a new and more successful technique?

ANSWER: At the moment it's impossible to answer your question conclusively. There are three reasons that argue against your suggestion. First, the present operations are at such an early stage of development that it's impossible to form a judgment about them. As far as I have heard about Marvin Mason's operation—and I use the phrase "as far as I have heard" advisedly—it was, like all new procedures, full of risks and accompanied by severe complications. We must therefore await further developments. Let me say this in principle: The heart-lung machine and open-heart surgery are already realities, but only in their inception.

Most of the machines in use at the moment show deficiencies which only time can remedy. They can be used for only a few hours because the contact of the blood with metal or glass damages the red blood corpuscles. Another problem is that during the operation the heart is not completely empty of blood. You see, the musculature of the heart is supplied with blood and oxygen by means of several coronary arteries. These arteries branch off from the aorta back of the junction with the heart. When the aorta is clamped off for hooking into the heart-lung machine, the branches of the coronary arteries are not clamped. The heart muscle itself has to be supplied with blood, you see. But after this blood has permeated the muscle it is discharged through a vein into the heart. Dr. Lillehei in Minneapolis has tried to eliminate this interfering bleeding. He incorporated into the heart-lung machine a second pump, which sends blood directly through the coronary arteries and afterward sucks it out again.

A further problem is that the heart continues to beat slowly after the circulation is attached to the machine. The beating interferes with the sureness of the operative procedure. In the meantime, methods are being explored for putting the heart completely at rest. They are partly based on the observation of the English physician Ringer, dating back to 1883. He found that animal hearts ceased to beat if immersed in potassium chloride, but that the beat resumed as soon as the blood stream washed away the potassium chloride. But this chemical procedure has its dangers, and I am sure that another method will be preferred, one that likewise derives from Dr. Lillehei.

Before having perfected his heart-lung machine in Minneapolis, Lillehei attempted, some eight years ago, to perform open-heart surgery by supercooling his patients. He based his method on the fact that a cooled body and brain need less oxygen, and consequently the activity of the heart can be interrupted for several minutes. If the cooling exceeded 82 degrees Fahrenheit, the heartbeat became erratic, and at still lower temperatures the heart stood still. Lillehei now simply cooled the blood that the additional pump of his heart-lung machine was driving through the coronary arteries. The heartbeat then stopped. After the operation the pump sent warm blood into the heart muscle and the heartbeat resumed. If that did not happen, or if the beat was abnormally irregular, he could restore normal heartbeat by electrical stimulation of the muscle. For this purpose an electric defibrillator is employed. To sum up: There are solutions to the existing weaknesses of the method, but they are not yet final and not yet generally accepted.

QUESTION: And what is the second reason for your caution?

ANSWER: It follows from the first. All the heart operations that have been made possible by the heart-lung machine are still in the developmental stage. This includes the repair of defects in the septum of the heart and the correction of stenosis, or narrowing of the entrance to the pulmonary artery—the principal repairs that have to be made in the case of blue babies. The use of plastic repair material is still very new. There are other sources of danger. Among these are the nerve nodes that regulate the normal heartbeat. These highly sensitive nodes are located in the vicinity of the septum. Pricking them with a needle is sufficient to injure them. In other words, it is not yet possible to judge whether the results justify abandoning the Blalock operation and in the case of blue babies switching to "open repair."

QUESTION: You mentioned a third reason.

ANSWER: Yes. In our conversation eight years ago I alluded to the possibility that the Blalock operation might keep blue babies alive until the heart-lung machine was developed and thus there would be a chance for removing the actual defects in a second operation. This chance has come, and in the operation on Marvin Mason it was taken. But all valid judgments will depend on how Marvin does—and how the others do who were operated on fourteen or fifteen years ago and can now undergo a second operation. But in general we do not yet know what pathological changes the Blalock operation may have produced in the intervening ten or fifteen years, and when these changes may have reached such a state that a second operation is no longer possible. We have no idea what the most favorable moment for a second operation would be. We do not know whether it may be too late for a twenty-five or twenty-six-year-old person, because his heart will no longer survive the surgical procedures. We also do not know whether we can venture open-heart repair in the case of a child of six or ten, because of the later body changes, and no one can predict what will happen to plastic materials which do not grow along with the growth of the body.

Every new step in medicine proves its value or its uselessness by the fate of the patients on whom it has been tried. That may sound inhuman, but it is a basic truth. We now know the fate of the blue babies who were operated on by Blalock's method. We have yet to see what will be the fate of those who have undergone open-heart surgery.

Barbara

Barbara Rosenthal was fourteen years old. Two years had passed since the operation in Baltimore, after which her parents left Buffalo and moved west to Beverly Hills, California. Leonard Rosenthal continued in business as before, and continued to prosper. But for him and his wife, Shirley, life still centered not around prosperity, but around their daughter.

She no longer differed from her friends and from the other Beverly Hills girls with whom she went to high school. The school was situated on the edge of the Twentieth Century-Fox studio grounds, in the midst of wide, parklike lawns. Barbara seemed as sturdy as other girls her age. But the memory of her years as a blue baby remained and sometimes filled her with anxiety and tension. Occasionally, when she was tired, a touch of blue would creep into her fingers or her lips. She knew nothing about the medical theories underlying the Blalock operation and had no notions about its limits as a remedial measure. Yet every memory of the past stirred inhibitions and aroused deep-seated fears. Frequently she would refuse to be driven to school, like most of the children, but walked a mile, even though walking was hard on her after so many years of having to forget she knew how. That walk to school was a form of reassurance to her. When she came to Baltimore for a checkup in November 1947, the doctors noted in their clinical report: "The mother . . . is considering the need for psychological support for her daughter."

But with each passing year the memories grew dimmer. At the age of eighteen she graduated from high school. She had long been interested in newspaper work and decided to study journalism at Berkeley.

None of her fellow students ever learned that she had once been a blue baby. By now she had all but forgotten it herself. Still, the sense of not being quite a normal person continued to motivate her unconsciously. It was manifested, for example, in her deliberately moving into a university dormitory that was situated high up on a hill, and then choosing a room on the top floor, with many flights of stairs to climb.

In Berkeley she met Richard Israel, one of the editors of the university newspaper. He was twenty-five, Barbara twenty-one. Richard had no reason to think that she had ever been severely ill. And Barbara always chose the hardest work among the machines in the print shop, as if to prove her strength. In 1957, when Richard proposed to her, she put him off for a while—as though she had a problem to settle with herself. Then she explained she had to tell Richard something that might change his wish to marry her. That was how he heard her story. She showed him the bluish sheen in the skin of her hands when they climbed a hill. Her courage deeply impressed him. At the end of the year they were married in Beverly Hills. Richard found a job on the *San Francisco Chronicle*, Barbara on the *San Francisco Examiner*. They moved to San Francisco and had a year of happiness and joyful work, without ever talking about blue fingernails or lips. Then—in 1958—Helen Taussig came to San Francisco for a medical convention. Barbara called on her and told her about Richard, her new life, and her hope of having children. Dr. Taussig warned her that she must not, that if she did she would be imperiling her own life and the baby's as well. Barbara told Richard about this conversation, but she concealed from him how much the incident had reawakened her sense of not being a normal person. The following year Richard got a job with the CBS Television Studio in Los Angeles. They moved to Hollywood and rented an attractive apartment on El Cerrito Place. Barbara went to work in the public relations department of the Cedars of Lebanon Hospital. They lived apparently happy with their work, their parties, and their friends. Then, in January 1960, there occurred a seemingly casual incident whose full importance Richard learned much later.

One day in January, Barbara attended a lecture by one of the well-known specialists who gave talks for the medical staff at Cedars of Lebanon. It was Barbara's job to make reports on these lectures. The lecturer was a heart specialist, and he talked about the Blalock operation and the experiences that had accumulated in the past fifteen years. For the first time Barbara learned that she had only a "temporary" repair inside her chest and that she was living "on reprieve." Moreover, at her age—twenty-six—the reprieve was very nearly over. For the first time, also, she heard about the advances in heart surgery and learned that the time was ripe to replace Blalock's makeshift operation by a genuine surgical repair of the heart.

At home she told Richard something about the lecture and the latest achievements in surgery. She did not mention that that one hour had re-awakened her entire past and that she was afraid she had heard her own death sentence. She went on to live as she had done before, with such courage that Richard did not notice her actual state of intense despair. But she consulted a number of doctors. Her anxiety intensified when, several months later, she again began suffering from shortness of breath and dizzy spells. She consulted a cardiologist, who referred her to Dr. Eugene Saxon, one of the thoracic surgeons at Cedars of Lebanon. In October 1960 she was given a series of intensive examinations. Dr. Saxon wrote in one of his reports:

"Indications for surgery: A 27-year-old cyanotic girl who in the last six months has noted daily dizzy spells and dyspnea upon exertion. X rays revealed venous congestion of the lungs. . . . It was felt that there were signs of deterioration and left ventricular failure, and it was thought that this may represent the patient's last opportunity for total correction. . . ."

In her uncertainty, Barbara thought of going to Baltimore for the operation. But she learned, as Marvin Mason had, that Blalock would not engage in open-heart surgery, and so she decided in favor of Dr. Saxon and the Cedars of Lebanon Hospital. Up to the last moment, however, she concealed her dizzy spells from Richard. She also concealed from him her knowledge that she had reached the end of the reprieve granted her in Baltimore, and that an operation had now become a matter of survival. She merely explained to him that she had become convinced of the progress of surgery and wanted the operation so that she would be a fully healthy woman, able to bear children. She arranged to be admitted to the Cedars of Lebanon Hospital on January 15, 1961.

Richard Israel to Jerry LeBlanc, 1970:

"Once in a while, from overexertion, particularly the last couple of years, she would get out of breath, but that was all. . . . Her biggest concern was that people would notice once in a while how the blueness crept into her finger tips. Sometimes there would be a touch of it in her cheeks. . . . There was never any sign that she was sick at all, and she didn't go in to be operated on because of a relapse or anything like that— she was healthy to the last day. . . . I think that the main reason was that she believed that if she had the operation, then she could have children. Yes, I'm sure that was it. I drove her down to the hospital on the day we had made reservations, and she walked in as healthy as you or I, carrying her little overnight case. I saw her in her room that last morning, and we expected everything to be all right."

The operation began at 8:20 A.M. on January 18, 1961. Dr. Eugene Saxon was assisted by Dr. Joseph H. Miller, Dr. Francis Buron, Dr. Joshua Fields, and Dr. Milton Marmer. Dr. Miller operated the heart-lung machine; Dr. Marmer supervised the anesthesia.

All the preparations had been made by 9:35 and the actual operation began. Saxon opened the thoracic cavity. He revealed the arteria innominata, which Blalock had connected to the pulmonary artery sixteen years before. It was well supplied with blood. But when Saxon exposed the pulmonary artery, he understood why Barbara Israel's condition had deteriorated to such a degree in the past year. The diameter of the artery had expanded to four or five times its normal size. Overburdening by the unnaturally increased supply of blood had actually bulged out part of the arterial wall, creating an aneurysm. Saxon removed the arterial diversion of the Blalock operation, and the assistants attached the heart-lung machine. Insertion of the catheters for the venous blood into the major veins, and of the catheter for arterial blood into the femoral artery, caused no difficulties.

Nevertheless, it was 1:36 P.M. when the heart-lung machine began to run and Saxon embarked on the decisive phase of the operation. He opened the pulmonary artery, intending to narrow it. Inside it he discovered a large blood clot which had probably been lurking behind the pulmonary valve for a long time. The pulmonary valve itself had only a tiny passage to the right ventricle. Saxon opened the valve, but when his groping finger attempted to penetrate into the ventricle he found that the whole connection between pulmonary artery and heart was virtually blocked by adhesions. In order to normalize the outflow of blood from the right ventricle to the lung he would have to open up the ventricle.

Dr. Marmer and Dr. Miller reported no unusual signs. Blood pressure continued to be normal. As soon as Saxon had finished narrowing the diameter of the pulmonary artery, he made an incision into the right ventricle. After twenty-seven years of having had to force blood through a tiny opening into the pulmonary artery, the overburdened ventricle was considerably enlarged. At this sight Saxon probably wondered whether it might not be too late, whether the heart muscle was still strong enough to maintain normal pulmonary circulation.

The defect in the septum between the right and left ventricles was large, slightly over an inch by an inch and a half. But Saxon succeeded quite speedily in closing this opening with fourteen stitches without injuring the nodes of the heart's nervous system. Immediately afterward he turned to the almost blocked entrance to the pulmonary artery and opened it wide, replacing the missing tissue by a Teflon patch. It was nearly 3:10 P.M. when he closed the right ventricle again. The heart rhythm was normal. This gave him hope that the operation would turn out well after all. He signed to Miller to restore the normal body circulation and turn off the heart-lung machine.

At 3:14 P.M. the pump was stopped. Barbara's heart at once began beating vigorously. It worked for a few minutes—and Saxon began to feel that all was well—but then the blood pressure suddenly dropped; the strength of the heart muscle diminished dramatically. At 3:18 P.M. Miller had to turn on the pump once more because the heart was failing. Circulation resumed. At 3:23 the pump was again turned off, but Barbara's heart worked for only a few minutes. At 3:26 Saxon and Miller had to resort to the pump for the third time. From then on there began a desperate struggle to keep the heartbeat going. From 3:45 to 5:40, Miller switched the pump on and off five more times. At the same time Saxon administered larger and larger quantities of heart and circulatory drugs. But neither digitalis, Adrenalin, nor calcium had the slightest effect. The right ventricle became flooded with blood. The heart did not have the strength to pump this blood into the pulmonary artery, becoming more and more swollen. When the situation appeared wholly desperate, Saxon considered opening the heart once more and restoring the hole in the septum, so that the blood—as had been the case before the operation—could discharge from the right ventricle into the left.

He had to abandon this idea. It was too late. The heart-lung machine had taken over the circulation too often. Barbara Israel's reflexes became fainter and fainter. After a last application of the pump at 5:40 P.M. her heart beat on its own for a few minutes. Shortly after six o'clock it stopped permanently. A few days later Saxon wrote to Helen Taussig and reported to her the death of the second of the three patients with whom the history of blue-baby operations had begun.

Marvin

In the spring of 1961, Marvin Mason had two experiences that made him surer than ever that his real life had just begun now, after his second operation. On the fringes of Hollywood's movie world he encountered Linda Weiner, a pretty black-haired girl who was called "Kippy" because she had been born on Yom Kippur, the chief Jewish holy day. The two fell in love. Almost at the same time Marvin was given his first small part, on the stage of the Rancho Park Theater in Los Angeles. It was a first installment on the fulfillment of his dreams.

During the rehearsals for *Inherit the Wind*, the play in which he was to make his debut, Marvin suffered a fall from the stage and hurt his knee severely. But he was so afraid of missing this first chance that after morphine injections to quiet the pain he had himself brought to the stage in a wheel chair. In this way he performed for three nights, until his fiancée persuaded him to go to a hospital and forget his dreams of stardom.

He underwent a knee operation, the third operation in his young life, and returned to his job at the Film Fair Company. Kippy and he were married in November, after he had told her about his earlier operations and asked her whether she could stand seeing the big scars on his chest for a lifetime.

Marvin was happy, but could not forget his aspirations. They would surge up every time he saw a well-known actor in the studio. And so in the summer of 1962 he secretly started looking for another part. After endless pleas and after receiving many promises that were not kept, he obtained the part of a minor hoodlum in *Detective Story*, which was being put on in a converted stucco building by a group called the Westchester Playhouse. Directors and actors alike were more or less unsuccessful aspirants, some of whom earned their livings at other jobs. They played only on weekends; there were no salaries. The chance to act was reward enough for the members of the cast. Marvin told Kippy about it only after he was sure of his part; then he admitted that the theater had him hooked. His wife accepted that. She accompanied him to rehearsals and was as happy as he at any word of praise that came his way.

No one in the troupe learned that he had been a blue baby. And no one suspected that he had any physical weakness, for he tried to work harder and be livelier than the others. In September he was given a second part. It, too, was only a minor one, but he thought of it as a step upward. This was the role of a young cadet in *The Dark at the Top of the Stairs*, a play that had opened in New York in 1957. The play deals with a family full of self-pity, into which Sammy, the cadet, suddenly bursts, calling on the daughter, Reenie. He leaves with Reenie on his arm—and does not reappear. In the third act the family learns that Sammy has committed suicide that same night.

Marvin had only ten minutes on the stage in the second act—dressed in a blue uniform, his cadet cap under his arm. But as he proudly walks off the stage with Reenie, the girl's mother remarks to her husband: "Why, that's the nicest young man I ever met." Even in New York this exit had evoked a burst of applause.

Night after night Marvin rehearsed with his partner, Elyse Silvers, the lovely sixteen-year-old daughter of the director, Jerry Silvers. They made a handsome pair. On opening night, Marvin, too, was given a big hand after his exit. Hot with pride and excitement, he unthinkingly stripped off his shirt in the dressing room. Too late, he noticed that several of the girls recoiled when they saw the scars on his chest. But he passed it off casually, remarking that the scars were from an old operation. A week later, on Friday, September 28, he made his fourth appearance on the stage. A few minutes after ten o'clock he stepped through the curtains with Elyse Silvers. The thunder of applause as the curtain dropped covered the sound of a fall. Silvers was standing at the theater entrance catching a breath of air when two members of the cast came running to him with the news that Marvin had collapsed. The director rushed back and found Marvin lying behind the curtain, his face purple. Jerry Silvers tried artificial respiration while someone asked whether there was a doctor in the audience. But there was none. A doctor in the neighborhood was called; meanwhile Silvers continued to try mouth-to-mouth resuscitation, although by now Marvin's face had turned almost black. The doctor arrived a few minutes later and sent for an ambulance. Marvin was taken to the Daniel Freeman Hospital, a few blocks away. By the time he was carried into the emergency room, he was already dead.

The sole consolation for Kippy, and for Ruth and Lewis Mason, was the probability that even as he was dying he had heard the closing line of the act: "That's the nicest young man I ever met."

During the night his body was taken, as are all victims of unexplained deaths, to the Los Angeles morgue. There Dr. Musgrave performed an autopsy and read in Marvin's chest the history of his disease. He could also read the story of the operation of January 1959, which had left Marvin convinced that his heart defect was now healed. Musgrave saw that the defect in the septum had not been completely closed. For Dr. Musgrave noted an opening in the septum about two-fifths of an inch in diameter. He concluded his report with the standard professional phrases: "Cause of death: Acute myocardial failure. Congenital heart disease (intraventricular septal defect)."

From a letter by Dr. Alfons Scheffold of Westwood (Los Angeles) dated February 15, 1971:

"I am only an amateur as far as the history of modern medicine is concerned. But during the past month I looked for the graves of Barbara Israel, née Rosenthal, and Marvin Mason. I was impelled by a sense of the fatedness of their lives. Today, approximately a decade after their deaths, medical authorities still do not agree about the part that Blalock's first operation on blue babies may yet have to play and whether or not it should give way completely to open-heart surgery. Blalock died on December 15, 1964, of a cancer that had formed at the stump of the ureter of his right kidney, which had been removed in a nephrectomy thirty-seven years earlier. Consequently, he is out of the fight. Helen Taussig, in her seventies but still not ready to retire, has tried to show by the examples of Blalock's first 750 blue-baby patients that it is wisest to use the Blalock shunt on younger children, thus aiding them to live a fuller life, and correcting their heart defects by operation only after they have reached the age of ten or fifteen. Opposed to her are a group of surgeons who hold that open-heart repair is best even for younger children; if absolutely necessary they think that even infants should be treated in this way. At any rate, we now have several ways to help those who twenty-five years ago were simply condemned to death.

"In their short lives Barbara Israel and Marvin Mason had made a possibly unique contribution to the history of medicine. They had experienced not one but two crucial phases in the development of blue-baby surgery. They had given their lives, but not in vain."

2 / Mary Richardson

Peter Bent Brigham Hospital, Boston, news release, May 13, 1960:

"The development and first successful use of a ball valve for the total replacement of a damaged aortic valve in the human heart was described today by a Boston surgeon at a meeting of the American Association for Thoracic Surgery in Miami Beach.

"Dr. Dwight E. Harken, Chief of Thoracic Surgery at Peter Bent Brigham Hospital, . . . told of the methods by which this new valve has been devised over a period of years. . . . It is made of materials which have been pretested for use in humans through laboratory research. The stainless-steel double 'birdcage type' valve is made of steel threads surrounding a silicone-rubber ball. . . . The first patient to be wearing this steel valve is an attractive young Florida housewife whose heart illness had shown no other hope."

In November 1958 the airport of Jacksonville, Florida, was still in the northern part of the city, and Bill Richardson had to leave his home in southeastern Jacksonville at 10:40 P.M. in order to catch the midnight plane to Boston. Bill was thirty-eight years old, of medium height, a vigorous, brown-haired man with a pleasant, friendly face. He worked as a truck driver for Texaco. Except for a trip to New Orleans, he had never left Florida, and in fact on this night he himself was not planning to fly. He was taking his wife, Mary, and her mother to the plane; he had picked the night flight because tickets for the older DC-7s that flew this route were cheaper.

Mary was seven years younger than Bill, and although she was now thirty-one he thought she looked just as pretty as she had in the summer of 1945, when he was still a city bus driver and Mary had got on his bus for the first time. Now, however, she was very pale and breathing rapidly. Her left hand, resting on the coat she had bought for the cold weather of Boston, looked thin and frail. But this only intensified Bill's feeling, which he had had since the day they first met, that he was Mary's protector.

Mary Allen had been eighteen at the time, working from eight to five-

47

thirty as a salesgirl in a department store. She lived in her parents' red bungalow on San Juan Avenue, only a few houses from the bus stop. But although Mary had so short a walk to the bus, she was out of breath when she dropped into the seat directly behind the driver. She was so pretty that Bill did not long resist the impulse to say a few words to her.

Mary's mother, a vigorous woman with the same auburn hair as her only daughter, had taught Mary to be careful about men in uniform. For since the war started the rather sleepy city of Jacksonville had changed completely. The pilots from the air force base on the St. Johns River and the sailors from the aircraft carriers in Mayport swarmed all over the city. But Bill was neither a sailor nor a flyer. He was well-mannered and thrifty, and had already bought himself a red Chevrolet convertible. A few weeks after they had exchanged their first words, he was waiting in his car outside the department store when Mary's working day ended. Bill noticed that she was exhausted when she left the store. But in those days the salesgirls had to wear dark dresses even when the Florida sun turned the department store into a hothouse. To Bill, that alone explained why Mary was so dead tired; and she always revived as soon as she sat down beside him in the car.

It was only two months later, when Bill proposed to Mary, that he learned she had "heart murmurs." Even at school she had not been allowed to go to gym with the other children. Yet none of the doctors in the vicinity had been able to discover anything particularly wrong with Mary. When she was nine the Allens had asked their new family doctor, Dr. Harold, to examine her. He was the first to hear a slightly abnormal heartbeat. But he assured her parents that she would outgrow it in time. There were thousands of people with such murmurs, he said.

Mary's parents liked Bill from the first. But since they were conscientious people, they thought it only right to tell him everything about Mary, including the heart murmur. Bill laughed away their scruples. He and Mary were married, and a daughter, Loxy, soon made them a family of three.

From the start they dreamed of owning their own home. In order to bring that dream closer, Mary continued to work after their marriage. During the early years, while they still lived with Mary's parents, Mary had also found time to help her mother in the household, to bring up Loxy, and to make her own clothes. Bill could only wonder how she managed all that after he discovered how often she suffered from weakness and shortness of breath at work. Bill himself changed jobs because he was better paid at Texaco, and the two went on with their savings program. Ultimately they bought their own home in a new development, surrounded by trees that gradually grew higher than the roof. But a shadow hung over their happiness. For by now Bill knew that in all the years of their marriage Mary had not been really well for a single day. Over those years he had taken Mary to as many as ten doctors, trying to find out why in spite of all her energy she had this weakness and this trouble breathing. Again and again they received the same answers: that Mary was imagining her symptoms, and that they certainly had nothing to do with heart murmurs.

Finally, in 1954, when Mary's shortness of breath grew worse after the slightest exertion, Bill read about a marvelous clinic in New Orleans, something like the Mayo Clinic in Minnesota that the papers were always so full of. It was called the Ochsner Clinic. Bill decided to use his next vacation to take Mary there. Bill drove the whole distance in one day. She stayed at the clinic for several days, and Bill waited confidently, expecting that the doctors here would at last find an explanation for Mary's condition. Since he had the habit of getting up around four o'clock in the morning, he spent many hours pacing back and forth outside the windows of the hospital where Mary lay. After several days he was called in by the doctors and told that their tests had discovered nothing that would account for Mary's complaints. On the drive home Mary asked him whether he thought that the trouble lay in her simply not being smart enough to explain to the doctors exactly how she felt. But Bill was convinced that the trouble lay with the doctors, not with Mary.

The past four years, since that trip to New Orleans, Mary's condition had gone steadily downhill. In the autumn of 1957, Bill found her unconscious on the floor of the garage. Perhaps she might have died if he had not happened to be nearby. But he had given up asking new doctors to diagnose her case, and it was sheer chance that had led Mary to Dr. King at the St. Johns Medical Building during the past summer. Mary had gone to see him because of an injury and had not even mentioned her spells of weakness. For some reason, though, he examined her with his stethoscope and abruptly said: "Well, young woman, I think you ought to look around for a heart specialist."

As Bill drove toward the lights of the airport, he thought of the excitement Mary had shown when she returned home from her visit to Dr. King. For the first time she had met a doctor who did not tell her that her sickness was all imagination, but, instead, said of his own accord that she was really ill. Bill had telephoned Dr. King at once; the doctor had repeated that he was certain Mary had serious heart trouble. When Bill asked in perplexity why none of the many doctors they had seen had ever suggested anything of the sort, he received no answer. But he had learned that doctors never criticized other doctors. And so he contented himself with asking for the name of a heart specialist. Dr. King recommended a

Dr. Hammer near Riverside Avenue, one of the most expensive neighbor-hoods in Jacksonville. But Bill was determined to pursue the matter, even if it took all his savings. Dr. Hammer examined Mary, ran some tests, and told her a few days later: "Mrs. Richardson, you are suffering from an aortic stenosis. You must have an operation, and soon."

Even now, while driving the last half mile to Imerson Airport, Bill and Mary still did not know what the words "aortic stenosis" meant. It was enough for them to have confirmation that Mary had never imagined her symptoms, that she was suffering from a real illness, which had a name and could be remedied by operation. Bill had asked about a surgeon, and Dr. Hammer had told him: "Among all the surgeons who are performing such operations today, I'd recommend Dr. Dwight E. Harken in Boston. If you agree, I'll write to him."

Dr. Harken had replied promptly, expressing great interest in Mary's case and saying that he expected her in Boston in the middle of November. Since Bill could not leave his job and Mary was by now much too weak to travel by herself, her mother would be flying with her. Dr. Harken's secretary had been kind enough to arrange for a room for Mary's mother in the vicinity of the hospital—and now the two were on their way.

It was after six o'clock in the morning when the Charles River and Boston loomed beneath the plane from Jacksonville. It was a gloomy November morning; Logan Airport spread out, a gray mass amid the gray. At this season Bostonians expected nothing else. But to Mary the leaden color of the sky and the raw cold of the morning seemed alien and oppressive.

She noted only dimly that her mother and she rode in a taxi for some time down narrow streets between rows of dark-red brick houses, break-fasted somewhere, and later stopped at a tall office building near Copley Square. As she was led into a large waiting room, Mary felt a more and more violent pain in her shoulders. It moved into her elbows and became so intense that she had to lie down on a couch and curl up into a position that made the pain slightly more bearable. She was still lying there when the door opened and a tall, powerful man in his forties entered. He had light hair and a round, somewhat florid face. He sat down at once on the edge of the couch, turned Mary around to face him, and said: "I am Dr. Harken. What's wrong with us?" Mary liked him instantly.

Dr. Harken had come to Boston from Iowa. People recognized him from a distance by the speed with which he walked, swinging his arms vigorously, or by his way of taking patients by the chin when he wel-comed them, or roughly embracing them in a paternal fashion. He began his studies in 1931 at Harvard and completed the major part of his medical training there. From 1942 to 1946 he worked as a thoracic surgeon with the American army in England. During this time he ventured to open the hearts of wounded men and remove bullets from the ventricles of the heart.

At his station there was a young sergeant who had survived a bullet wound in the right ventricle received in France. On August 25, 1944, Harken attempted to open the beating heart by a small incision and pull the projectile out with a forceps. But he lost his hold, and the metal vanished along with the blood stream into the right atrium. Nevertheless, the heart continued to beat, and there was no dangerous hemorrhage. Thus the operation refuted all the fears that had hitherto restrained surgeons from attempting to touch the heart. Harken sewed up the incision and on November 16 attempted a second operation. This time, also, the missile slipped from his forceps and slid into the right ventricle. There it lay in such an unfortunate position that the heart muscle was constantly rubbing against it. Hammer told the sergeant: "I'm afraid we'll have to leave it there." But the wounded man pleaded so fervently for another attempt that on February 19, 1945, Harken decided to risk a third operation. When he inserted his forceps into the ventricle, the heartbeat changed rhythm. There was a regular "shower" of extrasystoles. But after three minutes, the time it took to remove the projectile, the heart resumed its regular rhythm. Fifteen years later the sergeant was still alive, working as a farmer near Columbus, Ohio.

Similar experiences during the war determined Harken's future course. When he came home after the war, at the age of thirty-six, he brought with him the conviction that the heart was far less sensitive to surgical intervention than had been thought. Incisions scarcely affected it. Only displacements from its normal position seemed to bother it. Harken drew his conclusions. Two years after his return home (he was now operating at the old Mount Auburn Hospital and the venerable Peter Bent Brigham Hospital) he was among the first surgeons to open stenotic heart valves by thrusting instruments through the wall of the beating heart. Thus he laid the foundations for his subsequent lifework—cardiac valve surgery.

The pioneers of these days, who experienced so many failures and deaths in the course of their experiments, strike us today as gamblers. No doubt about it, there were ambitious men who found willing victims in desperate patients. Harken was a different type. Since he knew that it was possible to operate on the heart, he was simply incapable of standing by passively and watching patients with valvular difficulties of the heart die. He therefore took the risk of operating not only for valvular stenoses, but also for valvular insufficiency, as defective closure of a valve is called. In cases of mitral valve insufficiency, he made a small incision in the auricular wall. Then he tried to draw threads through the fibrous ring of the defective valve and bring these threads out through the heart wall again. As soon as he pulled the threads, the ring narrowed and the valve cusps were drawn closer together. In this way Harken hoped to diminish the gaps between the cusps, which no longer closed tightly. But two of his first three patients died; only the third survived.

In 1951, Harken hit on the idea of introducing a plexiglass ball into the left ventricle. It was suspended on a thread inserted through the ventricle wall just below the mitral valve and brought out through the other side. He hoped that at the moment the ventricle contracted to pump its blood into the aorta, the wall of the heart would push the ball against the mitral valve and so prevent the blood from going back into the auricle. The first operation of this type, on a thirty-six-year-old woman named Mary Dansereau, created a sensation in 1952. The patient was in such poor condition that she could no longer climb a single step in a flight of stairs. Harken noted: "Her family feels that her illness makes her a burden. She thinks her life is no longer worth living. . . . We proposed the insertion of a plexiglass ball, and she eagerly agreed to our suggestion." But the operation failed, as did seven more of the same type. Mary died on August 8, 1952.

However, he did not give up his basic idea. Instead of the ball he employed—in twenty-four more operations—a bottle-shaped device that was fastened by threads above and below the entrance to the valve. When the mitral valve opened and blood poured from the left auricle into the left ventricle, the device hung loosely in front of the valve opening; during the subsequent contraction of the ventricle, it was pressed against the leaky valve. Fourteen of twenty-four patients died. The remaining ten showed some improvement.

When the heart-lung machine made open-heart surgery possible, Harken leaped at the opportunity to repair mitral and aortic valves directly. In the case of the aortic valve, which has three cusps that act as "lids," the gaps between the cusps could sometimes be closed by suturing two cusps together. Along with this, the first experiments with such plastics as Teflon and Ivalon were undertaken; defective valve cusps were replaced by bits of plastic, or patches were added to the deformed edges of cusps. It remained a question for Harken how long this plastic would last inside the beating heart, how long the sutures would hold, whether blood clots would form, and how long the new valve parts would keep their shape without shrinking or curling.

Around 1957 or 1958, Harken began to feel that repairs of valvular insufficiency were still fraught with peril, even with open-heart surgery.

He therefore decided to construct an artificial valve that would do more than just repair the defective valve—it would replace it completely.

The idea was not new. Dr. Charles Hufnagel of Georgetown University Medical School had already spent several years after the war experimenting on dogs to check the retroflow of blood in cases of insufficiency of the aortic valve. In 1950–51 he constructed a small ball valve. It consisted of a plastic-coated metal ring the same size as the cross section of the aorta. In the center was an opening with a plexiglass ball in front of it. When this artificial valve was inserted into a tube like the aorta, it allowed a fluid like blood to flow freely one way, but if the flow came from the opposite direction, pressure would force the ball into the opening, effectively sealing it. To prevent the ball from being carried away by the fluid, Hufnagel fastened a tiny grating around it, thus limiting the area within which the ball could move. Hufnagel thought that this valve could assume the function of the natural aortic valve.

Six years before the introduction of the heart-lung machine, however, he could not conceive of removing the aortic valve of a dog and inserting an artificial valve. No animal would have survived the operation. He therefore implanted the valve in a part of the aorta that was accessible to him. He inserted it at the spot where the aorta turns downward, after the arteries supplying the brain with blood have branched off. Hufnagel knew that he could not interrupt the blood supply to the brain without unacceptable damage, but that he could temporarily cut off the blood to the lower part of the body. In several experimental animals he artificially produced aortal insufficiency, then clamped off the "descending aorta," opened it, sewed in his artificial valve, and closed the aorta again. The regurgitation of blood diminished by almost two-thirds. The greater part of the blood that the ventricle pumped into the aorta traveled beyond the ball valve on the initial impulse, and the valve prevented it from leaking back.

In 1951, Hufnagel tried this operation on one of his patients for the first time. The patient died, and another year passed before Hufnagel ventured a second operation. This time the patient lived. The noise produced by the valve as it operated was so loud that it could be heard at a considerable distance. But the patient felt revived, at least for a time. Hufnagel repeated this operation several times, although some of his patients died of blood clots that formed inside the ball valves. The operation depended so much on personal skill, however, that hardly anyone succeeded in reproducing it.

Harken was convinced that Hufnagel was on the right track, but that it was necessary to make a better valve which, with the aid of the heart-lung machine, could be inserted directly into the place of the defective natural valve. He fully realized how difficult it might be to construct a valve that could withstand the enormous burden borne by a normal heart valve, and withstand it not for months but for years. A valve opens and closes about 100 times per minute, 6,000 times per hour, 144,000 times per day, and almost 53 million times in a year. Nevertheless, Harken felt confident. His optimism was sustained by the rapid development of plastics so tissue-neutral that the human body would not reject them, but would enclose them with its own tissue. Another plus factor was the development of anticoagulant drugs which, if taken consistently, could prevent the formation of blood clots in artificial valves. In 1958 he teamed up with the engineer W. C. Birtwell of the Davol rubber company in Providence, and before long the two were able to try out several model valves in an instrument that imitated the human blood stream and the action of the heart valves. What they called their ball-birdcage valve consisted of a stainless-steel valve ring embedded in Teflon, a steel cage that held the ball fast, and a silicone-rubber ball.

Two hours after Mary Richardson had first looked into Harken's robust, friendly face, she was in a bed in Mount Auburn Hospital across the Charles River, a few blocks from Harvard University. Outside, sleet was falling. Her mother left to go to her room in the home of a family named Ford on Channing Street. Mary was alone. But she no longer felt despairing, for Dr. Harken had told her: "Mary, I believe every word of your story. We're not going to waste any time. We'll start a series of tests right away. I must warn you that some of them may be painful. But then we'll know what we have to do, and then we'll do something."

Mary Richardson's recollections:

"I didn't have any idea what it was all about, but I think the less you know, the better, sometimes. If I had known too much I might have been scared. As it was, I wasn't. I was just glad that finally I had been able to convince somebody that something was wrong with me and now they were going to do something about it."

In fact, her notions about heart diseases were of the dimmest. She also was unaware that many of the doctors she had previously consulted were not incompetent, but were simply of the traditional belief that nothing could be done about valvular defects of the heart, for which reason they preferred to conceal from their patients the hopelessness of their situation. She did not know what a heart valve was. She merely knew that Dr. Dwight E. Harken, a professor at Harvard University and more famous than any doctor she had ever met, believed her. That was the strongest psychological support she had in her situation.

During the following days all the tests, which included classification of the sounds of her heart, electrocardiograms, and X rays, confirmed the same diagnosis: Mary was suffering from stenosis of the aortic valve. But there were indications that the aortic valve was also insufficient. In order to make sure, Harken decided to undertake a test that for some years had permitted physicians actually to look into the left ventricle of the heart. The method had originated with the German physician Werner Forssmann, who in 1929 hit on the idea of introducing circulatory medicines directly into the heart. Experimenting on himself, he had inserted a thin rubber catheter into a vein in his arm and pushed it up the vein until the tip of the catheter reached the right side of the heart. During the Second World War, Dr. André Cournand and Dr. Dickinson W. Richards of Bellevue Hospital in New York had recognized the value of this technique for cardiac examinations. Using fine plastic catheters, they had followed the venous blood stream up from veins in the arm or leg as far as the right atrium and right ventricle of the heart. Later they had used the catheter to introduce dyes opaque to X rays into the right ventricle, and thus for the first time had obtained clear X rays of the heart in action.

These methods were for a while restricted to the right side of the heart. In order to examine the left side, it would have been necessary to introduce a catheter into an artery and push it against the flow of the blood. Since this seemed dangerous, the Swedish physician Björk devised another procedure. After local anesthesia a long hollow needle was inserted through the skin alongside the backbone and pushed toward the heart until it penetrated the wall of the heart and into the left auricle. Then a thin catheter was introduced through this needle, passed through the auricle and the mitral valve, and finally into the left ventricle. In this way it was possible to measure the pressures inside the heart, and to inject opaque chemicals so that the left ventricle and its valves would show up on X rays. The needle had to pass by the lung, esophagus, and aorta before it reached the left side of the heart, and during the earlier years severe injuries and deaths had resulted. Even the greatest skill on the surgeon's part did not altogether exclude complications. But there was no other way to examine the left side of the heart thoroughly. Consequently, Harken, too, had adopted this method.

Mary Richardson had no idea what was in store for her when the catheter examination began. Since she had already endured so much, she submitted to the examination of the right side of the heart without feeling any particular anxiety. But when she was placed face down on the table and the needle was inserted next to her spinal column, she fainted.

Mary Richardson's recollections:

"They stabbed me in the back. I went into shock, and all I remember after that was being in a daze. . . . I was so sick for two weeks that they wouldn't even let my mother in."

But since Dr. Harken had told her in advance that some of the tests might be painful, this experience did not alter Mary's admiration for him and her confidence that he was the only doctor who understood her and would help her. For Harken himself, however, the more or less unsuccessful catheterization meant that his diagnosis remained incomplete. What he had been able to discover lent support to his hunch that Mary was suffering from a combination of stenosis and insufficiency. He feared that Mary was one of those patients who could be helped only to a limited degree. Elimination of the stenosis would produce distinct improvement and prolong her life. But the development of the insufficiency could not be checked. He hoped, however, that the stenosis operation might tide Mary over until his ball valve was ready for use in human beings. He therefore decided to carry out the operation by the old-fashioned "blind" method, and to postpone major open-heart surgery until he could attempt a complete replacement of the defective valve.

As the month drew to its close, he told Mary that he would operate and try to relieve her heart defect on November 29. Mary and her mother were given no details about the diagnosis or the operation, nor did they ask, for they assumed that they would not understand the explanations. Mary's faith in Dr. Harken was so great by now that any decision he made had to be, in her mind, the right decision.

Mary Richardson's recollections:

"He treated me like a daughter, and through the years it's been like that. He's like having another father, that's what he seems like to me."

Mary's mother telephoned Bill and her husband. Both men took time off from work and arrived in a depressingly gray, chilly Boston on November 27. But Bill found Mary in a sanguine mood; she assured him that Dr. Harken was undoubtedly doing the right thing.

The operation took place on schedule on November 29. When Bill was allowed to see Mary in the recovery room a few hours afterward, he was aghast to find her with tubes in her nose, catheters and needles stuck into her arms and chest. Machines were humming steadily, and jagged lines moved across a screen, accompanied by a monotonous beep-beep-beep. But Bill calmed down when a nurse assured him that all was going well and explained that the beeps were reproducing Mary's heartbeat.

Sure enough, Mary was able to get up two weeks later. She was still in pain, since several of her ribs had had to be severed. But she assured Bill that she felt better than before the operation. And he could see for himself that she no longer suffered from breathlessness. On the day he and Mary's father had to fly back to Jacksonville to return to their jobs, Mary was climbing steps without breathing hard. After a total of seven weeks in Mount Auburn, she telephoned Bill that she was coming home, and that she felt well—so wonderfully well. Two days later, when she emerged from the plane, she was still pale from the sunless north, but Bill thought she was utterly beautiful and looked like a new person. Both were convinced that they were beginning a new life—and they did not complain when the bills from Mount Auburn swallowed up all their savings.

Mary Richardson's recollections:

"We had learned that health was more important than money. . . . So I was able to work half days again. I was full of nervous energy, and I soon forgot that Dr. Harken had told me before I left to stick to a salt-free diet and sleep a lot. . . . I now think Dr. Harken had me in mind for his artificial-valve operation right from the start, but it wasn't ready the first time I went in and he just wanted to keep me alive long enough to try the valve."

By 1959 the functional tests on Harken's ball valve were essentially complete. To test the valve for durability, a model was mounted on a rod that was pushed rapidly up and down by a motor. In three months this testing apparatus had subjected the valve to as many pulsations as a normal heart valve would receive in five years. At the end of the test period, the steel framework and the ball showed no significant signs of wear. But this mechanical test, of course, provided no information on chemical changes in an actual blood stream.

Moreover, no matter how tough the valve itself was, it would be useless unless it could be anchored in a patient's aorta as permanently as a natural valve. For this reason the steel ring at the base of the valve was embedded in Ivalon plastic, which is compatible with tissue. Harken intended to suture the Ivalon parts to the wall of the aorta with strong silk threads.

At the end of 1959, Harken was ready to attempt his first replacement of a human aortic valve. His first patient was a young man who had become an invalid because of rheumatic aortic valve insufficiency. His left ventricle was enormously enlarged and his death only a question of days. Harken opened the thoracic cavity and attached the heart-lung machine. Hypothermia brought the heart to a stop. Harken then opened the aorta with a Y incision. He removed the defective aortic valve, sutured the Ivalon patch of the valve to the wall of the aorta, and closed up the aorta. But when he stopped the hypothermia and warmed the heart again, he could not make it resume beating. The enlarged left ventricle filled with blood, but many years of sickness had left the muscles too weak to pump it into the aorta. The patient died on the operating table.

Mary Richardson at first refused to believe it. When her first spells of giddiness came on in the summer of 1959, she tried to think that it was due to a heat wave, or that she had been mowing the lawn too long. Shortly afterward, however, she began feeling breathless again when she climbed the stairs at the real-estate office where she worked. She stopped trying to deceive herself. So she had not regained her health; she had only received a reprieve, and she realized that Dr. Harken had foreseen this when he put his arm around her shoulders and told her she must let him know at once whenever she did not feel well.

She and Bill wrote to Dr. Harken. By this time it was autumn, and Mary's spells of weakness had increased to the point that she had to give up her job again. It was a relief to hear from Dr. Harken that he was coming to Florida for a convention in Orlando. Mary could meet him there and spare herself the flight to Boston. Bill and Mary could drive the 145 miles to Orlando in a few hours.

Mary Richardson's recollections:

"He told me I needed another operation, but he didn't say anything about the artificial valve; maybe he wasn't sure it would be ready in time. So we drove home. But there it got worse from week to week. I gained quite a few pounds—it was all water. . . . In January 1960 it was clear something had to be done. Dr. Harken had me come to Boston, to the Peter Bent Brigham Hospital this time. I arrived there on February 20. By then I was so sick that Bill and my parents flew with me because they were afraid Dr. Harken would operate at once, and they wanted to be there in case anything happened to me. They didn't talk about that, but I knew what they were thinking."

They took the midnight plane again. At the Peter Bent Brigham Hospital, Mary was placed in a twelve-bed ward—the family had to economize.

They were partly disappointed, partly relieved to learn from Harken's deputy, Dr. Warren Taylor, that Dr. Harken was out of town. But the preparations for the operation would take two weeks in any case. Rather than lose so much time from their jobs, Bill and Mary's father decided to fly back to Jacksonville during the interval.

Two days later, after Mary had undergone the first examinations, a tall, gray-haired man opened the curtain that hung in front of Mary's cubicle. He was Dr. Lewis Dexter, the hospital's chief cardiologist. Here was a doctor whose aura was of cool reserve, in contrast to Dr. Harken's warm friendliness. He announced a new catheter examination. Mary remembered the shock she had suffered in November 1958. But Dexter assured her that another method would be used, one that would cause her no pain. Nevertheless, she was fearful when she was taken to an examination room on February 26. The name "transseptal catheterization" meant no more to her than the name of its inventor, Dr. John Ross.

The method consisted of introducing a triple catheter into the femoral vein and pushing it up the blood vessel. The outside catheter entered the right atrium of the heart. The second catheter, inside it, penetrated the septum into the left auricle. The third, inside the other, was forced through the mitral valve into the left ventricle. Mary did feel the catheter moving through her body. But this time she was spared the stabbing sensation in her back. Finally she was told that an X-ray–opaque dye was going to be injected into her heart and that she would feel a kind of heat wave racing through her body. Fortunately, the wave of heat lasted only for a few seconds.

The results confirmed all of Harken's fears. Mary was suffering from a nonreparable aortic insufficiency. He and Dexter agreed that the only chance to save her was the installation of an artificial valve. Harken had not forgotten his first failure, and he had conceived a genuine affection for the brave little woman from Florida. But he thought that by now he had learned enough from the first case to have some prospects of success. Moreover, Mary was in much better condition than the young man who had died under his hands. Her left ventricle was scarcely enlarged, and Harken had reason to hope it would adjust to the sudden change of a new aortic valve. He decided that he would make his second attempt to implant his valve on March 10, 1960; but he allowed Mary to believe that she would merely be undergoing a repetition of her first operation. He intended to inform Bill Richardson about the novelty shortly before the operation.

On the morning of March 10, Bill and his father-in-law were the first to enter the waiting room near the swinging doors to the operating rooms. Meanwhile, Mary lay on the operating table, and Harken, assisted by Dr.

Soroff, Dr. Taylor, and Dr. Lefemine, began the decisive phase of the operation. Mary's body had been chilled to 82 degrees, and the ventricles of the heart were merely fluttering when he made a Y incision into the aorta. When the aortic valve was exposed, the destruction was plain to see. The brittle valve tissues were folded feebly into the ventricle when the pumping contraction ended, and blood poured back from the aorta into the ventricle. Nevertheless, this valve had kept Mary alive. As soon as it was removed, there would be only two alternatives: either the heart functioned with the new valve, or Mary would die. Here was another of those last moments before irrevocable decisions that Harken had faced so often in the course of his career.

Extirpation of the defective valve proceeded without difficulties. Harken was handed a ball valve and made the first sutures with strong silk thread.

Meanwhile, Bill paced the waiting room. Perhaps the hours of waiting would have been more intolerable if a stranger had not joined him and his father-in-law. She introduced herself as Mrs. Norma Lawson, of a Boston club called Mended Hearts. The members had survived heart operations themselves or were relatives of such survivors; they had all undertaken to stand by new heart-operation patients. Norma's husband, George Lawson, had been operated on in 1957. Since then he had resumed his travels as a salesman through the entire Northeast. Norma had heard about Mary's impending operation and had turned up—talkative and optimistic—to make the time of waiting easier for Bill and Mary's father. She, too, did not know what Harken was doing at the moment, but she told them about his other wonderful accomplishments and distracted them somewhat from their anxiety.

Harken completed the suture of the valve. He closed the aorta. Now came the decisive moment, at which he had lost his first patient. Warming began. When the temperature rose to 85 and then 86, then 87, all those who had gathered around the operating table and who had witnessed the first debacle looked in silent suspense at Mary's heart. The thermometer showed 88 degrees. One of the assistants held the defibrillator ready, to shock the heart if it failed to beat of its own accord. The temperature increased to 88, then 89. At that moment the heartbeat began, without any external impulse.

A few minutes later, Bill stepped to the door of the waiting room and peered out just as the swinging door was thrown open and Harken reappeared.

Bill Richardson's recollections:

"When I saw his smile, I knew it was all right. He had his chest thrown out this far, he was so proud. 'She's fine, just fine,' he called out. 'We put in a new valve and it's working beautifully.' "

Bill only wanted to know when he could see his wife. Harken advised him to go out with Mary's father and have a good meal. When they returned and he was allowed to enter the recovery room, he again saw the battery of machines he remembered from last time. Mary was surrounded by doctors and nurses. But she recognized him and smiled. That was enough for him. He still did not realize that she was the first human being whose aortic valve was made of steel and plastic.

During the following days Bill arrived at the hospital between four and five o'clock in the morning. He would sit for a while at the counter of Jim's Restaurant, only a few steps from the hospital, having his breakfast and listening to the radio until the hour when he could be admitted to the hospital. Word had meanwhile gone round that he was the husband of the patient from Florida in whom Harken had implanted the first artificial heart valve. Sometimes young doctors or nurses would pause to chat with him, and from them he gradually learned what a new heart valve was and why the operation on Mary was such a sensation.

Mary herself still had no idea what had been done to her. But now and then she heard a curious sound inside her chest.

Mary Richardson's recollections:

"The first thing I remember was waking up and hearing this funny click. I asked Dr. Harken what it was and he just laughed at me and said: 'There's no noise there at all.' But I still heard it."

Harken succumbed to the illusion of many doctors who have not themselves suffered their patients' illnesses and can never really empathize with the patients' sensations. On the basis of his technical experiments he was convinced that the valve could not be heard. But it was audible to Mary and remained so. Nevertheless, it was some time before she found out what was producing the clicking sound she heard inside her chest. For ten days she suffered from a slight fever, and Harken was beginning to worry about infection. Temporarily, her heart began to race. But both symptoms disappeared after treatment with antibiotics and digitalis. In order to prevent the formation of blood clots, Mary was given dicoumar and regular blood tests.

Mary was recovering so well that Bill and her father went home after two weeks. Shortly after these members of her family had left, Mary finally found out that she had been the subject of an unprecedented experiment. Day after day unknown doctors appeared at her bedside and applied their stethoscopes to her chest. When she asked Harken the reason, he at last sat down beside her and carefully explained the kind of operation she had undergone. His explanations agitated her so much that for several days she kept listening to the clicks inside her heart. When she was allowed out of bed and began walking around, it took days before she felt sure that the clicking would not stop when she moved—that, in other words, she could rely on her artificial valve. By the beginning of April, however, she had grown accustomed to it. And on April 2, when she and her mother were summoned to the ground floor of the hospital, she suddenly found herself confronting a group of photographers and a nurse who held a Harken valve in her hand. Mary was photographed with the valve. That was how she first saw the strange little ball in a cage that was keeping her alive. Next day she boarded the noon plane for Florida, climbing the steps without assistance.

At the time this first successful patient of Harken's flew home, she scarcely had any idea of her importance to him and to the future of the artificial heart valve. Her trouble-free convalescence encouraged Harken to undertake at once a third implantation of the ball valve, in a twenty-eight-year-old patient. The operation itself went smoothly, but as in his first case he did not succeed in restoring a regular heartbeat. Ten shocks were needed before the heart began to beat at all. Only a few days later it stopped altogether. Harken experienced the same disastrous failure with his fourth patient. Even twenty-two shocks did not restore the heartbeat after implantation of the valve. He assumed that his defibrillator was not strong enough to do the work with a single shock, and that the succession of shocks destroyed the heart muscle. Then his fifth patient, a man of forty-nine, died during the operation. This time the cause was fatal hemorrhages from the sutures between the aorta and the valve.

Only the successful example of Mary Richardson kept Harken from despair. He hoped to do better by increasing the strength of the defibrillator and by improved methods of suturing. On June 7, therefore, he operated on a forty-seven-year-old workman named Alfred Gallo from Franklin, near Boston. Since 1955, Harken had been treating Gallo, with the collaboration of the man's family doctor, Pastorello, for valvular insufficiency. But, as usual, he had not been able to prevent progressive deterioration of the heart. On March 18—elated by his success with Mary Richardson—he had proposed implantation of a valve. But Gallo hesitated until June before he gave his consent. This time the operation proceeded without complications. Gallo's heart began beating after a single shock, and a few weeks later he returned home. This happy outcome convinced Harken that the series of misfortunes was over; at brief intervals he undertook his seventh, eighth, and ninth valve operations. But his seventh patient died of an infection after four days. With the eighth, hemorrhaging from the sutures could not be checked. The ninth died of circulatory weakness. By the end of 1960, Harken was again so discouraged that he decided he must wait and watch the development of his two surviving patients in order to determine whether further operations were justified.

For the second time Mary Richardson felt her return home to be the symbol of a new life. She soon noticed that the artificial valve in her heart could not work as efficiently as the kind that nature provides. She also learned the limits of her own capacities. But then she began to live—almost like a normal person. At first she worked around the house, and then in the garden. Soon afterward she returned to her job. Bill received a contribution from the Florida State Vocational Rehabilitation Department to help pay the hospital bills, but the amount was not enough, and so the family needed every penny they could earn.

Some time later Norma Lawson of the Mended Hearts Club sent Mary clippings of newspaper articles about her operation. Mary was most impressed by the point made in most of the articles that the lives of thousands of other persons with diseased hearts depended on her survival. If she proved by living that the artificial heart valve would function, Dr. Harken and other surgeons would have the courage to continue their work. Mary began to feel that fate had assigned her an important mission.

Punctually, twice a month, she went to see Dr. Hammer. He examined her heart and blood and supplied her with digitalis and dicoumar. She now understood clearly why she would have to take dicoumar for the rest of her life. It was essential to prevent the formation of blood clots around the new valve.

In the late autumn she flew to Boston because Dr. Harken and Dr. Dexter wanted to determine the condition of her valve. It gave her a curious feeling, half sadness, half triumph, to hear from one of the interns that all but one of the other patients who had received an artificial valve had died, and that her visit was restoring Dr. Harken's courage. So she really had a mission. In the spring of 1961 she traveled north once more for another examination, and returned with the news that Dr. Harken was very pleased with her. The same friendly intern assured her that his confidence in the artificial valve had been so far restored that he intended to undertake new operations. Her sense of mission deepened.

In June the Mended Hearts Club invited her to Boston for the celebration of its tenth anniversary at the Sheraton Plaza. Everyone was eagerly awaiting her, she was told; and Dr. Harken would also be present. In spite of the expense, she and Bill decided to go. Mary made herself an evening dress. When she arrived at the Sheraton Plaza on June 3, she proved to be one of the prettiest of the women. Her face glowing, she listened to the discussions between Dr. Harken and other doctors on the future of heart surgery. When the banquet was over and the music began, Bill asked whether she would like to try dancing with him once more, after so many years. She replied: "No, Bill. The first dance is for Dr. Harken. I must show him that I can dance again. I want everybody to see it." She went over to the speakers' table, took Harken's hand, and drew him onto the dance floor. The doctor, ordinarily so robust and self-assured, seemed timid, as if he did not trust his own work. Then he let her lead him, while everyone watched the pair. Mary felt the click-click inside her chest grow unusually loud, and for a moment she had a touch of breathlessness. But she ignored it. She walked Harken back to his table and returned to Bill, to risk still another dance with him. Later, a short, quiet man was brought to her table and introduced to her as Alfred Gallo, the only other survivor among Dr. Harken's heart patients. She also danced with Gallo and proudly faced the cameras directed at them.

After Harken had observed Mary Richardson for a year, he decided to venture a further series of operations. But it turned out that his valve and the suture method were still imperfect. Three of the patients survived, but four died of hemorrhages from the sutures connecting the aorta with the valve. Under these circumstances, it was a considerable shock when Mary Richardson, Harken's foremost success so far, was thrown into a perilous crisis that was likewise caused by the valve sutures.

It actually began as early as the autumn of 1961, with spells of weakness and breathlessness. At first Mary and Bill were thrown into a panic. At night Bill would listen to the soft clicking within Mary's heart; it could be heard distinctly in the stillness and darkness. In January 1962, Dr. Dexter came to Jacksonville for a lecture. He heard about the relapse and informed Harken.

Mary was compelled to give up working. But after the first shock was over, she remembered her mission—to stay alive at all costs. For the first time she began making a regular practice of reading articles on heart diseases, in order to inform herself. She learned that Dr. Harken was not the only man in the field by now. A Dr. Starr at the University of Oregon

Medical School, in Portland, collaborating with an engineer named Edwards, had constructed a similar heart valve. Dr. Starr's first patient had died. But his second, a man named Philip Amundson, had received one of Starr's artificial mitral valves on September 21, 1960, and was still living; he was fifty-two years old. In January 1961 a blood clot had formed at the valve, causing a stroke, but Amundson had since recovered. On October 27, 1960, Dr. Starr had operated on a young Chinese girl, Amanda Chiang, who had reached Oregon from Formosa after an adventurous voyage. She, too, was living, was married, and now worked in San Francisco. The more Mary read, the firmer grew her determination to survive and show that her Dr. Harken was the real pioneer of artificial heart valves and had the longest-living patient.

When she received word that he was expecting her in Boston for an examination, she set out on April 24 with Bill and her mother. Now she was no longer ignorant. When Dr. Harken said she would have to undergo a third operation, she asked him this time to describe it. Harken admitted that in his preceding operations he had not yet had enough experience and had not drawn the sutures tightly enough. The threads had loosened, producing a new valvular insufficiency; he would have to repair that. The seams had to be tightened. For several days after hearing this, Mary had the feeling that the artificial valve was hanging in her heart by only a single thread, and she was anxious for the operation to take place as soon as possible.

But Harken had not forgotten the fatal hemorrhages in his last operations. He wanted to have enough blood of Mary's blood group available to be prepared for all contingencies. As it turned out, obtaining the blood was no problem. One of the Richardsons' neighbors in Jacksonville went from house to house, and in a few days so many donors offered blood that the blood bank in Jacksonville was able to send forty pints to Boston.

The new operation began on the morning of May 3. Harken opened the scar of the previous operation and enlarged it. When the aorta was exposed, he saw to what extent the sutures had loosened. He decided to insert new Ivalon patches, to sew strong threads around the valve through the aortal wall, and to draw the tissue right up to the valve ring. A first ring suture proved insufficient, so he added another, but this still did not stop the existing leaks. Harken therefore sutured the valve with a third thread. Even then it was not completely leakproof. But he had done what could be done.

Then—a few minutes after the repair work was apparently finished—the pattern of the electrocardiogram suddenly changed. The heart began to race. Immediately thereafter ventricular fibrillation began, and the blood pressure dropped until it was no longer measurable. Harken, who had already removed his gloves to leave the closing of the operation wound to his assistant, reached in with bare hands. By massages and injections he tried to restore the action of Mary Richardson's heart.

Bill Richardson's recollections:

"We were waiting in the lobby hoping that everything was going well. But suddenly we were called to Dr. Harken's office. I said to myself: Oh-oh, this is it. We had to pass the operating-room suite on our way. A nurse came out and I stammered: 'How is she?' She said: 'It was touch and go, but it's getting better.' It was an agonizing wait in the doctor's office. At last Dr. Harken came in, and the first thing I noticed was that he had blood on his hands, Mary's blood. He told us: 'She's all right, she's going to be all right, you needn't worry.' He explained what had happened and said Mary would have died if they had stitched up her chest before it happened. But after five minutes of heart massage and three shocks they'd pulled her through. But he was so shaken he said he would never operate on Mary again."

Harken was deeply shaken, and probably not only because Mary had almost died on the operating table. He knew now that the repair had been only partly successful and that Mary faced an uncertain future. Bill, however, was persuaded that even though Mary had barely escaped death, she was now all right again. At the end of seven weeks she returned to Florida —proud that she had come through all dangers and could continue to live for her mission. An additional piece of good news came from Dr. Harken: this time a scientific foundation would be paying all the costs of the operation.

A year of confidence was to follow. The couple refurbished their house. They often worked until late at night, Mary painting the doors, Bill the walls. Then her daughter, Loxy, married, and Mary was alone more often. But she felt so secure that she did not fear solitude. She continued to read whatever she could about artificial heart valves, and so she learned that in 1962 more and more operations like her own were being performed. Toward the end of the year she heard that Dr. Harken was coming to Orlando to show a medical convention a film that had been taken during her second operation. She asked whether she and Bill could come to see the film. Dr. Harken gladly agreed, and so Mary saw the famous operation on herself. It was a color film that had not been produced like ordinary medical films for television or the movies—with as little blood as possible shown. This film showed the extremely bloody reality. But Mary was by now so accustomed to operating rooms and hospitals that the film did not upset her. Rather, it strengthened her sense of pride in being an important link in a chain of development that had begun in March 1960.

In the spring of 1963 she flew to Boston, for the first time all by herself, because Dr. Harken had suggested another checkup. To her dismay, she learned that she needed still another operation.

This was a totally unexpected blow. She felt neither tired nor ill. But Dr. Dexter's tests showed that the reinforcement of the sutures, undertaken only a year ago, was already beginning to give way. It was only a question of time before a complete aortic insufficiency developed. As Mary understood it, Dr. Harken wanted to act before that point was reached, and all that was involved was a new "reinforcement" of the valve. Harken, however, feared that the plastic parts and sutures of the first valve might have become so worn out that every attempt at a fresh repair would be hopeless. He therefore planned to implant a completely new valve.

Mary went home for a while. On September 3, 1963, she returned to Boston with Bill and her mother for a fourth operation. Mary was the calmest of them all. She had grown used to living in a sphere in which hospitals and operations were not frightening, but were necessities in the struggle for survival. Bill, on the other hand, remembered that Dr. Harken had said he would never operate on Mary again. He told himself that Harken could have changed his mind only because Mary was on the brink of death anyhow.

On September 10 he and Mary's mother waited once more in Peter Bent Brigham Hospital. They kept fearing every minute that they would be summoned to Harken's office, as had happened last year. But after several hours the doctor appeared with a cheerful expression and told them that everything was all right. He had implanted a brand-new valve in Mary's heart.

Three weeks later they were able to return to Jacksonville.

By the time of the fourth operation on his first patient, Harken had accumulated so much experience that he no longer had any doubts about the future of the artificial heart valve. Most of the technical difficulties had been overcome. The fact that in Mary Richardson's case it had been possible to implant a valve twice, within a relatively short interval, naturally strengthened his faith in the surgical possibilities of heart-valve surrogates. Only the necessity to combat blood clotting continually remained a problem, but time alone could decide how long dicoumar and similar anticoagulants were effective and how reliable they were.

Now followed perhaps the happiest years in Mary Richardson's life. They began in October 1963 and lasted until Good Friday in 1968—and

Mary "lived" every single day of the time. She flew to Boston three more times. Each examination revealed that her new heart valve was "in perfect order." There was no signs of any loosening of the sutures. None of the tests indicated any tendency toward the formation of blood clots. Nevertheless, Dr. Harken warned her every time that the danger existed. Mary never forgot to take her dicoumar tablet, and to have Dr. Hammer check her blood twice a month. Otherwise, the single thing that reminded her of the valve in her chest was the clicking noise. But that sound had become a part of her life. While she was on the plane to Boston in April 1967 for a checkup, she read an article about the number of persons who had received artificial valves in the past seven years. No less than 18,000 valves of the type Dr. Starr had developed in Portland had been implanted. But after she finished the article she began thinking about one curious sentence: "after use" 2,800 valves had been returned to Dr. Starr so that he could examine them for signs of wear. This could only mean that the people who had worn those valves had died, even though the valves themselves showed virtually no traces of any failure in their materials. All the same, this half-hidden reference to the still existing faults of the valves did not frighten Mary. She had experienced some of the faults herself, but she was still living, and she felt sure there would be more and more survivors of valve operations and that some day the valves would be foolproof.

After returning from this last flight to Boston, she had an experience that showed her how closely her life was connected with the valve.

Mary Richardson's recollections:

"I was sitting on the couch here in the living room one day, and I guess I had started to get up too quickly, or made some quick move, and my heart stopped. I can feel every beat, so I felt it stop; I knew what had happened. And you know, just instinctively I hit myself on the chest. I don't know what made me do it, but it was just natural, like you'd hit a television set that doesn't focus, and when I hit it, it started working again, just like that."

Later, Mary thought this incident might have been a forewarning. On Good Friday morning in 1968 she and Bill drove to the nearby shopping center. They were back home by eleven o'clock, carried their bundles into the kitchen, and talked about Easter presents for their grandchildren, Jimmie and Debbie. Then Bill drove back to the shopping center to get a haircut. When he returned three-quarters of an hour later, he saw Mary's feet protruding from the open kitchen door. He found her lying immobile on the floor. In despair, he called a neighbor for help. The neighbor found that Mary was still breathing and telephoned for an ambulance, and she was rushed to the nearest hospital. There it turned out that after eight years, in spite of all the dicoumar and all the tests, a blood clot had formed in her aortic valve. It had reached an artery of the brain and produced paralysis of her left side. Mary was only forty-one years old. But the stroke was so severe that she had to be carried when she was brought home seven weeks later. Her left arm dangled slackly; her left leg was supported by heavy splints. Still she was determined not to capitulate to the deadliest threat to artificial heart valves—blood clots. In 1969, Bill took her to Warm Springs, Georgia, 275 miles from Jacksonville. There, in five weeks, she learned to move her leg in a light support, to dress herself, and to comb her hair. When she returned home, she removed the leg support.

She was no longer able to fly to Boston to show Harken that she was still alive. But she could hope that someday, with Bill's help, she would be able to enter a plane again. This hope was shattered in 1970 when Bill came down with such severe arthritis in his hands that he, too, needed an operation. Yet even now Mary would not admit defeat. In 1970 she and her heart survived an abdominal operation, and in 1971 the severing of several nerves that had been causing her increasingly intense pain in the shoulder ever since the stroke. When the writer Jerry LeBlanc called on her that same year, to find out how the first person with an artificial heart valve was doing eleven years later, he noted in his diary:

"Mary Richardson, blue-eyed and pale-faced, walks very slowly, delicately, yet with a kind of grandeur about her. Even though her left side has been paralyzed by a stroke since 1968, she limps along with a look of triumph about her, a small smile coming through despite what is an obvious struggle for her, just moving around. She emanates a sort of gratitude for the very act of human existence. Each beat of her heart is a victory for her, one senses. When it is still in the room you can listen for the click and hear it, a rhythmic beat like the tapping of a pencil on a desk, a dull click. I know Dr. Harken says you can't hear it and the patient can't feel it, but I heard it and she says she can feel it."

In medicine complete victories are rare. Harken and his successors were not granted any complete victory with their artificial heart valves. But tens of thousands of persons are now living with such valves, like Mary Richardson. There have been many variations of Harken's 1960 model; undoubtedly the Starr-Edwards valve has attained the widest distribution throughout the world. The purely surgical act of implantation has become routine. From substituting a single heart valve there has developed, in cases of severely diseased hearts, the replacement of several valves. But surgeons are still confronting the problem of blood-clot formation. That is the reason for efforts to use natural valves from cadavers or animals, or valves made of tissues from other parts of the body, instead of the artificial valves. On the basis of experience so far, such valves seldom result in blood clots. But they do not last as long. One must wait to see whether artifice or nature ultimately proves truly successful. The struggle to reach a decision has just begun.

The Kidney Patients

The artificial kidney, which ten years ago was still in the experimental stage, nowadays keeps countless people alive throughout the world. Kidney transplants, a perilous adventure a decade ago, today form part of surgical routine and save thousands from death, allowing them to lead a normal, productive life. Physicians such as Dr. Kolff, who invented the artificial kidney, Drs. Merrill, Murray, Hamburger, Kuss, who did so much to further kidney transplantations, are known the world over. But neither the artificial kidney as we know it today nor a kidney transplant could function without the courage of the patients whose bodies first accepted the dialysis solution of the artificial kidney or the natural kidney of another person. For all those who witnessed this chapter of medical history, these early patients are the pioneers and forerunners for the countless rescued lives of today. Their fate and their tragedies are more moving than those of us medical men. We owe them our knowledge, our experience, the prerequisites to success.

—Dr. Hans Winter, 1967

1 / Sofia Schafstadt

Paul Lester Gronstein in a lecture on "Wonders of Medicine,"
Prague, July 1937:

"Even the greatest miracles we think we have achieved are patchwork. The true miracles are nature's. One of the greatest is the kidney. Look at these kidneys from a cadaver. Each weighs no more than 120 to 150 grams. Each looks like a large bean. But these two ridiculous beans perform an incredible amount of work.

"Our hearts pump the blood in a continual stream through our kidneys. Their most vital task is to filter the blood and the body fluids contained in it. They must remove all the poisonous wastes deposited in the blood in the course of our metabolism. They do this by means of a filtering system consisting of innumerable microscopic filtering tubes, the glomeruli. If all the glomeruli in a single pair of kidneys were placed end to end, they would cover a distance of from 80 to 100 kilometers. As many as 1,800 liters of blood pour through this filtering system in twenty-four hours.

"Among the wastes removed by the kidneys are urea, creatine, uric acid, and salt. This refuse is passed on through the ureter to the bladder and excreted as urine. Out of the 1,800 liters of filtered body fluids, between 1.5 and 2 liters of waste-laden urine leave the human body daily.

"Our kidneys have still another task, that of maintaining the water content of our bodies at the same level, no matter how much fluid we take in. Thus they prevent a surplus of water from becoming established in our tissues and producing dropsical swellings.

"Finally, the kidneys do a third job. We all need certain chemicals in order to live. Among these are electrolytes such as potassium, sodium, and calcium. An excess or deficiency of these chemicals harms our organs. If there is an excess, the kidneys filter it out of the blood. If there is too little, they restore the balance. In this way the kidneys decide health and illness, life and death. Nature is aware of the importance of their function, for if disease incapacitates one of the kidneys, the other is able to take over the full work of its mate.

"But if you were to ask me how and why each of these curious 'beans'

73

is capable of performing such a tremendous amount of work, I would have to admit that I don't know. I know only this: The human being whose two kidneys are destroyed by malformations or diseases is hopelessly condemned to death. And there are many such diseases and malformations. They extend from changes in the ureter, which block the outflow of urine and so destroy the kidneys, to mysterious inflammations of the glomeruli—glomerulonephritis, as it is called. We are helpless to do anything about inflammations of this type. The filtering function is then paralyzed. The metabolic wastes accumulate in the blood. The electrolytic balance is lost. The end of the trail is the poisoning of the body through its own waste products, uremia. This disease kills its victims slowly, and the process is often accompanied by violent symptoms: tremendous increase in blood pressure, unbearable headaches, blindness, mental confusion, and finally convulsions that end in a fatal coma. And we must look on helplessly."

His name was Jan Bruning. He was only twenty-two years old, the son of a small farmer from a village near Groningen, in Holland. In October 1938 he lay in bed in the Groningen university hospital. High blood pressure made his face ruddy. The accumulation of urea in his blood was so enormous that crystals of urea penetrated his skin, producing an intolerable itching. He vomited up all food. The retinas of his eyes were changing; the world around him was darkening.

One Sunday, the last Sunday in October, he no longer recognized his mother—who had come to Groningen in a silk Sunday dress, wearing a white lace cap she had made herself. He had become blind.

Three days later he lost consciousness, and twenty-four hours later he was dead. The cause of death was recorded as: Final stage of chronic glomerulonephritis—uremia. That year there were thousands of others throughout the world who died in the same way. Only one factor was different—the doctor who watched over that death.

The doctor's name was Willem Kolff. He was also a young man of only twenty-seven. His wife and friends had nicknamed him "Pim." Pim had three distinguishing characteristics: a soft heart, not yet inured to medical routine; a fondness for the technical problems of medicine; and a kind of obsessiveness in the pursuit of ideas. When the hospital administration of Groningen put Jan Bruning into one of the four beds assigned to Willem Kolff, it was unwittingly making a fateful decision. Bruning was Willem Kolff's first patient to die of uremia, and Kolff never got over the fact that this boy had had to die. The doctor had still to learn to accept death without emotion. Kolff also could not get over having had to tell the lace-capped peasant woman that her son could not be saved.

Willem J. Kolff twenty-seven years later in Annals of
Internal Medicine:

"I had to tell her that her only son was going to die, and I felt very
helpless. Gradually the idea grew in me that if we could only remove 20
grams of urea and other retention products per day we might relieve this
man's nausea, and that if we did this from day to day life might still be
possible."

That was how it began. During the last few days before Jan's death,
Kolff ransacked the Groningen university library. He searched for information on some technical way to replace the filter tubes of the kidneys.
Would there not be some material or apparatus that could be used to
purify human blood of waste products if the blood were channeled out of
the body through such a filter and back into the body?

Kolff found that other doctors and technicians had entertained similar
ideas. In 1913 the Americans Abel, Rowntree, and Turner had attempted
to construct an "artificial kidney" employing a blood filter. But they could
find no material capable of performing the filtration of the natural kidney.
In 1925 a man named Haas had likewise experimented with blood purifi-
cation. He, too, had failed.

None of these experimenters had found a suitable filter material. Nor
had there been any way to prevent the blood that they pumped through
their filters from coagulating as soon as it left the body of the animal they
were experimenting on.

That was about the limit of the information Kolff found in the library.
But thirteen years had passed since 1925, and in the past year the drug
heparin had become available—a drug that controlled the property of
blood to coagulate. The question of the blood filter remained.

Three weeks after Jan Bruning had been laid to rest in his home village, Kolff met one of his teachers, Professor Brinkmann. Brinkmann
taught biochemistry in Groningen. He showed Kolff a remarkable new
material called cellophane, a recently imported cellulose product from
Germany that could be made into extraordinarily thin membranes. Several
factories were producing sausage casings from it. Brinkmann had discovered important biochemical uses for cellophane. If two fluids of differing
chemical concentrations were separated by a layer of cellophane, an exchange of chemicals took place through the membrane: molecules of
chemicals that were present in greater quantity on one side moved to the
side of lesser concentration. Blood corpuscles, on the other hand, were too
large to pass through the cellophane membrane.

During Brinkmann's demonstration Kolff kept thinking of Jan Bruning and his death from nephritis. He asked himself whether cellophane might not be the material that Abel, Rowntree, Turner, and Haas had vainly sought. He bought a supply of cellophane sausage casing and filled a piece 45 centimeters long with 25 cubic centimeters of blood. To this blood he added 100 milligrams of urea, sealed both ends, and tied the casing to a wooden holder. He then suspended the tube in a vessel containing saline solution, which has the same concentration of salt as normal human blood, but no urea, and kept it in gentle motion.

When he withdrew the tubing from the vessel fifteen minutes later and measured the urea content of the blood, he found that all the urea had been transferred to the saline solution. Surprised and delighted, Kolff started to calculate. If instead of 25 cubic centimeters of blood he filled a 10-meter cellophane tube with 500 cubic centimeters and somehow rocked it in a saline solution, it should be possible to remove 2 grams of urea from the blood in fifteen minutes.

Willem J. Kolff twenty-seven years later:

"I built or had built several apparatuses. . . . None were constructed well enough to be clinically applicable. On the 10th of May, 1940, the German armies invaded the Netherlands. . . . The head of the Medical Department, Professor Polak Daniels, and his wife committed suicide as soon as it was known that the *Waterlinie,* the inundated defense line that had protected the provinces of Holland through previous centuries, proved to be no sufficient deterrent for German parachute troops. . . . Whereas other members of the staff had shown marked impatience regarding my plans about an artificial kidney, Polak Daniels had allowed me to go ahead without ridiculing the idea. His death left a vacancy . . . and the Germans, instead of following the recommendations of the faculty, appointed a Dutch national socialist with a German name, Kreuz Wendedich von dem Borne, to become the Professor of Medicine. On the day he arrived I left, and consequently had to look for a job, which I found in the city of Kampen. Kampen is one of the oldest cities of the Netherlands, situated where the river Yssel runs into the old Zuider Zee."

Kampen—it meant brick buildings, low houses, cobbled streets, people occasionally still clattering over the cobbles in wooden shoes, factories, a secondary school, and an old-fashioned eighty-bed hospital—a small town of 23,000 people under German occupation. There were a few German military offices, spies, strict controls of all aspects of life, confiscations, labor permits, ration cards, and, finally, hunger, cold, and the black market.

When Kolff, his wife, Janke, and his children, Jakob and Adrie, moved into a modest house on Jan van Arkel Straat, only five minutes away from the hospital, the doctor had primarily two things in mind. He wanted to have nothing to do with the Germans. And he wanted to create a laboratory where he could continue to develop his artificial kidney. He needed hardly any furniture (grateful patients later made a sofa for him), but he had to have his apparatus and his boxes filled to the brim with cellophane sausage casings.

Kolff was able to set up his laboratory, and obtained his first laboratory assistant, Mieneke van der Ley. A young assistant, Dr. P. S. M. Kop, was assigned to him, and he found an excellent head nurse, Ter Welle, and two eager student nurses named Raab and Grieteke van den Noort. Some members of the municipal administration in Kampen began to wonder whether they had done well to bring Kolff to the city as an internist. For they learned that he had cleared out Room 13 of the hospital, renamed it 12a for superstitious reasons, and installed therein the peculiar apparatus he had brought from Groningen, something he called the artificial kidney. Moreover, it was rumored that he left his patients to his assistant, Kop, while he tinkered with the apparatus in Room 12a. Other rumors had it that he had made friends with Hendrik Berk, director of the Kampen enamel factory, and had coaxed Berk into building more artificial kidneys. Kehrer, the hospital surgeon, spoke irritably or scornfully about Kolff's "playing with kidneys."

Under the eyes of the German authorities, who expected the factory to concentrate on war production for them, Berk built a larger artificial kidney, which for the first time had the benefit of expert technical advice. In October 1942 it stood in the middle of the mysterious Room 12a. Kolff had meanwhile trained Mieneke van der Ley in all the standard kidney tests and had installed a second laboratory assistant, Willy Eskes, in an adjacent laboratory. He had aroused Grieteke van den Noort's interest in his apparatus and hired a Dutch medical student, Bob van Noordwijk, as a further assistant on the project—the Germans having barred the young man from the university because of his socialist ideas. Altogether, Kolff had exercised so much charm and persuasiveness that virtually everyone in the hospital, including Andries Sybrands, the gatekeeper, was willing to help him with his artificial kidney whenever he needed help.

Willem J. Kolff's recollections:

"When the time came for me to pay for the first rotating-drum artificial kidney, it was realized that only work done for the German Wehrmacht could appear in the books of the company. Consequently Berk Enamel Works forgot to charge for the artificial kidney.

"The principle of the rotating-drum artificial kidney is very simple. Twenty meters of cellophane tubing are wrapped around a horizontal drum. If you imagine a little bit of blood sitting in the limp, wet cellophane tubing anywhere around the drum, that blood will certainly sink to the lowest point of the drum. If the drum turns around slowly, the blood inside the cellophane, continuously seeking the lowest point of the cellophane, would be compelled by gravity to run through the cellophane from one end of the drum to the other. Since the lower half of the drum is immersed in a large bath with dialyzing fluid, we have fulfilled the important requirement that both blood and rinsing fluid must be in continuous motion. Of course, the blood has to get in one end of the cellophane wrapped around the drum and then out the other end, and this was best done by leading it through the hollow axle of the drum. . . . During the first treatments we had some trouble with the rotating couplings. I went to see the local car dealer and took over the idea that Henry Ford had used in constructing the seal of the water pump of his engine. The packing around a rotating joint good enough for a Ford automobile would certainly be good enough for an artificial kidney."

Hendrik Berk's recollections:

"I built the artificial kidney in 1942. Six months after delivery Kolff hooked the first patients to the machine. Later I heard about how many people had subsequently died from the 'kidney.' . . . As builder of the apparatus, that news depressed me deeply."

Actually it was not quite six months later that Kolff, in 1943, made his first experiments to test the effectiveness of his kidney on nephritic patients.

Through the winter he worked in Room 12a preparing for the tests. He and his assistants and the nurses became accustomed to working evenings and nights, when their regular duties were over. There were plenty of problems that remained unsolved. With nephritic patients, it was not only the urea disposal but the entire electrolytic equilibrium of potassium, sodium, calcium, and magnesium that was out of kilter. The composition of the dialysis bath had to be just right if the blood's electrolytic level was to be diminished or increased. Kolff personally weighed the chemicals and prepared a wide variety of dialysis solutions.

Another problem was how to hook the cellophane tubing to the patient's blood circulation. A glass tube could be introduced into an artery, connected by rubber tubing to the cellophane skin, and returned by similar rubber and glass tubing to a vein. But what would happen to the blood in the tubes? Would it form clots and therefore kill the patient as soon as it was returned to the blood vessels?

Kolff did have heparin at his disposal. But the drug was new and known to cause severe shock reactions in many patients. Kolff had no idea what the dosage should be to prevent coagulation as the blood made its long journey through his artificial kidney. Also, there was as yet no drug to counter the anticoagulant effect of heparin. Dangerous hemorrhages might occur at the point where the tubing was inserted, since the patient's blood would no longer have the ability to clot. At the time there was talk about a certain protamine sulfate that showed promise of counteracting heparin. But this drug was just beginning to be tested.

From the notes of a deceased assistant of Kolff:

"Toward the end of the winter of 1942–43 we brought our first patient into the 'kidney room.' His name was Boele, Gustav Boele, I think. He was a Jew of advanced age who had spent his entire life in Holland. If I recall rightly, his entire family had been transported by the Germans to a Polish death camp. He had been hospitalized for many months and we managed to keep him from deportation.

"Boele was suffering from hypertrophia of the prostrate, which should have been operated on earlier. But the German invasion and the isolation of the Jews had prevented proper treatment. As a result of the prostate tumor, his urethra was displaced. The urine had backed up to the kidneys and so produced a chronic inflammation accompanied by uremia.

"His mind often wandered. When coma ensued, Kolff decided that here was so desperate a case that only his machine could rescue the man. He did not dare to insert a cannula into the old man's brittle arteries. Instead, he used a venepuncture needle to remove 50 cubic centimeters of blood from one of the arm veins, ran this blood through the artificial kidney, and injected it back into Boele's vein after filtration. It was a highly circumstantial process. But Kolff hoped in this way to remove the deadly urea wastes from a liter, perhaps from two, three, or four liters, of blood.

"Boele, however, did not come out of the coma. He died showing no effects from Kolff's experiment. At least it was granted to him to be buried in his homeland, not cremated somewhere in Poland."

A few weeks later, on March 16, 1943, one of the few ambulances still allowed the Dutch for the civilian population brought a young woman to Kampen. Her name was Janny Schrijver. She was twenty-nine years old, had been working as a cleaning woman, and was suffering from glomerulonephritis. Her father, an old peasant, came along to the hospital. When

Kolff saw her for the first time, she was sitting up in bed, propped against pillows, struggling for breath. She was a simple person who had never really grasped what was wrong with her. She had worked until she collapsed. Now she complained about the mad racing of her heart, about the terrible pressure on her chest—as if a sack of grain were lying on her, taking her breath away. Her mind became confused. Her blood pressure was 245/150. It was obvious from the condition of her eyes that her sight was going. The urea level had already reached 1.69 grams per liter, as against the normal amount of 0.45 to 0.5 grams.

It was clear that she would fall into a fatal coma within a few days. Since she was doomed in any case, Kolff decided to try his machine for the second time. He took Janny's father aside and tried to explain in the simplest possible terms what he proposed to do. "Janny's blood is poisoned. We want to take part of her blood out of Janny's body, run it through a machine that will remove the poison, and return the blood to her body. You may stand by if you like and watch to see that nothing wrong is being done to her."

The old man trusted Kolff because he spoke to him in rustic dialect. But he wanted to know whether Kolff was sure this thing would help.

When Kolff replied that he could not be sure, that he would only try to do his best, the old man said: "Then let the minister come first. Afterward you can try it."

And so the Reverend Gastman of Kampen came and stayed for a while by Janny's bed—never imagining how often in the next year he would be coming to the beds of dying persons before Kolff took them into his kidney room and tried out his machine. Then Sybrands, the doorkeeper, wheeled the patient into Room 12a. She lay on a narrow bed that Kolff had designed because the door to 12a was too narrow for ordinary beds.

Janny was scarcely aware of her surroundings by now. The room was bare, equipped only with the implements that belonged to the artificial kidney—containers of dialysis solution, an instrument table, and a blackboard for keeping track of the progress of the treatment, the changes in the patient's condition, and the results of the blood tests, which were to be taken at regular intervals.

A number of bricks were distributed over the floor. In previous experiments it had developed that the cellophane tubing, even if it was turned with great caution, tore easily. Then the blood in it flowed into the dialysis solution, at once forming a bloody foam that overflowed the tub and spilled out on the floor. In this third year of the war, neither Kolff nor his associates possessed watertight shoes. When the tub began to overflow, they took refuge on the bricks so they could remain dry-shod while repairing the cellophane tubing.

In this macabre environment, Janny Schrijver lay half unconscious. In her case, too, Kolff did not dare attach her arteries and veins directly to the machine. First he injected heparin in such amounts that in after years he shuddered—the dose was almost ten times what future research would prove necessary. Then he waited. He wanted to determine whether any reactions Janny Schrijver might show during the coming treatment were due to the heparin or to the operation of his artificial kidney. Only after he had seen that there was no stronger reaction than chills and fever did he take a tenth of a liter of blood from one of Janny's veins and fill the cellophane tubing of the machine with it.

The motor that turned the drum began to hum. Slowly, the blood moved through the bath from cellophane loop to cellophane loop. Everyone prayed that this time there would be no mishaps—no break in the cellophane, no leaks, no bloody foam spilling on the floor. After twenty-two minutes Kolff poured the blood into a glass infusion vessel, from which it flowed through a vein and back into Janny's circulatory system. Ten times he repeated the procedure, until he had laboriously, in the course of many hours, run through the machine a liter of blood and returned it to the patient.

Kolff's assistants watched every reaction, checking the blood pressure, testing samples of blood for urea, creatinine, uric acid, and phosphates. They worked late into the night, and repeatedly found that the blood leaving the artificial kidney was actually free of urea. But the filtered quantity was much too small to influence the patient's condition.

The following evening, therefore, Kolff and his associates were back in Room 12a, gathered around Janny Schrijver to undertake another, lengthier treatment. On March 18 they dialyzed 1½, on the following day 3½, then 4½, and finally 5½ liters of blood. Each dialysis was a matter of many hours, removing the blood, filtering it, and injecting it back into the body.

The puncture needles that Kolff inserted into the veins were well worn. New needles were no longer obtainable in Holland. Many of the needles in the hospital had been used and resterilized hundreds of times. Some were rusted on the inside, and in spite of the heparin tiny blood clots formed on these particles of rust. Worse still, Kolff had to puncture more and more veins. No one had thought of the possibility, but it now became evident that before long there would be no usable undamaged vein left in Janny Schrijver's body. On the other hand, there were now the first signs of improvement in Janny's condition. The urea level suddenly stopped increasing. It did not drop, but held at 1.64 grams. Simultaneously, the very high blood pressure began to fall.

For the first time Kolff felt a sense of confidence. Unfortunately, further tests showed that the long period of nephritis had severely damaged

Janny's other organs. Her heart was suffering from chronic pericarditis. Moreover, she was subject to creeping infections which were especially hard on her in her wretched condition. But fourteen days passed without any worsening of the uremia. Contrary to all expectations, Janny was still alive.

At this point Kolff decided on a further step which would avoid this continually interrupted, painfully slow, and imperfect method of treatment. He would try to connect Janny Schrijver directly to the machine and have her blood flow through it from one vein and back into another vein. On April 4, as he and his assistants watched blood flowing for the first time directly into the cellophane tubing, through the machine, and back into Janny Schrijver's vein, they all had the feeling that they were living through a historic moment—in the midst of the war, in an occupied town that hardly anyone outside of Holland had ever heard of.

All of them were braced for some kind of disaster. They took turns watching at Janny Schrijver's bed. But nothing happened—no fatal shock, no sepsis caused by bacteria that had somehow got into the dialysis bath and entered Janny's blood. The urea levels came down. In the days following April 4, Kolff performed four more dialyses. By the fourth he was successfully passing 20 liters of blood through the machine. The urea level dropped below 1 gram. Janny recovered somewhat; it became possible to talk with her, and she spoke quite rationally about her home. But the improvement lasted for only two days. Then the urea level rose steeply again, and Janny sank back into her coma. Hastily, she was brought to Room 12a. Again 20 liters of blood were passed through the machine; again she improved and spoke rationally—but only for two days. Within forty-eight hours the metabolic wastes in the blood had reached a dangerous level. Kolff labored desperately. Twice more, by many hours of dialysis, he brought Janny Schrijver back from the threshold of fatal coma to temporary consciousness. But on the twenty-sixth day of treatment, after the twelfth dialysis, what Kolff had feared at the end of March happened: he could find no uninjured usable vein on Janny's body by which she could be attached to the artificial kidney. In somber silence, Janny was brought back to her ward for the last time. Mieneke van der Ley, who week after week had been examining an endless succession of blood samples, could only report that the urea level was rising rapidly. Within a very short time, it reached 6.4 grams. Shortly after that last test, death came to the poor patient.

Kolff himself performed the autopsy, assisted by Sybrands. The dead woman's kidneys were extremely shrunken; they weighed only 67 and 80 grams. Was this outcome a defeat, proving that the idea of the artificial kidney was wrong? Had he merely tormented a dying woman for weeks with useless venepunctures and heparin chills, without really helping her? At a time when tens of thousands of persons were daily being shot, gassed, blown to bits by bombs, charred in burning cities, or were dying of epidemics and hunger, the question seemed academic. It was depressing to have lost his patient, but Kolff refused to see this as the final word. The experiment had shown, after all, that it was possible in principle for an artificial kidney to assume the functions of natural kidneys, even if only briefly—for the present. On April 16, when the family came to recover the body of the dead girl, the peasant father knocked on Kolff's door. He did not talk about fault. He said: "I know you tried everything. I've come to thank you."

Kolff made a weary gesture. But the old man said he had come not only to express his thanks; he also wanted to know what he owed the doctor. Kolff tried to wave this aside. The old man insisted. At last Kolff mentioned the sum of 60 guilder. And Janny Schrijver's father took out his purse, paid the money, and went to bury his daughter.

Willem J. Kolff twenty-seven years later:

"From March 17, 1943, until July 27, 1944, fifteen patients were treated. Of these fifteen patients only one survived. This patient . . . might not have needed the artificial kidney. . . . I sometimes wonder what would have happened to this project if I had done it not in the Netherlands but in some location in the United States, and if having treated fifteen patients . . . I could not have claimed a single therapeutic triumph."

From the notes of a deceased assistant of Kolff:

"Today it is difficult to cast one's mind back to the circumstances in which we went on with our project after the death of Janny Schrijver. I wonder whether anyone would be prepared to do this sort of thing today. There were many nights when Kolff himself never left the hospital. He slept on a stretcher and lived mostly on zwieback and tea, for he was suffering from gastric trouble.

"The doctors in the vicinity of Kampen would normally let patients with chronic glomerulonephritis die at home. Kolff asked them to send him the patients they could no longer help. In time we saw more and more such patients. But all came too late. The doctors did not send people until they were dying, on the theory that although Kolff could not help them when they reached this stage, at least he could no longer harm them.

"Frequently the patients died before we even had time to connect them to the machine. With our inadequate instruments, it was a lengthy procedure before we could start the blood flowing through the machine. After we lost our tenth patient, Kolff switched to opening arteries and veins with a small incision and inserting larger glass cannulae, from which rubber tubes led to the artificial kidney and then back to the patients. But since the patients came too late and their blood vessels had already been damaged by uremia, the walls of the arteries often collapsed after the most minor surgery. Soon we were unable to obtain rubber tubes, because all rubber had been confiscated for the German army. To save rubber we had to use glass tubes, but these caused the formation of clots, in spite of the heparin.

"We had all reached a nadir of depression by the time Kolff, in his efforts to obtain support, invited a number of influential medical men and persons in the municipal government to watch a treatment with the artificial kidney. On this occasion, a rip developed in the cellophane tubing. The sight of the hapless patient and the idea that the blood was running out of his body into a primitive machine severely tried the nerves of the laymen—and possibly of the doctors as well. But to have the machine break down and flood the floor with bloody foam—that was too much for the outsiders. The whole cause seemed to be lost. At such times Kolff was so upset that he would forget to remove the surgical mask from his face and to the astonishment of the townspeople would bicycle home with it on.

"What was most depressing was the implication that nothing could be done for patients with chronic nephritis. Since their kidneys would never be able to function, they would have to be attached to the machine at regular intervals for the rest of their lives, in order to remove the metabolic wastes from their blood. But this could not be done more than ten or twelve times. For soon not a sound vein or artery was available.

"Consequently, Kolff began pinning his hopes on patients who were suffering from an acute inflammation or failure of the kidneys due to infectious disease or poisoning. In cases such as these, he was convinced, the kidneys could recover and resume their work if the burden on them was temporarily relieved by connecting the patients to the artificial kidney and keeping them alive until the recovery process was completed.

"A fresh struggle began. Kolff tried to persuade the doctors, who had been sending him only their dying chronic patients, to let him have patients with acute kidney failure. His pleas and arguments proved vain, and possibly we would have given up if chance had not brought such a patient to Kampen on April 24, 1944.

"He was a relatively young man, an enormously overweight baker whose name, if I remember rightly, was Termeulen. In his case, too, the doctors had waited until he was uremic and unconscious before they decided to let Kolff have a last desperate try at keeping him alive. The urea level in his blood had reached the tremendous value of 7.04 grams. Strictly speaking, he was as good as dead; he seemed just another example of 'too late.' But this was a case of acute kidney failure, and Kolff summoned our whole team.

"We attached Termeulen to the artificial kidney for fourteen hours, taking turns watching over him. During the night we found it hard to keep our eyes open because the sound of the motor was so lulling. Every three hours Mieneke van der Ley and the other laboratory assistant changed the dialysis solution, replacing it with a fresh one.

"Ultimately, we passed 120 liters of blood through the machine. The artificial kidney had filtered Termeulen's blood twenty-four times. And during this period 263 grams of urea, a good half a pound, were absorbed by the dialysis solution. As a dried powder this quantity later filled a whole sugar bowl. The urea level in Termeulen's blood dropped from 7.94 to 1.92 grams.

"To our delight, Termeulen awoke from his coma and asked for the latest newspaper. On April 28, Kolff connected him to the machine for the second time and removed the urea that had again accumulated. Meanwhile, Termeulen's own kidneys actually began functioning again. They excreted urine. On April 29 the quantity excreted rose from hour to hour, and we began hoping for our first tangible success. But then came the relapse. Once again it was too late. Termeulen's general resistance had been too greatly undermined. Three days later he died under our hands.

"From the summer of 1944 on, it became impossible to transport severely ill patients. There were no longer any automobiles or ambulances available for the purpose. In order to be able to treat patients nevertheless, Kolff had several more artificial kidneys built and installed in other hospitals in Holland. The difficulties of building them were far greater than in 1942, for the Germans kept a close watch on even the smallest workshop. A cooper made the rollers for us out of wood.

"Kolff transported one machine to The Hague, taking it part by part. Another was smuggled to Amsterdam. There a school had been converted into an emergency hospital. The doctor in charge let Kolff set up his machine in an unused room, and promised to inform Kolff as soon as a suitable acute kidney case came his way. He kept his word, and Kolff took one of the few trains to Amsterdam. There he found a young woman, Greta Cleef by name, I think. She was only thirty-three, had survived an attack of scarlet fever, but was left with acute nephritis. Unfortunately, this had not been diagnosed early enough, so that Kolff was once more confronting the old problem of too late. The urea level was already 5.3 grams. The patient was unconscious.

"Kolff was alone; none of our team had been able to accompany him.

But he strove so hard for success that he remained awake for almost thirty hours straight, carrying out all the procedures himself.

"His difficulties began with an old trouble he had already encountered in Kampen: the patient's bed could not be moved into the room in which his machine stood because the door was too narrow. With hammer and saw, Kolff himself took out the doorframe. He brought the patient into the room, prepared the dialysis bath, connected Greta Cleef's blood vessels to the machine, and let it run for eighteen hours. During the night, after ten hours of dialysis, the patient awoke from her coma. In the morning, when an exhausted Kolff removed the tubes, she was fully conscious and talked about her family. The urea level had dropped to only 1.57 grams. The edema that had disfigured her body had literally shrunk.

"By afternoon Kolff was full of hope. Greta's own kidneys were excreting 400 cubic centimeters of urine. But the following evening she suddenly developed pneumonia with high fever. She died in the course of the night. Kolff returned to Kampen in a state of utter exhaustion.

"After each such experience he was depressed for days. There could no longer be any doubt that the artificial kidney was effectual. Yet Kolff knew that he must have at least one surviving patient who had been saved by his machine if he were ever to attract the attention of influential scientists to his work.

"On July 27, 1944, he was forced to abandon all further work on the artificial kidney. The Allies had landed in Normandy, and the Germans intended to defend Holland to the last, since their rocket installations were on Dutch soil. Kampen and Kolff were right in the middle of the final assault. Tens of thousands of Dutchmen were being transported to Germany. Many of them passed through Kampen, and we tried at least to save the sick ones and get them to an emergency hospital where they would be reasonably safe.

"In addition, the hospital was crowded with refugees. Emergency beds had been set up in all the corridors. The artificial kidney was pushed off in a corner. Kolff could not attempt to use it again until after the first British troops appeared in Kampen. But by then it was battered and beyond repair. While several workmen labored to build a new machine, Kolff wrote a preliminary report on his experiences with it: *De kunstmatige Nier* ('The Artificial Kidney'). It ended with the sentence: 'We must admit that all patients so far treated died. But in so-called hopeless cases we saw some small improvement several times, and we were able to delay death for considerable periods in a number of cases, despite total kidney failure. . . . I do not doubt that sooner or later I shall be able to treat a patient of whom I can say: he is cured. And without the artificial kidney he would certainly have died.'"

.   .   .

In fact it was only a few months before such a patient came his way.

Wherever the Germans left an occupied country, harsh and often merciless vengeance followed. It struck all those who had collaborated with the Germans, or who had expressed sympathy, friendship, or love for a German.

In Holland such retribution struck 126,000 men and 24,000 women. Among these women was Sofia Schafstadt, a widow, since remarried, sixty-seven years old, who was accused of having collaborated with the Germans for four years. A Dutch tribunal condemned her, her daughter, Elisabeth, and her son Jan to long prison sentences.

In the summer of 1945, Sofia Schafstadt was a prisoner in the old barracks at Kampen, which the Germans had used for Dutch slave laborers. Now it was filled with arrested collaborationists.

On September 3, 1945, an ambulance sped from the barracks to the Kampen hospital. On the stretcher lay Sofia Schafstadt, unconscious, running a high fever. Kehrer, the surgeon, diagnosed inflammation of the gall bladder, jaundice, kidney failure, and uremia. What urine was still being passed was dark brown. The patient's blood pressure was 250/160. She now reacted only to painful stimuli or to being loudly shouted at. Obviously her gall bladder should have been removed days earlier, before its toxic secretions caused the kidney failure. But in the final weeks of the war 20,000 Dutchmen had died of hunger; others were still dying of the consequences of privation. Against that sort of background, what did the sickness of a collaborator amount to?

Because an operation seemed too dangerous, Kehrer prescribed heavy doses of sulfanilamides to fight the infection. Because of the kidney failure, he consulted Kolff, who found large quantities of albumin in the patient's urine, and in her blood a urea level of nearly 2 grams. By September 6, however, the fever was slowly dropping. But then the treatment with sulfanilamides had to be abandoned because the kidneys were unable to excrete the drug and were thus being further damaged by it. On September 9 the urea level exceeded 2 grams. Sofia Schafstadt could produce only a few incomprehensible sounds from her parched throat. Kolff was sure that she was sliding into the fatal uremic coma he had seen so often, and that it was high time to undertake dialysis; otherwise he would once more be applying the artificial kidney too late.

Kehrer, however, decided on September 10 to try another cystoscopy, on the chance that some mechanical obstacle might have caused the kidney failure. He was able to insert a catheter up into the kidney only on the right side. On the left side the instrument stuck fast in the ureter.

The urea level rose and rose. Kolff kept pressing for the patient to be transferred to the "kidney room." He prepared his machine, while all his associates, who had shared so many disappointments with him, hoped against hope that this time the experiment might go better. On September 11, when the urea level reached 4 grams and there was no longer any sign of kidney function, Kolff was at last permitted to transfer the patient. Kehrer himself was so doubtful about it that he called in Sofia Schafstadt's family, so that they might see her for the last time.

Accordingly, her three children appeared at her bedside shortly before the treatment began. Their presence reflected something of the history of Holland in that period. Her son Jan—a prisoner in the penal camp at Amersfoort—was permitted out only because Sofia Schafstadt's second son, Henk, who had a record of opposition to the Germans, personally guaranteed the return of his brother to the penal camp after the hospital visit. The patient's second husband did not come. He, too, had been against the Germans; the couple's marriage had broken up, partly because of political disagreements, and only hostility remained between them. It was a somber gathering at the bedside of an unconscious woman in the shadow of death.

From the recollections of Sofia Schafstadt:

"I don't know how I was brought to the hospital. . . . I had violent pains in my joints. The first thing I thought was: maybe I broke an arm. All I knew was that I was in the hospital. In the morning two nurses took care of me. . . . They handled me roughly and it was terribly painful. The pain brought me to. I heard one blonde nurse saying to me: 'You don't have to scream like that. You weren't so gentle either when you were giving the orders.' . . . My answer was: 'You horrid brute.' "

The scene in Room 12a was familiar by now: the unconscious patient, the humming and splashing machine. Kolff, his face gaunt and furrowed, Dr. Kop, Grieteke van den Noort, thin and dark-haired, Mieneke van der Ley, Willy Eskes, and Sybrands. But the world around them had changed. The Germans were no longer there. Kolff had obtained a few improved instruments and better heparin from the British. Otherwise, the room was much as it had been during those unforgettable years 1943 and 1944.

The machine ran for 11½ hours. At the start Sofia Schafstadt was shaken by violent chills. She had to be kept warm with hot-water bags. Two hours later her breathing assumed that loud, irregular rhythm which for centuries had been recognized as the sign of severe kidney disease. Was it too late again?

The suspense mounted. The blackboard on the wall was soon covered with chalked notations on the dialysis bath, the blood pressure, urea levels. The bath solution was renewed several times. Then, at last, the urea level began to drop. The blood pressure sank. Even the dangerously high accumulation of creatinine diminished. As the night advanced, the blood pressure was lowered to 160/80. The urea level came down to 1.21 grams. Eighty liters of blood had passed through the machine when Kolff switched it off and had Sofia Schafstadt moved to a small private room.

He himself stayed at the hospital, waiting. He was both hopeful and inwardly steeling himself for a fresh disappointment. But on the morning of September 12 the patient stirred. She opened her eyes, shortly afterward regained full consciousness, and spoke her first distinct words. They sounded strange and macabre in the present situation, for they evidently expressed what Sofia Schafstadt had been brooding on during her illness. "Now," she said in a low but clear voice, "now I'm going to divorce my husband."

To Kolff those words were an encouraging sign of reawakening life. But a few hours later he had to recognize that the crisis was not yet over. The patient's kidneys began secreting urine, but hesitantly and slowly. The urea level rose again to 1.72 grams. Seized by new doubts, Kolff began preparing for a second dialysis. Then, without warning, the balance swung the other way. The kidneys worked faster and faster. Soon a purifying flood of urine began to pour from them. The urea concentration dropped at last to normal levels. By September 18 the full natural kidney function had been restored.

Kolff, and all the others who had gone through so many disappointments with him, felt a moment of indescribable elation. Later it might seem profoundly ironic that the first patient to be saved by the artificial kidney was one of those collaborationists whom Kolff had despised throughout the war because they had taken the enemy's side. But at this moment political and human aversions vanished. Kolff had only one idea in mind: he must not lose Sofia Schafstadt. She was his first living demonstration.

From the recollections of Sofia Schafstadt:

"As long as I live I'll never forget my gratitude to Dr. Kolff. It's only because of him that I am alive and able to write these lines. . . . Hardly anyone visited me. On St. Nicholas Eve I was sad. Everybody received packages except me. But Dr. Kolff played Santa Claus. . . . That was typical of him. If only all doctors knew . . . what miracles a friendly word can do for a patient."

.   .   .

Kolff tried to keep Sofia Schafstadt in the hospital as long as possible. But the time drew near for her return to the barracks in Kampen. As a last resort, the doctor paid a call on Commandant Oudshoorn, who was in charge of the barracks—and discovered that he knew the man. During the war Oudshoorn had been hunted by the German police. Kolff had saved him by giving him injections that temporarily turned him into an invalid. Kolff explained the special importance of Sofia Schafstadt's life and his fears that she might die in camp. Oudshoorn promised that he would bend every effort to procure a special dispensation for the woman.

Oudshoorn kept his word. Sofia Schafstadt's son Henk came to take his mother to his home in The Hague. There she recuperated rapidly. By 1946 she was taking long walks and beginning to ride her bicycle. She never again complained of kidney difficulties. In 1951 she developed symptoms of a disease of the pancreas, which, however, had no relation to her former kidney trouble. She underwent an operation and went to stay with her second son, Jan, for her convalescence—he had obtained an early release from prison in 1949 and had settled in the village of Bilthoven. There his mother died that same year, at the age of seventy-three.

Kolff made certain revisions in his article, *De kunstmatige Nier*, which was being printed in a medical journal. To the concluding paragraph, where he had written that all his patients had died, but that sooner or later his method would prove successful, he added the sentences: "After the first part of this article was set, such a patient actually came to me. . . . The patient was in such desperate condition before treatment with the artificial kidney that we expected her imminent death. With this patient we have in fact provided proof that it is possible to save the life of persons with acute uremia by use of the artificial kidney. . . . She gave us the decisive impetus to continue along the road we had set out on."

From the notes of a deceased assistant of Kolff:

"Sofia Schafstadt truly became a milestone. Even after her survival Kolff could not get full endorsement of his artificial kidney in Holland. Among others, Professor Borst, the most prominent kidney specialist in our country, who had spent a long time in a German prison camp, had many reservations. At a convention in Utrecht, at which Kolff was trying to explain the potentialities of the artificial kidney, Borst countered with some weighty criticisms. With the somewhat grim humor he was given to, Kolff replied: 'Like all Dutchmen I rejoice that Professor Borst has been freed from the concentration camp. . . . That was a great day for Dutch medicine. But as far as the artificial kidney is concerned, he might have stayed there a while longer.'

"In the United States, however, Kolff's papers aroused so much interest that American physicians invited him to a convention at Atlantic City. From there he went to the Peter Bent Brigham Hospital in Boston, where a young doctor named John P. Merrill was anxious to experiment with the artificial kidney. Kolff had no machine to give Merrill, but he could provide him with sketches. These sketches formed the basis for the first rotating artificial kidney that was put to work in Boston.

"In 1950, Kolff left Europe for good and settled in Cleveland, Ohio. His active mind was already turning over the possibilities of other artificial organs, such as an artificial heart. But he was also concerned with further ways of helping victims of incurable kidney diseases. The most daring of these ways was the idea of replacing a diseased kidney with a healthy one from another human being: the idea of kidney transplantation."

2 / Ruth Tucker

Dr. Isidor Duclos in a lecture in Brussels, December 1969:

"The real father of transplantation was the Frenchman Alexis Carrel. Between 1900 and 1920, working at the Rockefeller Institute in New York, Carrel envisioned replacing incurably diseased organs by operation. He began by severing the blood vessels of dogs and then fitting them together, with a suture he invented, so tightly that the connection healed permanently and the blood was able to flow unhindered through the vessels.

"This blood vessel suturing, or anastomosis, formed the essential basis for transplantation of organs, since all organs live and die by their blood supply. In other words, it must be possible to fit an organ into the blood vessel system of the animal or human being destined to receive it.

"Alexis Carrel performed his first kidney experiments on dogs. He severed the artery and vein that connected one kidney to the animal's circulatory system, and then severed the connection between kidney and bladder, the ureter. He next took out the kidney, connected it to an artery and a vein in the throat of the same animal, and ran the stump of the ureter into a bottle. Amazingly enough, the displaced kidney began working at once, as soon as blood flowed through it again. It resumed its filtering activity and secreted urine as if it were in its normal place in the intestinal cavity. After a few weeks, however, the organ failed; it did not have sufficient protection from infection in its new site.

"Carrel's next feat was to operate on two dogs simultaneously. He removed a kidney from one animal and implanted it in the second animal. In this case, too, the transplanted kidney resumed its normal activity. But this time it functioned for only a short time. Then it broke down without external infection, and sometimes with dramatic speed; it was as if the recipient would not tolerate the foreign kidney in its body.

"Carrel repeated this type of experiment again and again. Finally he came to the conclusion that every living organism must have a defensive mechanism against tissue from other organisms, even those of the same species. He did not, however, clarify the mystery of this mechanism.

92

"An American named Williamson continued Carrel's work during the twenties. He transplanted the kidneys of his animals to the abdominal cavity, rather than the neck, connecting them to the pelvic blood vessels. In the course of his experiments he discovered that even the kidneys of dead animals could be transplanted to living animals and would resume their function, so long as the transplantation was undertaken within two hours after death. But such kidneys, too, were quickly rejected by the host body. Williamson in his turn could not solve the mystery of rejection. Yet he felt sure that someday it would be possible to transplant kidneys between healthy and sick human beings."

Time, *July 3, 1950:*

TRANSPLANTED KIDNEY

"Last week in Chicago, trying a desperate experiment on a woman doomed to die because both kidneys were hopelessly diseased, doctors performed the first human kidney transplanting on record.

"Both the mother and sister of Mrs. Ruth Tucker, 49, had died of the disease. . . . There is no known cure for polycystic kidneys, an ailment in which cysts form and destroy the normal kidney tissue. After talking things over with her husband, Mrs. Tucker agreed to let Dr. Richard Lawler, 54, staff member at the hospital, try a transplant."

Ruth Tucker was a housewife from a South Chicago neighborhood, Evergreen Park. The neighborhood did not live up to its name; it was an area of small houses and ugly utility poles lining gray streets. The Tucker home, 2549 West Sixty-second Street, was a modest but well-cared-for place. Here, in the spring of 1950, Ruth Tucker was living with her husband, Howard, and her son, Bill. Howard Tucker was a railroad worker. Bill, who had fought with a tank division in Europe, had only recently returned home.

In the middle of May, Howard Tucker took his wife to the Little Company of Mary Hospital, which belonged to the order of the same name and enjoyed an excellent reputation. Its staff included doctors from Cook County Hospital and the Loyola University School of Medicine. Among them was the urologist Patrick H. McNulty. Ruth Tucker had come to consult him.

Ruth Tucker was a courageous woman, but by this time she was at the end of her strength. For a long time she had been suffering from abdominal pains. She had already gone to several other hospitals. A gall bladder operation had only made her condition worse, it seemed to her. She had always done her own housework, but in recent weeks her pains, especially in the left side of her abdomen, had become so violent that she could scarcely take care of anything in the house.

As the details of the story came out, McNulty began to suspect a particular disease. Ruth Tucker's mother and a sister and an uncle had all suffered from a mysterious ailment. In the course of years they had repeatedly had spells of improvement, so that they thought the trouble had been overcome; but each time it would take a worse turn, until at last they died of it.

Ruth Tucker forthrightly told McNulty: "I've had enough of people telling me it's nothing serious. I want to know the facts, even if there isn't anything that can be done about what ails me."

Within a few days McNulty had confirmed his hunch. He gave Ruth Tucker the information she had asked for: "You have polycystic kidneys. Both are affected, but the left kidney particularly." That kidney was almost completely riddled with cysts which had destroyed its ability to function. It had grown to the size of a loaf of bread, and was the cause of the pain. The right kidney was also cystic, but was still functioning. Albumin excretion was small and the urea level in the blood only slightly raised. But there was no known way to prevent the continued formation of cysts. The disease would develop slowly, with temporary stages of seeming improvement, and would move on inexorably to the end. No one could say how long Ruth Tucker had to live. At best, a few years. The only way to give her relief from pain was to remove the useless left kidney.

After a short pause, Ruth Tucker said: "Good. Then go ahead and operate."

Patrick McNulty had seldom encountered a patient so resolute. In connection with the operation, he talked to Richard H. Lawler and James W. West, both surgeons, and mentioned this appealing quality of courage.

Lawler was fifty-four at the time. Despite his routine work in surgery, he had not abandoned the idea of exploring undiscovered country in the world of science. He had long given thought to organ transplantation and had discussed his ideas with West. Only recently he had read several papers by the American scientist Markowitz, who had been experimenting on transplantation in dogs. Markowitz had learned that transplants between dogs of the same type and sex, but particularly of the same blood group, would resist rejection for an unusually long time. There are, however, no such fine blood-group distinctions in animals as in men. Perhaps, with the more refined methods of blood-group comparison available for humans, it might be possible to carry out a kidney transplant successfully, provided that both type and blood group were carefully matched in the recipient and the donor of the kidney.

Lawler had often thought of attempting the operation foreshadowed by Carrel's experiments on animals: the transfer of a healthy kidney from a deceased person to a fatally ill patient for whom there is no other chance of salvation. When he heard about Ruth Tucker and the hopelessness of her condition, the idea sprang to his mind again. If Markowitz were right, and if, among dying patients in the Little Company of Mary Hospital, Lawler could find a woman of the matching blood group with healthy kidneys, one of which might replace the left kidney in Ruth Tucker's body, the worst that could happen would be rejection of the transplanted organ. Since Ruth Tucker's right kidney was still functioning, she would be in no worse plight than after the removal of the left kidney, which had already been decided on. If the experiment succeeded, it could only help the patient.

After Lawler had discussed these ideas with McNulty, he went to see Ruth Tucker. Sitting by her bed, he felt at once that McNulty had not exaggerated in speaking so warmly of her courage. And so after a while he asked: "Have you ever heard of the experiments on dogs where a sick kidney is replaced by a healthy one from another dog?"

"No," Ruth Tucker replied. But she grasped the point at once and asked how the operations had turned out.

Lawler tried to explain. "It depends on finding a kidney that matches the patient's. The specialists who have dealt with the matter think it may be easier to determine this in human beings than in animals. But nobody has tried it yet."

She eyed him keenly and asked where the kidney would come from. He replied that it could be taken from a person who was dying of another disease and might consent to have a kidney removed immediately after his death, as had long been the practice with the cornea of the eye. She showed no shock, but objected: "But then the kidney would be dead."

"No," Lawler said, "not if it were taken immediately. We've had proof of that from the operations on dogs."

Once more she gave him that keen look. Then she said: "Would that mean a chance for me?"

"No one can predict. But it might."

"So you want to try it on me?" she said acutely.

"Yes," he admitted, and explained his motivations, the prospects, and the dangers he could foresee.

She considered a moment. "I must talk it over with my husband," she said.

By the following day, the Tuckers had made their decision. "We've agreed that you should go ahead," Ruth Tucker announced stoically.

Like so many others who had long cherished a plan and suddenly found themselves on the point of carrying it out, Lawler and West were beset by doubts. They began to wonder about the possibility of a fatal shock resulting from the introduction of foreign protein into a human body. Would not a foreign organ bring on such anaphylactic shock?

At the same time, they once more reviewed all the technical aspects of kidney transplantation in a human being. They decided against attaching the kidney to the pelvic blood vessels as Williamson had done in his animal experiments several decades before. Rather, they would implant the donor kidney in place of the diseased left kidney, connecting it to the arteries and veins that had hitherto supplied the patient's own kidney. They would also have the ureter empty into the bladder. That involved considerable risk, since adhesions could form on the sutures, possibly preventing outflow through the ureter; such a complication might require a second operation. But the risk was worth taking. The most difficult problem seemed to be to find a potential donor resembling Ruth Tucker in physical characteristics and having the same blood group—AB Rh-negative.

It was June 17 before Lawler found a suitable donor. She was dying of cirrhosis of the liver. When Lawler approached her twenty-four-year-old daughter, explained his intentions, and asked for her consent, she hesitated briefly and then gave it.

An hour later the donor was dead. She was taken into the operating wing together with Ruth Tucker. Here Richard H. Lawler, James W. West, Patrick H. McNulty, and two assistants, Edward J. Clancy and Raymond P. Murphy, were waiting. West proceeded to remove a kidney from the dead woman, while Lawler simultaneously performed the nephrectomy on Ruth Tucker's left kidney.

From the recollections of Dr. James W. West:

"We didn't know what would happen; neither did anyone else. We were confident we wouldn't send the patient into shock, and we were hoping it would work."

From the operation report by Dr. Richard H. Lawler:

"On June 17, 1950, the patient was brought to the operating room and the left polycystic kidney was removed. A kidney removed from a white woman forty-nine years of age, with identical blood type, who had just died from hemorrhages from . . . cirrhosis of the liver, was transplanted into the host. In preparation for the transplantation, the donor's kidney, immediately after its withdrawal from the body, had been bathed in saline solution and the blood expressed by gentle pressure and aspiration. Heparin plus saline solution had then been injected into the artery and vein. . . .

"When the clamps were removed, the vessels filled immediately with blood and the color of the kidney changed from bluish brown to reddish brown. The ureter was then anastomosed to the host's ureter."

From the recollections of Dr. James W. West:

"The operation proved two things. It showed that transplants were feasible and that the patient would not go into anaphylactic shock."

Two hours after the operation Ruth Tucker awoke in her room. A few minutes later she asked whether everything was all right. She was told yes, and dropped off to sleep again. She did not know that no fewer than forty doctors, most of them from Cook County Hospital, had come to watch the operation. Inevitably the first reporters heard about it a few hours later. Soon afterward headlines and stories appeared.

Chicago Sun-Times, June 19, 1950:

WOMAN DIES, KIDNEY MAY SAVE LIFE OF 2ND

"A healthy kidney was removed from the body of a dead woman and used to replace the diseased kidney of a dying woman in a historic 90-minute operation by two teams of doctors in Little Company of Mary Hospital. . . . The patient . . . is Mrs. Howard Tucker, 49, of 2549 W. 62nd."

During the days that followed, Ruth Tucker recovered with a rapidity that amazed all her doctors, and made them more and more optimistic. On the fifth day after the operation she began feeding herself and reading newspapers attentively. On the seventeenth day she was able to sit up in bed. On the twenty-first day she attempted her first steps. Excretion of urine, which before the operation had amounted to 250 cubic centimeters at most—far below the norm of 1,500 to 2,000 cubic centimeters—reached amounts as high as 4,700 cubic centimeters.

On August 10, when Ruth Tucker entered the X-ray room on her own two feet, she herself could recognize in the X-ray pictures that both her own remaining right kidney and the new left kidney had filled with the X-ray–opaque dye and had passed it on to the bladder. There was absolutely no indication of any rejection of the kidney, such as Carrel and Williamson had reported in their animals. Only the place where the ureter of the new kidney was connected to the bladder showed, in the X-ray picture, a slight constriction due to cicatrization. Here, then, certain of the fears of the doctors were proving true. If the scar tissue continued to form, there was danger that it might some day obstruct the outflow of urine and destroy the new kidney by blockage.

Ruth Tucker guessed from Lawler's expression that something was wrong. And since Lawler understood her wish for candor, he explained what had happened or could happen. She asked what could be done about it, and he replied that he would have to operate again. As in all such matters, she came to a quick decision. On August 21 she lay on the operating table again. When Lawler and West exposed the left ureter and the transplanted kidney, they discovered an accumulation of pus around the kidney, which had to be drained. It would not have been advisable to go on and eliminate the constriction of the ureter. But the new kidney itself had retained its normal size and appearance to such an extent that Lawler could feel the first human kidney transplant was a success. He decided to postpone correction of the ureter constriction for a few months. During this time Ruth Tucker could return home to her husband and son.

This time, too, before Ruth Tucker left the hospital, he told her the full truth. He explained that the operation had to be postponed and that he wanted to examine her at intervals to determine the most favorable time for the new operation. On August 26, Ruth Tucker returned home to Evergreen Park.

She felt so relieved and well that next day she set out on a vacation trip with Howard. They drove nearly 300 miles to Jasper, Indiana, where Howard's brother, Ray, and his family lived. Ray worked for the American Legion. During the Tuckers' visit the legion was having a celebration. Ruth convinced all their friends that a miracle had been performed on her in the Little Company of Mary Hospital. She took part in all the festivities, danced, was hailed as the woman with the new kidney, and wrote Lawler a long letter of gratitude about it all.

On November 4, 1950, Lawler published his first official report in the *Journal of the American Medical Association*. He concluded with the confident observation that there had been no signs of rejection. His confidence increased when Ruth Tucker came in for checkups in October and December. She reported that she felt as well as she ever had in her life. She had gained twenty pounds, was driving her car again, and was going out evenings with Howard. When she visited Lawler again in January 1951 she asked whether the other operation was still necessary at all.

But then, in February and March, the excretion of urine steadily diminished. Lawler assumed that the cicatrization had advanced to such a point that it had become a serious obstruction and it was high time to carry out the long-postponed third operation. Ruth Tucker accepted his verdict with the same courageous equanimity she had shown throughout. On March 30, 1951, Howard took her to the hospital. The operation was set for April 1.

In the presence of West, McNulty, Clancy, and Murphy, Lawler opened the almost-healed incision of August 21. After eight months, now they would be able to see the implanted kidney again and determine whether it had changed. Possibly they were all inwardly prepared for an unpleasant surprise. Nevertheless, it was a shock when the bed of the left kidney lay exposed before them.

The kidney they had transplanted seemed to have vanished. Only after looking carefully did they find a shrunken remnant which was no longer functioning, obviously no longer producing any urine. Ruth Tucker's organism—like Carrel's and Williamson's dogs—had fought a secret defensive battle against the foreign tissue. The mysterious mechanism of this defense had not been propitiated by physical resemblance and identity of blood group. The host body had obviously attacked the transplanted kidney and destroyed it.

Lawler could not know when this had happened. At that moment he and the others would not venture to say whether the kidney had ever really functioned. Perhaps the amazing improvement in Ruth Tucker's condition had been due only to the removal of the diseased left kidney. Perhaps the right kidney had drawn on all its reserves and managed to make up for its absent twin.

But these were questions that could not be answered. Lawler broke off the operation. There was no sense proceeding with the correction of the constricted left ureter. Lawler now had another decision to make. What should he tell Ruth Tucker when she came out of the anesthesia? Should he destroy her confidence, which was perhaps a major contributory factor to her good condition? How could he know whether the right kidney, which had obviously performed amazingly well, might not continue to work for a long time to come—much longer than had been expected—before it succumbed to the inevitable development of further cysts? For the first time he told his patient a comforting lie.

A few days later Ruth Tucker returned home for the second time. She did so firmly believing that she was the first person to carry a functioning kidney taken from a dead body. Lawler hoped that she would be able to spend a few happy years. But he evidently forgot something that seemed unimportant in his world of medicine—that, in fact, had no place in that world. He forgot about the publicity the operation of June 17, 1950, had provoked. He forgot that Ruth Tucker was not one of his many unknown patients. And apparently McNulty also forgot.

On May 22 the telephone rang in the Tucker home at 2549 West Sixty-second Street. When Ruth Tucker answered, a reporter asked whether she was the Mrs. Ruth Tucker in whom Dr. Lawler had implanted a kidney in the summer of 1950. When she said she was, he asked whether she had heard about the forty-sixth annual meeting of the American Urological Association, which had just been held at the Palmer House in Chicago. Rather surprised, she said she had not.

But she did know Dr. Patrick McNulty?

Yes, she said, of course she knew him.

Well, then, the reporter went on, he would like to have her reaction to a lecture that Dr. McNulty had delivered to this meeting on her case. Although her name of course had not been mentioned, there was no doubt that it was her case.

Interested, but with no trace of uneasiness, Ruth Tucker asked what McNulty had said.

The reporter quoted McNulty: "The operation was a failure. The grafted kidney is not functioning and never has. It has shrunk to the size of a hazelnut. The reason is that the donor's tissues were incompatible with Mrs. Tucker's."

Ruth Tucker took only a moment to compose herself. Then she said: "The doctors have always told me everything because they know I can take bad news. . . . It's still there, it hasn't floated, and I can feel it, and if it's only the size of a hazelnut, it's the biggest hazelnut that ever grew."

That was all Ruth Tucker had to say. But the same press that had made her into a heroine of medicine showed no mercy. Next day that press proclaimed that her confidence was based on an illusion.

Chicago Tribune, May 23, 1951:

"The first attempt in history to transplant a kidney from one human to another has ended in failure . . . it was revealed Tuesday. . . . The failure was reported by Dr. Patrick H. McNulty, consulting urologist in the disease. He appeared before the public relations committee of the American Urological Association which was holding its 46th annual meeting at the Palmer House. Inability of tissues of one person to be compatible when transplanted to another was given as the reason for the failure. The committee, composed of top experts in the field, pledged that no more such operations be attempted until science uncovers new knowledge about the biological compatibility of tissues and organs. The operation was performed on Mrs. Tucker on June 17, 1950, at Little Company of Mary Hospital. . . . Several weeks ago an exploratory operation was performed and found that the organ had shrunk from the size of a grapefruit to a small hazelnut."

· · ·

The *Chicago Tribune* reporter added these reassuring phrases: "The experts said the remnants of the kidney would continue to waste away but would not harm the patient" and "A normal life span was predicted, however, for Mrs. Ruth Tucker, 2549 W. 62nd." But Ruth Tucker was not a woman to be fooled. At any rate, when a reporter from *Time* magazine also called her, she declared: "What a way to get your death sentence— from a newspaper reporter." She continued to insist, however, that she could feel the new kidney. No one outside her family ever learned what her emotions were that day.

On September 1, 1951, Richard Lawler published a second scientific report in the *Journal of the American Medical Association* in which he frankly informed the world of medicine that the transplant had been a failure. It is hardly likely that Ruth Tucker ever saw this report. In December 1954 she developed pneumonia which was related to her chronic kidney ailment. She overcame this first attack. But a few months later, on April 21, 1955, she succumbed to a second attack that proved stronger than her courage and will power.

3 / Jacqueline Cado

France-Soir, *January 24, 1951*:

"New Miracle of Surgery in Créteil Hospital
"First time in Europe. The kidney of an executed man (taken from his body ten seconds after guillotining) has been implanted in twenty-two-year-old Jacqueline C."

The light in the death cell at the Santé Prison in Paris was switched on at 5:15 A.M. on the morning of January 12, 1951. It illumined the pallid faces of two prisoners, Nedelec and Estingoy, who sat chained to their beds. Both men were waiting for the day of their death—one having waited six months, the other eighteen months. Nedelec, the first to awaken, leaped to his feet crying out: "It's not my turn yet, not mine. . . ."

Nedelec knew quite well it was not his turn. The night before, the guards had given his cellmate, Jean Louis Estingoy, a strong sedative. In the past eighteen months, Nedelec had seen several cellmates led to the guillotine, and all had received the same sedative on their last night. Nevertheless, Nedelec did not drop back on his cot reassured until the four guards who had entered the cell turned their backs on him and went over to Estingoy.

Behind them appeared State Prosecutor Raphael, Judge Goletty, and the state-appointed defense attorney, Maître Burger. Raphael had prosecuted the murder charge against Estingoy; Burger had defended him; Goletty had passed the death sentence upon him on June 13, 1950. By French law they were all to be the witnesses of Estingoy's death.

One of the guards lifted the blanket from Estingoy and shook him until he awoke. When the guard unlocked his chains and pulled the coarse woolen smock off his body, Estingoy began to understand. Numbly, he let the guards put on his own shirt, which he had worn up to the time of his arrest. Then he fell to his knees, crawled over to the toilet, and writhed in cramps. The guards held him tightly until he calmed down. Then they pushed him out of the cell past the waiting officials and down the labyrinth of corridors. They stopped on a landing where the prison priest waited beside a table with two burning candles and gave Estingoy the opportunity to take communion.

Maître Burger, a powerful, heavy man, briefly supported himself against the cold wall of the corridor. The sight of Jean Louis Estingoy reminded him all too clearly of the weeks before the trial. Estingoy's dull, absent look reinforced his conviction that here was a mentally unbalanced man going to the guillotine.

Estingoy had murdered a child. Of that there was no doubt. But to Burger's mind he was also a mute, bewildered human wreck. The man who knelt coughing by the wretched altar, because he had choked over the host, came from the vicinity of Poitiers. From 1940 to 1945 he had been a prisoner of the Germans. Upon his return home he had found his wife with another man, and never recovered from this disillusionment. Later he became a maintenance man for a church in Paris; while there he had scrawled pornographic words on the church walls. In 1946 he had been taken to the Sainte-Anne mental hospital, but had been discharged as cured a year later. After that he became an attendant in the Centre Alexandre Lugnet, a home for unwed mothers, where the murder had taken place.

The gruesome altar scene was over. The guards pushed Estingoy into a chair and gave him a cigarette. "Would you like some rum?" Estingoy shook his head absently. But they held an old mustard jar filled with rum to his mouth. "Drink, it's better that way. And hurry up."

Burger took a step toward the prosecutor and judge. Should he make one last protest to Raphael and Goletty, reminding them of his plea for mercy, which the judge had rejected? Estingoy's crime had undoubtedly been horrible. Among the "fallen girls" in the Centre Alexandre Lugnet he had found himself a mistress—Denise Vorroy, the mother of four children. When he asked her to marry him, she repulsed him angrily. "You're crazy. Do you think I'm going to marry a madman?" In revenge, on August 18, 1947, he had hurled Denise's oldest child, Pierre, three flights down the stair well. Then he had fled. He had been caught in Chaumont.

"Are you ready now?" the guard growled. For the first time that morning Estingoy spoke audibly. "Let me at least finish my cigarette."

"Then hurry up—we've only another half minute."

Burger felt the cold of the wall against his shoulder. Probably the death sentence could be laid not to the court but to the psychiatrists. He had tried in vain to make them say that Estingoy was mentally ill. But they had gone on affirming the prisoner's sanity because they did not want to admit that his release from Sainte-Anne had been an unforgivable mistake.

The guards hesitated no longer. They opened a curtain that had concealed the sight of the dark, cold prison yard and pushed Estingoy out into the arms of several men who served as assistants to Desfourneaux, the executioner. Desfourneaux himself stood near the guillotine, beside him the round-faced court physician, Dr. Paul, in his white smock. There were also a few journalists present to report the murderer's end. It was the usual dreary picture, but today it was somewhat different.

At the door to a room on the left of the prison gate waited three other men in white physicians' smocks. They wore surgeon's masks over their faces. Maître Burger did not know them. But he assumed that one of them must be Dr. Marceau Servelle. That was the name he had been given at the time he learned that Estingoy's death was to be something more than the usual extinction of a murderer. He was to have a share in a scientific sensation, the first transplantation of a kidney in the Republic of France.

Burger felt increasing nausea as Desfourneaux's assistants seized Estingoy and thrust him under the guillotine. As Estingoy's head fell into the basket, the cigarette was still glowing between his lips. What followed next took place with ghostly speed.

The doctors vanished into the room next to the gate. Two guards hastily carried the basket with Estingoy's head into the same room. A reporter murmured to another: "Now they're going to cut out the corneas for the eye clinic. But that isn't our affair. The big story is coming. When they take the body into the room, Servelle is going to extract the kidney for the girl in Créteil. We must get into that room. Try to remember every detail. If they don't allow any pictures, I must at least have a drawing."

The coroner gave a sign. Two attendants picked up the headless corpse and carried it to the room beside the gate. There Dr. Marceau Servelle stood at the telephone. Someone was holding the receiver for him.

Servelle was thirty-six, a tall, lean man with a high forehead, light blue eyes, and a thin, expressive mouth. The call had already been put through to the Créteil Hospital, the connection made with his wife and assistant, Dr. Mireille Servelle. "It's done," he said. "Prepare the patient for the operation."

Marceau Servelle had long been one of the outstanding young surgeons in Paris. He had told the already half-blind girl in the small white hospital room that the decisive hour was at hand, without mentioning that she was to receive a murderer's kidney. Then he had planned everything so that his wife and another assistant would have the right side of the patient's pelvic cavity already open when he arrived at Créteil after the execution.

It was 5:45 A.M. when he removed Estingoy's kidney. In his animal experiments he had discovered that a kidney turned blue-gray and soon suffered irreparable injury when cut off from the donor's circulation. But if it were washed in saline solution and placed in a vessel of the same solution, it could be kept alive for a short time. He therefore began the washing at once, and placed the kidney in the vessel of saline solution he had brought with him.

The streets were still quiet; there were no traffic delays as he approached the Place de l'Italie. Servelle increased his speed when he reached the Boulevard de la Gare. He could be sure that Jacqueline Cado at this moment lay under anesthesia on the second floor of the hospital, and that Mireille and his assistant, Rougeulle, had exposed the pelvic artery and vein and prepared the bed for the kidney.

Jacqueline must have been a merry girl before the disease began, for even now she was a sweet-tempered person, in spite of phases of profound despair. Her parents, both schoolteachers, had moved from the village of Treglamus and bought a house in the old town of Dinan. Eugénie Cado had opened a bookshop on the ground floor while François Cado continued to teach school. All in all, theirs was a peaceful house and a peaceful, close family. There were eight children, all of whom seemed to be following what was beginning to seem an old-fashioned ideal: to read and to teach.

The story of Jacqueline's sufferings could be read in the dry, objective language of her case history. She had been a frail child since her birth in Treglamus in July 1928. For that very reason, in all likelihood, she became the darling of the family. No one suspected that she had been born with only one kidney.

As she grew up, her health improved. At the age of thirteen, when the Germans were occupying France, she was in the *lycée*, delicate and slender as were all the Cados, a girl with a small face, brown curls, and brown eyes. Along with her brothers and sisters and friends, she had witnessed the Germans parading into and out of the village, and at sixteen had hailed the arrival of the Americans and British. But just at the moment the war was ending and life should have begun for her, she was taken ill. She was on the point of graduating from the *lycée*. Suddenly she withdrew from all games. Headaches tormented her so terribly that she would collapse over her schoolbooks. No one had doubted that she would pass her final examinations without difficulty. But she failed.

In 1945 she tried to surmount the hurdle of the examinations again. Once more she failed—and was desperate, incapable of understanding what was happening to her. Her father and mother thought of the old remedy so often recommended in their own childhood: a change of air. François Cado took his daughter to the country, to Gourin, where he himself had been born and where he knew the mayor and the teachers. Jacqueline worked as a teacher's aide in a school. For a short time she was able to laugh with the children and enjoy herself. But after a few months she collapsed again.

In 1946 she returned home, very quiet and withdrawn. She would have good days, which she spent in her mother's kitchen learning the arts of the housewife, for of course she would marry eventually. She had bad days, which she spent sitting in her bedroom at the rear of the house, looking down into the small garden. In 1948 she terrified her mother by crying out: "I can't read any more. I can't make out small letters." This was a cruel blow for a girl who had grown up with books.

This time a doctor in Dinan, who took her blood pressure and examined her eyes, suspected the cause of her fatigue, her pains, and her failing eyesight. Her blood pressure was 180/100, tremendous for a twenty-year-old girl. A few days later François Cado took his daughter to Paris, to see Professor Lemaire, internist at the Hospital Saint-Antoine.

To Lemaire, the diagnosis was clear after a few days' examination: chronic nephritis accompanied by dangerously high blood pressure, anemia, edema, and enlargement of the heart. With Jacqueline and her parents Lemaire used the usual assurances and evasions, and in fact for the first few days he himself still hoped that only one kidney might be affected. The possibility that Jacqueline might have had only a single kidney from birth did not occur to him. It was only after the first X rays had been developed that he recognized how hopeless her case was.

Servelle was now crossing the Seine bridge. He followed the left bank toward Ivry and Alfort. The cold fog that coated the windows of the car reminded him of that January day in 1949, almost two years ago, when he had seen Jacqueline for the first time. Lemaire, with a last flicker of hope, had sent her to him.

There were cases in which the second kidney, though present, was cut off from the blood circulation by congenital malformations of the blood vessels. Such a kidney would not show up on X rays. The only way to tell was by opening the abdominal cavity. Lemaire had asked Servelle to undertake such an exploratory operation. If there were such a "sealed-off" kidney, that might account for the high blood pressure. Sometimes surgical removal would improve the blood pressure, stop the headaches, and save the eyesight.

In May 1949, Servelle and Mireille had performed this exploratory operation on Jacqueline. But they had found only a gravely diseased single kidney that could not be removed without killing the girl. Servelle could do nothing but sever the connection between the diseased kidney and Jacqueline's sympathicus nerve. Sometimes such operations had a favorable effect upon high blood pressure.

But in Jacqueline's case the attempt had failed. The blood pressure persisted, with destructive regularity, in the range of 180/100; the quantity of urea in the blood steadily increased. It was the usual clinical picture of a slow but certain death.

The road to Alfort and to Route Nationale 19 was almost deserted. Servelle reached Highway 19, the direct route to Créteil and the last stage of his drive.

At that time, in the early summer of 1949, Servelle had already been carrying out experiments on animals at Professor Simonnet's Ecole Vétérinaire. He was only beginning, had no more than a vague prospect of future success, and could scarcely conceive of applying his discoveries to human beings. Jacqueline Cado—still unaware of her true condition—had returned to Dinan. But she was too intelligent to be deceived much longer. She was a girl who lived among books. It was impossible to prevent her from finding out by reading what she was suffering from. And François and Eugénie Cado, who had learned only half-truths from Lemaire, could not be prevented from discovering the whole truth in the same way. As it happened, during this period they read a magazine article about kidney transplantation, but the procedure sounded utterly incredible and nothing in which they could place any hope.

In the summer of 1950, Jacqueline was suddenly seized by a longing for the sea. In July her parents took her to the seashore. She sat among the dunes and waited for a miracle that did not happen. Steadily she became more emaciated. Her legs twitched convulsively, and her eyes were so weak that she seemed to see the surf only through a veil. In despair, her parents took her back to Lemaire at the Hospital Saint-Antoine in Paris.

During those summer months in which Jacqueline herself became convinced that she was near death, the Cados had seen accounts in French newspapers of the Tucker operation in Chicago. Indeed, they could scarcely have missed such headlines as those in *France-Soir:* KIDNEY OF A DEAD WOMAN TRANSPLANTED TO A SICK PERSON FOR THE FIRST TIME. OPERATION IN CHICAGO SEEMS SUCCESSFUL. Suddenly the fantastic article they had read the previous year seemed closer to reality.

At first the Cados merely asked Lemaire his opinion of the matter. He replied that he had seen the reports and had just been discussing them with the editor-in-chief of *Le Monde,* who wanted to do a big story on transplantation. From the surgical point of view, it was undoubtedly a fantastic undertaking. From the medical point of view, he believed that the attempt was premature; he doubted whether the reported success would be lasting.

And so the parents had left. But after sitting for several hours by Jacqueline's bed, helplessly watching as their daughter visibly faded, they had called on Lemaire once more. Eugénie Cado in particular could not stop thinking about that operation in Chicago. She asked Lemaire whether in spite of his doubts he could not give her the name of a French surgeon who would have the courage to follow the example of the Americans. Her persistent pleas at last softened Lemaire. He recalled that Servelle had long been occupied with the possibility of kidney transplantation and had already undertaken experiments on animals. Servelle had, in fact, forewarned him that he would someday ask him for a suitable patient from Saint-Antoine—in return for which Lemaire would have exclusive rights to publicize the event in *Le Monde*, and to report on the first kidney transplant in France, or even in the world.

And so Lemaire had referred the Cados to Servelle, whom they already knew from his first operation on Jacqueline. And then, in Servelle's office, there had begun the quiet drama of the Cados' struggle for a last chance for Jacqueline, a chance, no matter how slim.

Servelle had now reached Créteil. He turned into the Avenue de Verdun and up the curving drive to the hospital door. A doctor and several nurses were waiting there.

"Is everything ready?"

Everything was ready. Jacqueline's parents had been informed and were on the way to Créteil. Quickly, the vessel containing Estingoy's kidney was carried into the hospital. It was 7:55 A.M. when Servelle entered the operating room. The others were waiting: Mireille, Dr. Rougeulle, Dr. Delahaye, the nurses, and an attendant. Delahaye, the anesthetist, signed to Servelle that everything was going well. Jacqueline was asleep. Her face, usually flushed from high blood pressure, was pale. But she was breathing evenly. The right iliac fossa had been opened, and the pelvic arteries and veins were visible. Servelle worked swiftly. The vessel he had brought was opened. The dead man's kidney, which was now bluish gray in color, was placed in the pelvic cavity. At 8:25 A.M. the kidney vein was anastomosed to Jacqueline Cado's iliac vein, at 8:35 the kidney artery to the iliac artery. A moment of suspense followed. But then Servelle saw what Lawler had seen before him: as the clamps were opened and the blood poured in, within seconds the kidney regained its natural color. Apparently it had suffered no damage from its removal at the Santé and its long ride; it came to life.

In his experiments with animals, Servelle had never connected the ureter of the transplanted kidney to the bladder, but had simply brought it to the outside through an incision in the skin, inserted a drain, and led the drain to a glass vessel. In Jacqueline's case he did the same. He knew quite well that he would be making life difficult for his patient. But he thought that in this way he could better check the functioning of the implanted kidney. And if the risky operation really succeeded, there could always be a second operation to connect the new kidney to the bladder. He left the diseased kidney in place for the present, in order not to prolong the operation needlessly.

By nine o'clock, it was all finished. The attendant wheeled Jacqueline Cado back to her small white room, where her parents were waiting by the window.

During the first twenty-four hours the patient did not fully awaken from her sleep. Servelle waited impatiently for Estingoy's kidney, which had shown such distinct signs of life, to assume its natural function of excreting urine. Two nurses, Mère Marie-Thérèse and Cécile, took turns watching the drain from the ureter. Would it begin to drip? Would the kidney excrete?

They had to be patient for several hours, but suddenly the first drops appeared at the tip of the drain. Drop followed drop, until at last there were 30 cubic centimeters. That was only one twenty-fifth or one thirtieth of the excretion of a normal kidney in a twenty-four-hour period. Nevertheless, the nurses felt enormously cheered.

Late in the evening Jacqueline awoke for the first time since the operation. She recognized her mother; then she asked softly: "Do I have a new kidney?" And when Servelle, who happened to be in the room at the moment, nodded, she fell asleep again.

François and Eugénie Cado, elated and filled with new hope, left to spend the night at nearby Villeneuve-Saint-Georges, where the mother-in-law of one of their daughters lived. They planned to stay there so that they could visit Jacqueline every day and perhaps, in a few weeks, take her home with them. Next morning they returned to Créteil and resumed their waiting.

On the second day the quantity of urine increased. Estingoy's kidney excreted 50 cubic centimeters. Then—on the third day—there was a sudden complication. Jacqueline began to breathe heavily. Professor Soulié, a cardiologist whom Servelle called in for consultation, diagnosed a pulmonary edema. Jacqueline was given oxygen, heart stimulants, and infusions of glucose; and after some very anxious hours the accumulation of fluid in her lungs vanished. The kidney itself seemed unaffected by this crisis. On the fifth day it excreted 75 cubic centimeters, on the seventh day 80, and by the ninth day its excretion amounted to 90 cubic centimeters—still only a fraction of the performance of a healthy kidney. Nevertheless, Servelle and his associates regarded every smallest increase as a positive sign. And François and Eugénie Cado waited, patiently hoping.

On January 24, the twelfth day after the operation, Jacqueline sat up in bed for the first time. She declared that her head felt clearer and that she could see better. She was even able to eat something, although only creamed soup and stewed fruit.

On January 27, the fifteenth day, the quantity of urine increased to 120 cubic centimeters. Toward noon, when Servelle entered the patient's room, she was eating baked calf brains. For the first time her brown eyes glowed with something of their old look, and she said: *"Je mange de votre cervelle."* Everyone laughed at her pun on the name Servelle and *cervelle*, the French word for brains. Eugénie Cado burst into tears of joy. Five little words had become a magic spell that promised everything.

For the first time since the operation Jacqueline Cado began thinking beyond the immediate present. Obviously she had decided that she was going to live, for she thoughtfully regarded the dripping drain that protruded from her pale skin. Finally, her voice quivering, she asked whether she would always have to go around with this instrument and perhaps would never be able to associate with people outside her family again. Mère Marie-Thérèse reassured her, explaining that the drain would be removed if the kidney continued to work as well as it was now doing. By evening Jacqueline seemed considerably cheered and listened attentively as her mother sat by her bed, reading to her.

The mood in the hospital on January 28 was a confident one. But in the course of the day there was suddenly a total change. Jacqueline was overcome by a numbing weariness. Servelle and the other doctors suspected that excessive excretion of salt was the cause. They injected 250 cubic centimeters of physiological saline solution. But to their horror the injection produced so violent a shock that Jacqueline lost consciousness. On January 29 she was so weak that François and Eugénie Cado sat, totally distraught, by her bed. The change seemed all the more incomprehensible because the new kidney continued to function. They could see that for themselves. The miraculous kidney excreted 268 cubic centimeters on January 30, and on the following day this actually rose to 600 cubic centimeters. Why, then, was Jacqueline nevertheless sinking into a stupor before their eyes? Servelle could not answer the parents' questions. He ordered blood transfusions and—in the stubborn belief that Jacqueline was still suffering from saline deficiency—a second subcutaneous saline injection. But even as the injection was being given, Jacqueline suffered a second shock. On the night of February 1 she received her last transfusion. But her breathing was weaker, her heartbeat barely audible, and at four o'clock in the morning she died.

France-Soir, *February 2, 1951:*

"Jacqueline's death still unexplained. . . . The girl had already been taking nourishment. The kidney was functioning normally. . . . The doctors suspect that she died of another cause. . . . At the moment, nothing is known."

Servelle was tormented by the question: why? Although he personally performed an autopsy on the dead girl, he could not discover the answer. He found Estingoy's kidney to be its natural size and color, but he did not open it up and give the tissue to a histologist for careful examination. Instead, he looked for the answer in some accidental, unfortunate complication. He wrote: "Before the operation our patient was in a desperate general condition. In a patient subject to less strain the consequences of the operation would not have been so extreme. Our observations show that the transplantation of a kidney from one person to another is quite feasible. We believe that this method has a great future before it."

Meanwhile, François and Eugénie Cado accompanied Jacqueline to the small, treeless cemetery of Dinan. From the day of the funeral Eugénie Cado withdrew into her own home. Her personality changed completely; she lost all interest in the outside world and began spending her days in the total isolation of her thoughts and memories. Only her children suspected that she was wrestling with the question of whether she had been wrong to believe in the American operation. Five years later it was said in Dinan that she had "followed Jacqueline, dying of a broken heart."

4 / Marius Renard

From an unpublished anonymous letter to a Paris newspaper,
May 1952:

"More than a year has now passed since a pitiable young woman, Jacqueline Cado, became the needless victim of a needless experiment: kidney transplantation. You reported on this supposed triumph of medicine, which ended in a grave in the cemetery of Dinan. You would be performing a great service to humanity if you were to report how many other patients, in spite of the ominous example, have since been sacrificed on the altar of surgeons' ambitions. The matter has been hushed up, but on that same January 12 on which Jacqueline Cado underwent her operation, Professor Dubost, Dr. Oeconomos, and several other Paris physicians rushed ahead to follow the course of the American, Lawler. They, too, secretly secured the kidney of an executed murderer and transplanted it into an unfortunate twenty-four-year-old woman.

"The only name that has been given in the technical journals is Madame G. For twenty years she had been slowly dying of renal tuberculosis. She had at last reached the stage at which her sole possible release was by death when the kidney was grafted onto her. In doing this the physicians merely inflicted new sufferings upon her—and she died sixteen days afterward.

"Dr. René Küss and his colleague Teinturier were also apparently fired by the American example. From January 1951 to April 1951 they transplanted, without publicity, kidneys into five patients. They took these kidneys from other victims of renal diseases who had to have a kidney removed. None of the kidneys they transplanted was healthy. They even transplanted a tuberculous kidney. Not a single transplant saved the patient's life. All died. . . . Among them, Joseph K., who was fortunate enough to expire during the operation.

"At the same time, as I have learned from American friends, several American doctors in Boston likewise could not rest until they had tried to imitate their colleague Lawler. Among these were Dr. David M. Hume, Dr. John P. Merrill, and others, all members of the staff of the Peter Bent Brigham Hospital in Boston.

112

"From April 1951 to date they have implanted kidneys from cadavers into six dying patients. They did not even take the trouble, as the French surgeons did, to insert the new kidneys into the patients' abdominal cavities. Instead, they simply incised a pocket in the patient's thigh, stuck the kidney into the pocket, connected the femoral blood vessels, and directed the stump of the ureter into a flask. None of these kidneys actually functioned. They were not accepted by the bodies of the recipients. Four of the kidneys had to be removed because of the intense pain to the patients. When will our colleagues give up this game of experimenting on human beings? And when will they realize that dying, too, can be a mercy?"

Professors C. Dubost, N. Oeconomos, A. Nenna, and P. Milliez, 1951:

"We therefore believe that every kidney transplant in human beings is condemned to failure. We must advise against the attempt."

In a village of a thousand inhabitants, everyone knows everyone else. In Berthecourt, forty-seven miles northeast of Paris, everyone knew Marius Renard.

Marius was the elder son of the cabinetmaker Robert Renard, forty-five, born in Paris, and of his wife, Gilberte. He was a vigorous, merry-faced boy of sixteen with a shock of dark hair. The family lived in the old part of Berthecourt, in a brick house with a fortresslike door, surrounded by a small walled garden. His father was usually in his workshop in the cellar, his mother usually in the kitchen. There was another child in the family, a boy ten years younger than Marius.

Since the age of fourteen Marius had been going by train every day to Beauvais, 8½ miles away. Here, in the capital of the Oise Department, he served his apprenticeship under master-carpenter Homer. Sometimes he went to Beauvais on his bicycle, for bicycle riding was his passion. He preferred it to everything except the occasional family outings to the coastal village of Le Crotoy, where his parents owned some land and he could dream of a house and a life with the fishermen.

There was not the slightest indication that in December 1952 young Marius Renard would become the center of a violent emotional storm sweeping all of France.

On December 16, at two o'clock in the afternoon, he was working on a building in the rue Gambetta in Beauvais. As he was carrying boards up to the fourth floor, he lost his balance and plunged to the street. Bleeding and unconscious, he was carried the few hundred yards to the Hôtel-Dieu, the dreary old hospital of Beauvais. An intern took charge of him and found three broken ribs and two fractures of the pelvis. But above all there was severe contusion of the right side of his groin.

Marius was placed in one of the high-windowed, medieval wards. But when Robert and Gilberte Renard arrived from Berthecourt and wandered through the hospital corridors looking for Marius, they learned, to their alarm, that he had already been taken to the operating room and that Dr. André Warin, the surgeon, was preparing to operate on him. Distraught, the parents lost their way repeatedly in the hospital's unfriendly corridors. At last they found Dr. Warin, a huge bull of a man. Robert Renard tried to find out what had happened to Marius. He was given no information.

Robert Renard in an interview seventeen years later:

"I went up to him and tried to say something. But he bellowed at me: 'I have nothing to tell you. I know what has to be done here.' "

Warin operated. He found Marius's right kidney swollen and bleeding through a rent in its stem. The simplest way to end the hemorrhage was to remove the entire right kidney. Warin did so, ordering a transfusion of blood group O Rh-positive. He assumed Marius would have no difficulty getting along with only his left kidney.

When next day a nurse reported that Marius Renard was no longer excreting a drop of urine, a catheter was introduced into the boy's bladder. Only a few drops of blood were discharged. On December 20, when there were still no signs of renal activity, Warin grew uneasy. He got in touch with Dr. Michon of the urological division at the age-old but celebrated Necker Hospital in Paris, and asked him to take in Marius Renard and determine the reason for the absence of urinary production.

Robert Renard in an interview seventeen years later:

"This person didn't even think it necessary to talk to us. Whatever he had to say, including the news of Marius's transfer to Paris, he had other doctors or nurses tell us."

On December 21 an ambulance took the boy to Paris. His parents went, too, Gilberte sitting beside the stretcher, Robert in his own car. And once again the two parents wandered, uncertain and uninformed, through hospital corridors—this time the dreary corridors of the Necker, a short distance from the Gare Montparnasse.

Immediately after Marius's arrival, Dr. Michon tried to insert a catheter through the bladder into the left ureter and thence into the left kidney. He thought some obstacle might have formed in the ureter, blocking the flow of urine from the left kidney. In spite of all his practiced skill, he was not able to get the catheter all the way up. He then waited a day, hoping the blockage would clear of its own accord. But on December 22 Marius still did not excrete one drop of urine. It was as if he had no kidney at all.

A blood examination showed that the urea level in his blood had already risen to 3 grams. Michon hastily called in Professor Jean Hamburger, the forty-two-year-old chief of the Necker's internal division for renal diseases. Hamburger, after further examinations, began to suspect that Marius might have had only one kidney from birth and that Dr. Warin in Beauvais had removed this single kidney. He immediately ordered that Marius's fluid intake should be sharply reduced; he was to have only as much fluid as his body could excrete through the pores, without a functioning kidney.

The first X rays on December 23 showed no shadow of a kidney. But in order to make sure, Hamburger and Michon subjected the boy once again to the painful procedure of a catheter examination through the bladder. They injected X-ray–opaque chemicals into the ureter, took new pictures —and Hamburger's suspicion was confirmed: there was no left kidney, merely a stump of ureter that came to a blind end.

Necker Hospital as yet had no artificial kidney, and even if it had, the use of one could at best only have prolonged Marius Renard's life until his veins and arteries had, as usual, become worn out from the frequent connections.

Marius himself was still conscious and accepted everything that was being done to him with a mixture of astonishment, pain, and blind faith in the doctors. He did not know that the X rays had sealed his death sentence. Meanwhile, Robert and Gilberte Renard continued to wait in drafty corners, or to sit by Marius's bed during the brief visiting hours. When Marius asked: "Why are they sticking that tube into me?" they could not answer. They could only say: "Dr. Michon and Dr. Hamburger are the greatest specialists in France. Everyone says so. They'll make you well."

Evenings, they drove out to relatives on the Boulevard de Ménilmontant to sleep for a few hours. Early every morning they reappeared at the gate of the Necker and made their way across icy courtyards, through corridors, and up steps to their son's bedside. A friendly young intern named Antoine gave them reassuring evasions. They did not realize the full horror of what had happened until December 23.

Robert Renard in an interview seventeen years later:

"Even before Hamburger told us the truth, we had guessed something. While we were waiting in the hall for the outcome of some examinations, the door suddenly flew open and several doctors came out. One of them—

later somebody said it was Dr. Michon—said indignantly to the others: 'It's beyond belief, what he did to the boy.' "

The following day Hamburger took it upon himself to tell the parents the truth. He invited them into his office. They sat there looking at him, trying to read the expression in his thin face and in the blue-gray eyes behind strong glasses. Robert Renard, a tall, strong man, sat with hands in his lap and anxiously questioning brown eyes under bushy brows. Beside him was his wife, Gilberte, small, motherly, her normally rosy, amiable face now pale and drawn.

Robert Renard in an interview seventeen years later:

"Professor Hamburger told us that Marius no longer had any kidney, and that he could not live. What could we do? Bring suit against Warin? There was nothing we could prove. And doctors stick together when it really comes down to it. But that a doctor—a doctor is only human and can make mistakes—that this Dr. Warin to this day has never come to us to tell us that he made a mistake and that he's sorry—that's something I'll never understand."

From a letter of Dr. Ramon Franco Ansello, December 1953:

"It is a major question, how long the development of kidney transplantation would have been quiescent from 1951 on if young Renard had not fallen from a scaffold. Especially after the failure of the transplants of January 12, 1951, Hamburger was deeply discouraged, even though animal experiments had turned up a new phenomenon. Dr. Oeconomos in particular had shown that transplanted kidneys often functioned for an unusually long time if the donor animal was closely related to the recipient —for example, if the donor was a mother or a father. But in the desperate situation of young Renard, Hamburger would hardly have wanted to venture a new step into the unknown if a modest, simplehearted, loving mother had not happened to read a newspaper piece about a child saved by his mother's kidney. Marius's mother implored Hamburger to undertake an operation, and so pressingly that he at last overcame his doubts and reluctance."

From a report by Jean Hamburger in La Presse Médicale, 1953:

"Unusual circumstances led to consideration of an attempt at kidney transplantation. . . . The mother insisted on sacrificing a kidney in order to save her child."

From a report by Dr. L. Michon:

"The child's mother has not merely proposed, she has absolutely insisted that one of her kidneys be removed and an operation attempted, no matter how uncertain the prospects."

From the manuscript of a French reporter, April 1953:

"The decision to make another attempt at kidney transplantation, which was taken while the halls and wards of Necker Hospital were being decorated for Christmas parties, aroused in all the participants a feeling that it was not only a desperate decision, but possibly a historic one as well. Yet it was—romantic, trite, and sentimental though this may sound—primarily a mother's decision, made by Gilberte Renard. According to my sources, in Berthecourt, Gilberte Renard had recently read a story in a local newspaper (probably it was *L'Oise Libérée*) that centered around the transplantation of a kidney to a child otherwise condemned to death, just like Marius. The child's mother had sacrificed a kidney, and a daring surgeon had transplanted the kidney into the child and thus saved its life.

"During the night after Hamburger told Gilberte Renard the whole truth, this story came back to her. She could not rest until she had sought out the doctor the following morning and made her proposal. Shyly and uncertainly, she asked whether she could give up one of her kidneys for Marius—as had been done in the story. Hamburger listened to her suggestion without interrupting. Then he tried to explain to her that the story had been no more than a writer's fiction, and that in reality the state of kidney transplantation was entirely different. He told her that all efforts to transplant kidneys into other human beings had failed. The kidneys had been rejected like any other foreign tissue, and in all probability an attempt in Marius's case would likewise fail and could not prevent the boy's death."

But Gilberte Renard refused to accept this verdict. In her despair she would not listen to reasonable arguments and the voice of experience. She held fast to the miracle of the newspaper story. Marius would inevitably die otherwise? she asked. Yes, Hamburger replied, there was no way they could help him. And couldn't she herself live with one kidney? Hamburger agreed that she could. Then why, for the mercy of God, wouldn't they make the attempt? Wasn't there a chance that it would succeed this time? Had it ever been tried, putting a mother's kidney into her own child?

Hamburger had to concede that as far as he knew it had never been tried. And even as he said so he abruptly thought of the results of Oeconomos's animal experiments, which had shown that the kidneys of animals' mothers when transplanted to their young could function longer than other transplanted kidneys.

Gilberte Renard had arrived at the same conclusion without benefit of experiments. Hamburger had just told her that a kidney from a foreign body would be rejected. But the mother was not a foreign body to her child—she had brought Marius into the world. She had carried him in her own body—so why shouldn't he accept a kidney of hers and live with it?

Hamburger was confronted with a maternal logic that had nothing to do with scientific logic. He could not help himself; the idea took hold of his mind. It was true that no one had yet attempted to transplant a mother's kidney into her child. Might not this situation open up new prospects? Could he reject it and thus refuse to take so vital a step along a path that might lead to success? Moreover, in all previous kidney transplantations the organs had been taken either from cadavers or from severely ill persons. No one had yet ventured to graft a healthy kidney from one living person to another, and no such opportunity as this one had ever been provided before. What was more, in all previous known kidney transplantations the recipients had been severely ill, with years of exhausting ailments behind them. There had never yet been a recipient like Marius, a boy who was without a kidney but who was still physically strong, with the resistance and will to live of the young.

Gilberte Renard's appeal placed so unexpected and powerful a temptation before Hamburger that he began to waver. Hesitantly, he told her that he would think the matter over once more. He knew that if he acted at all, he must do so quickly, before uremia destroyed Marius Renard's resistance. But he still hesitated, and conferred with his colleagues Michon and the surgeons Delinotte and Vaysse. Then he ordered a determination of Gilberte Renard's blood group. It was B Rh-positive. So she fitted the blood group of her dying son.

Hamburger made his decision on a frigidly cold day, the day before Christmas.

Robert Renard in an interview seventeen years later:

"They decided to do it. But we had to sign a paper that everything was being done voluntarily and that if the operation failed we would make no claims against the doctors."

As Christmas Eve approached, the urea level in Marius's blood rose to 4.5 grams. Once the decision had been made, the doctors set the date for the operation on Christmas Day. Hamburger and his assistants, Dr. Richer and Dr. Antoine, and the surgeons Dr. Oeconomos, Dr. Michon, Dr. Delinotte, and Dr. Vaysse, feverishly began their preparations. Gilberte Renard was to be admitted to the hospital on December 25 and tested to determine whether her kidneys were quite healthy, for there was always the possibility of some abnormality that would exclude a transplant. In the operating section of the hospital, two adjacent rooms were prepared so that simultaneous operations on Gilberte and Marius could be undertaken. Thus the movement of the kidney from mother to son would take place over the shortest possible distance.

In spite of his increasing uremia, Marius Renard was fully conscious on Christmas Eve. He now knew not only that he had lost a kidney, but also that "something was wrong" with the other. Never in his days of health had he given a thought to the fact that human beings have two kidneys, and even now he did not suspect how close to death he was. It had been decided to tell him shortly before the operation only that he would have to undergo surgery in order to "get well again."

When Robert and Gilberte Renard came to his bed on Christmas Eve, they found him looking baffled at the coming and going of the doctors and nurses, who had to carry test tubes from the ward some 300 yards up and down stairs and through freezing inner courts in order to reach the Necker's laboratories, which were housed in ancient former stables. "They're taking so much trouble," he said, with a dawning sense of his own importance. "Like I was a president or a general." His mother was tempted to tell him everything, but she remained silent, as she had been told to do.

Next day, Robert Renard took his wife through the weather-beaten portal of the Necker on the rue de Sèvres into a wing of the hospital opposite the Laugier Pavilion, which was Dr. Hamburger's province. Gilberte was given Bed 29 in the women's ward; immediately, the X rays and kidney tests began. Renard went on to Marius to offer an excuse for his mother's not coming to see him. He said she had a very bad cold and that the doctors had forbidden her to visit because she might infect Marius. Marius believed this story. He had meanwhile been told that he would undergo surgery in the evening, but he was quite calm. "Tell Mama it's good because then I'll be back home soon," he said.

Later Renard waited at his wife's bedside until the results of the tests showed that there was no obstacle to the removal of one of her kidneys. Then he was sent away, and took himself to one of the small cafés near the hospital to wait out the next few hours.

Shortly before 7 P.M. attendants placed Marius and Gilberte Renard on stretchers almost simultaneously and took them to the operating wing.

There all the preparations had been completed for the first kidney transplant between a mother and son.

There were two teams of surgeons in the operating rooms, one to remove Gilberte Renard's kidney and the other to prepare Marius to receive it.

It was a long way through the mazelike hospital. The attendants carried Marius more than a quarter of a mile, placed him in eight different elevators, and crossed wind-swept courtyards in the biting cold. Marius's mother, wrapped only in blankets, was being taken along the same path, and the two parties nearly met in the course of the journey. Fortunately, someone realized the possibility at the last moment, and an encounter was avoided.

Finally Marius Renard reached the operating wing. At the same time Gilberte Renard was placed on the table. At 7:10 P.M. Delinotte opened her left side. He chose the left kidney because it usually has the ampler blood vessel connections. He exposed the kidney and prepared everything so that only the blood vessels and the ureter had to be severed in order to lift out the kidney and transplant it. In contrast to all the previous operations, the kidney was to remain connected to the circulation of the donor up to the very last minute. Thus the period during which it was not being fed by "living blood" would be kept to the minimum.

At 8 P.M. Vaysse began the operation on Marius Renard. Hamburger had learned from the history of the 1951 patients that it was dangerous to conduct the outflow of urine from the new kidney through the skin, for the kidney was thus vulnerable to infections from outside. He was convinced that the natural path to the bladder must be restored, even though this might lead to subsequent complications, such as an adhesive narrowing of the suture. For this reason, even before the operation a long catheter had been introduced through Marius's bladder into the stump of the ureter that was left after the fateful operation in Beauvais. The ureter of the transplanted kidney was to be connected with the bladder through this tube.

The operation that followed—opening Marius's right side, exposing the iliac artery and vein, embedding the mother's kidney in Marius's iliac fossa, and suturing the artery, vein, and ureter—proceeded with clockwork precision. Only fifty-five minutes passed between the time of the kidney's separation from Gilberte's circulatory system and its connection to the iliac blood vessels in the boy.

Servelle's experience was repeated in this case: the purely technical aspect of kidney transplantation was not especially difficult. Marius was given a blood transfusion, and by midnight the entire operation was completed.

Once again attendants carried the boy and his mother through drafty corridors, open staircases, those eight elevators, and interior courtyards that were now even colder. They took Marius to a small room separated by panes of opaque glass from the large ward in which he had previously lain. It would be easier to keep a close check on him here.

When the boy vanished behind the opaque glass panes, he was still deeply unconscious. He therefore did not notice that the catheter in his bladder suddenly began to drip, and in a totally different fashion from what had happened with Jacqueline Cado. The drops of urine appeared at the end of the catheter in more and more rapid succession. The mother's kidney was functioning with unexpected, almost inconceivable strength. During the first twenty-four hours it produced no less than 3,200 cubic centimeters of urine—so extraordinary a quantity that an amazed Hamburger became imbued with a confidence he had not felt up to the moment the operation was finished.

"The kidney is working—working magnificently." Those were the first words Gilberte Renard heard when she awoke from her long sleep after the operation.

It is still a mystery exactly how the Paris newspapers discovered what had taken place on Christmas night 1952 in Necker Hospital. By the time the operation was in progress, however, many persons inside the hospital knew that a healthy mother was sacrificing a sound kidney for her dying son. Attendants, nurses, employees, even patients might have talked. Before Hamburger, alarmed by the sudden appearance of reporters, could order a tight lid on all information, it was already too late.

A simple kidney transplant alone would have sufficed to lure the reporters. But the fact that for the first time in the history of medicine a mother was giving up one of her organs for her child, and that both mother and child had survived the operations, contained all the elements of a genuine sensation. It appealed to the basic emotions of people. Unknowingly, Gilberte and Marius Renard became the centers of interest to millions throughout the world.

On December 26, Marius was still too dazed to know what was going on. In the time since December 16 the boy had suffered a fall, broken ribs and pelvis, a kidney extirpation, several catheter examinations, the loss of his entire kidney function, thirst and pain, and finally more anesthesia and a second, still more difficult kidney operation. With closed eyes, he lay on his hospital bed, feeding tubes in his nose, the catheter in his bladder, broken bones and operation wounds still unhealed. Only now and then, when he awoke from his doze, did he become aware of all the white smocks around him hour after hour, checking his blood pressure, checking his urine, taking samples of his blood, or supplying him with medicines and fluids through the tube that protruded from his nose.

For the next four days, he remained dimly conscious. Only occasionally did he hear a voice saying: "You're doing fine—don't talk—you're doing fine."

During that same period Hamburger, despite his initial skepticism, began to be increasingly hopeful of a happy outcome to the experiment. The splendid kidney function continued, settling down after some oscillations to a normal quantity of 1,500 cubic centimeters daily. The transplanted kidney removed so much urea that the almost-fatal urea level dropped to 1.80 grams.

Gilberte Renard, recovering swiftly, asked every time she opened her eyes: "How is the boy? Is my kidney functioning?" And Robert Renard, arriving at the hospital early every morning, would ask the same question. After a few days, he no longer needed to ask. The news of the transplant had spread through the entire place. As soon as he entered the door, attendants and patients would rush up to him and report that the kidney was functioning wonderfully and everything was going beautifully.

On December 29, the father was at last allowed into the small room behind the opaque glass panes to see his son. He was shocked by the boy's appearance. But at Marius's bedside he met Dr. Antoine, the intern who had been so friendly to him and Gilberte from the beginning. Dr. Antoine assured him that Marius's new kidney was working better than Professor Hamburger had dared to hope, and that everybody felt confident now.

That reassured him. Then the boy said: "Where is Mama? Why can't Mama visit me?" And Robert Renard realized that Marius still did not know what had happened. He looked to the doctor for help. Antoine took him outside and told him that Marius had not yet been informed, in order to avoid exciting him. Probably his condition was good enough by now for him to be told the truth; if Professor Hamburger agreed, he, Antoine, would tell the boy. That same evening the doctor brought Gilberte Renard a slip of paper on which a few words were feebly scribbled—feebly, but in Marius's own hand: "Thank you, Mama. . . . I'm fine. Now I know you gave me a kidney."

From that moment on Gilberte Renard insisted so forcefully on seeing Marius that, on December 31, Dr. Oeconomos allowed her to be placed in a wheel chair and wheeled cautiously to the Lefort ward, at the end of which her son's room lay. Upon entering the ward, she started when all the patients sat up in bed and suddenly began clapping, as though receiving a heroine. She smiled uncertainly, and was relieved when the door to Marius's room closed behind her. He lay with the nasal tube, which somewhat distorted his face, parallel to the window, and the white hospital bed made him look even paler than he was. He was too tired to say much more than "Hello, Mama." But she fondled his hand, firmly convinced that he would soon be well. Then she was wheeled back to her ward.

On December 31 the kidney functioned with astonishing regularity. The urea level continued to drop. The first complication did not appear until January 1. Then Marius's temperature rose. He complained of pain in his right leg, and shortly afterward the leg began to swell. The doctors considered the possibility of a venous thrombosis and administered the anticoagulant drug heparin. Thereupon the swelling slowly diminished. On January 4 there came a sudden onset of fever. Marius complained about difficulty in breathing, and an accumulation of fluid in the right pleura was found. The infected site was punctured and 300 cubic centimeters of bloody fluid drained.

During this period the kidney, unaffected by any of these complications, continued to function reassuringly. The blood pressure, however, rose surprisingly. Robert Renard, who was now visiting Marius several times daily, was far too honest a man to conceal his anxiety when he came to his wife's bedside. She insisted that she be taken to Marius once more. This time she walked to the Lefort ward, merely leaning on a doctor's arm. Again she was touchingly greeted by applause from the other patients. Again they called out to her that Marius was doing well. And, in fact, she found him wide awake and looking alert. He said to her: "Mama, I think your kidney is just fine."

Back in her room, Gilberte suddenly exclaimed: "I was so affected I forgot all about wishing him a happy new year." She had no idea that this remark, under the headline WORDS OF A HEROIC MOTHER, would be published next day in many newspapers all over Paris and France. Among the other newspaper headings were:

"Astounding Operation at Necker Hospital."

"After a Remarkable Mother's Sacrifice."

"Ten Days of Struggle against Death. If the boy with transplanted kidney lives, French surgery will have won a remarkable victory."

"Operation Mother Love."

Millions of mothers were now demanding to hear more about Marius and his mother. Untold numbers were waiting for fresh news. Journalists could no longer resist the temptation to supply this demand. Robert Renard, taciturn, pale, exhausted by his daily trips to the hospital, suddenly found himself surrounded by reporters whenever he entered or left the gate of Necker Hospital. At first, surprised and happy that others were taking an interest in his son's fate, he answered their questions. He was happy, moreover, that he had good things to tell about Marius and Gilberte.

From newspaper accounts:

"Gladness speaks in the eyes of Robert Renard, this solicitous father who has closed his workshop in order to spend his days by the bedside of his dear ones."

"Last night we accompanied Robert Renard to Necker Hospital, where he went first to his wife's, then to his son's bedside. . . . The latest news that this doubly anxious father had to give us was decidedly good. . . . The boy's temperature is only slightly above normal. 'He wanted me to feed him,' Monsieur Renard told us. 'I gave him his bouillon a spoonful at a time and fed him his vegetables bit by bit.' "

Overnight Gilberte Renard began receiving telegrams from all over France, and letters declaring: "We are praying for you." For the first time in his life, Robert Renard saw pictures of himself, of Marius, and of Gilberte in newspapers. When he took cabs between the hospital and his lodgings, rather than drive his own car through the Paris traffic, the cabbies recognized him and refused to accept payment. These were totally new experiences for him, and so Robert Renard imagined that even the reporters were displaying human sympathy. He could not understand why the doctors begged him to give out no more information, or why they had the hospital gates guarded by policemen. He began to understand only after photographers disguised as male nurses forced their way into the ward and smashed the glass panes of the door to Marius's room in order to take pictures of the boy. When Marius awoke in fright at the sound of shattering glass, Robert Renard began to realize that he had come from provincial Berthecourt into a world in which humanity existed side by side with a rapacity for sensation, and genuine sympathy was accompanied by cold business calculations.

A few hours later Marius had another crisis. For two days a bout of diarrhea forced the helpless boy to call for the bedpan until he was totally worn out. His face grew smaller from hour to hour. One of the male nurses, who had a son the same age as Marius, took over the task of changing the mattress of Marius's bed. He carried the old mattress through endless corridors and courtyards to a shed where beds were kept, and carried a fresh mattress back the same way to the Lefort ward.

This relapse passed without any change in the functioning of the kidney. But then, on January 8, blood suddenly appeared in Marius's urine. Was the kidney itself failing now, putting an end to all hopes?

It took two days for the doctors to discover that the bleeding had been caused by a displacement of the catheter over which the ureter had been sutured. When the catheter was removed, something happened that struck Robert Renard as a kind of miracle. When he entered Marius's room he found his son sitting up slightly for the first time. Laughing, Marius reported: "Papa, I can do it myself again."

From the next day on—from January 11—he began to recover with such rapidity that even the optimists were surprised.

The reporters from Paris and the French provinces had now been joined by the first correspondents from Germany, Italy, England, even the United States. They could not get through the police blockade. But they did not give up, and in some mysterious way they continued to obtain information about what was going on inside the hospital.

From newspaper accounts:

"Toward noon Dr. Oeconomos and Dr. Antoine entered Marius's room. 'Little man,' Oeconomos said, 'today you're going to get up out of bed.' . . . They helped him to sit up. Then they lifted his by now thin legs over the edge of the bed and straightened him up. 'Is everything going round and round?' Cautiously, the boy shook his head: 'No.' 'All right, then let's try to walk a few steps.'

"Marius's face was anxious, and he clung desperately to the two doctors as they supported his first few steps. Oeconomos and Antoine had him walk around the bed once and then rest. Next they led him to a small table and sat him down. He was breathless and took some minutes to recover. Later a nurse brought his lunch: potatoes, green beans, honey, and stewed quince. He fed himself for the first time, eating slowly, his hands shaking. But feeding himself reminded him that at home they often had wine with their meals. 'I'd like some wine,' he said. Dr. Antoine was both surprised and delighted by this request. He had a tiny glass of wine brought. Marius drank only a few drops. Then the doctors took him back to bed, where he fell asleep at once."

The account of this event unleashed something like a wave of rejoicing in millions of readers. Robert Renard heard of the incident later that afternoon. When Marius awoke, he saw his father by his bed and sent to ask Dr. Antoine whether he might show his father that he could walk. Permission was granted, and for the second time the boy was lifted out of bed. Robert Renard watched his son take a few steps. Afterward, Dr. Antoine accompanied the father to the women's ward to tell Marius's mother: "We're more pleased than we ever dared hope we would be."

Next day it became evident that the experiment of getting the boy to his feet had done no harm to the kidney, aside, perhaps, from a slight excretion of albumin. Optimism increased. Marius began to request newspapers, and finally wanted to see his brother, Christian.

On January 13, Robert Renard brought the six-year-old to the hospital. Marius demonstrated that he could now stand and walk a few steps. He also showed his brother the flowers, gifts, letters, and telegrams he had received from all over France.

The kidney continued to function. The urea level in Marius's blood dropped to 0.8 grams, and this improvement held on the fourteenth, the fifteenth, and the morning of the sixteenth—by now twenty-one days after the transplantation. Then, only a few hours later—at four o'clock in the afternoon—the excretion of urine suddenly decreased. This might have been chance. But a few hours later it ceased altogether. By ten o'clock that night Hamburger was so alarmed that he called a conference among the doctors. The urea level was rising again, and Marius's temperature shot up to 102. The doctors still refused to believe that after so many weeks all their hopes could be shattered so rudely. They considered it likely that some constriction had developed at the suture of the ureter, preventing the outflow of urine. By eleven-thirty, when not another drop of urine had appeared, they decided to operate—to open up the transplant area once more in order to determine whether the ureter was blocked or the kidney itself was undergoing changes.

Robert Renard had been with Marius when the disaster began to be evident. Hour after hour he had waited while the boy's spirits flagged and he slowly deteriorated. When Dr. Antoine at last took the father aside and explained that they would have to operate again in order to determine the cause of the sudden worsening of the boy's condition, Robert Renard turned his head away without a word.

Report from the special correspondent of L'Oise Libérée, *January 18, 1953:*

"The unfortunate father was present when the child was being moved to the operating room and could barely control his feelings. The tormented boy uttered a single cry: 'I don't want to die.' As he was wheeled into the operating room he was heard to cry out once more: 'I don't want to die.' Since then there has been no information on the unfortunate boy's condition, because the surgeons have maintained silence. . . . According to rumors, despite the operation by Dr. Oeconomos and Dr. Vaysse the kidney has not begun to work again. Marius's father and his grave mother are broken with grief. The father was sobbing and staggering from sorrow. . . . In the corridors leading to the boy's room, everyone is talking in whispers. According to the latest information, the urea level has risen to 2.9 grams."

.   .   .

From the account in *L'Oise Libérée* it was clear that efforts to block the access of reporters to the hospital had been relatively ineffective. No one could determine the channels through which information flowed—presumably from nurses, students, laboratory assistants, patients. But whatever the source of the information, it was extremely close to the truth.

When Vaysse and Oeconomos examined the transplanted kidney on the night of January 16–17, they were horrified. They found no adhesions or any other developments that might have blocked the ureter. But the kidney itself had changed in a gross and terrifying fashion. It had swollen to about double its original size. Its surface was bloodshot. By dawn on January 17 the doctors had to face the facts; there was no longer any possibility of self-deception. Examination of tissue samples had revealed severe damage to and radical changes in the kidney tissues.

One of the doctors, who still did not want to give up, spoke of the possibility of suppressing the mysterious power that was rejecting the kidney if only the boy could be kept alive for a while longer. Mightn't they try to control the mysterious rejection process with drugs like cortisone, which had just emerged from the pharmaceutical laboratories?

The idea was based on no experience; it was an expression of sheer irrational hope. Hamburger nevertheless ordered this drug therapy to be started with an intravenous infusion of 200 milligrams of cortisone. No one as yet had had much experience with this new hormone. But possibly—just possibly—it would work a miracle.

The patients in Lefort ward lay awake watching the door behind which lay the boy to whom their own hopes also clung.

On January 18, still not a drop of urine was excreted. The urea level rose to 2.3 grams, the blood pressure to 180/110. When the cortisone proved useless, further attempts were made with antibiotics and antihistamines. These likewise produced no improvement.

When Robert and Gilberte Renard visited Marius, the boy merely murmured: "I'm so tired, and I can't see you clearly."

Meanwhile, newspaper accounts of the crisis had produced a new torrent of letters and telegrams. More than a hundred persons, in Germany as well as in France, in total ignorance of the medical problems, prompted by hysteria, suicidal impulses, thirst for adventure, or a desire to make themselves important, offered to come to Paris and donate a new kidney for Marius Renard. Outside the hospital, the swarm of reporters increased steadily. Policemen arrested hospital attendants who were observed in conversation with the journalists. But Hamburger's struggle against publicity was already lost. Almost every detail of Marius's condition somehow found its way to the outside.

On January 20 the urea level rose to 4.5 grams. Since all the drugs had been ineffective, Hamburger decided to exchange all of the dying boy's toxic blood for healthy blood, in order to gain time. Fourteen donors were brought to the hospital from various parts of Paris. In the course of three hours, five liters of blood were removed from Marius's system and exchanged for five liters of fresh blood from the donors. The concentration of urea dropped. On January 21 and 22, Marius recovered slightly. During a brief moment of alertness he indicated that he still hoped to survive. He whispered: "I know I'll never be a carpenter. But maybe I can move to Le Crotoy and sell fish. I know the fishermen will help me. . . ."

A few hours later the urea had reached the same level as before the exchange of blood. Hamburger and his colleagues decided on another desperate effort to gain time. Since the hospital did not have an artificial kidney, he would try a method that would use the intestines as a substitute for the filtering function of the kidney. The procedure was equivalent to cruel torture for the boy. It required introduction of a tube through the nose and esophagus down to the duodenum, and a second tube into the intestine, in order to achieve a slow-acting rinse with a dialysis fluid.

On January 23, Marius withstood this procedure, too. But it meant only a brief postponement of the end. The "intestinal perfusion" scarcely affected the concentration of urea. Soon the level rose to 5 grams.

By now Hamburger was exhausted and could no longer summon up any hope. Wearily, he looked at Robert Renard, who for the first time had been given permission to spend the night at Marius's bedside. Somberly, he told him: "It is hard to be a father, but, believe me, it is often just as hard to be a doctor."

Shortly afterward the urea level reached 5.5 grams, and at one o'clock in the afternoon on January 27 the French radio reported the first official statement by the doctors. It was one of total capitulation: "In the present state of our knowledge we would not attempt a kidney transplant again. The most favorable premises existed for this operation. Since it has not achieved the hoped-for result, we do not think such operations will succeed in the near future."

Meanwhile, Marius Renard sank into a coma from which he did not awaken.

Report of L'Oise Libérée:

"Monsieur and Madame Renard are exerting their last ounce of will to keep going. They were at the dying boy's bedside, but he was no longer able to see them. After a while Dr. Antoine came up to the unhappy mother, placed a gentle hand on her shoulder, and led her out to the corridor. The father followed, with a last long look at the bed.

" 'You must have still more courage,' Antoine began; then he paused, choked by his own feelings. 'As for our little Marius, I promise you that I will not leave him alone for a moment and will see to it that right up to the end he doesn't suffer.'

"And so the grief-racked mother, leaning on her husband's arm, left the hospital for the first time. Dr. Antoine stayed behind with Marius and tended him as he had promised up to the moment the boy succumbed painlessly to his disease."

Marius Renard died shortly before midnight on January 27, 1953.

Paris-Match, *January 1953:*

"Marius Renard was one of the greatest adventurers of our time. . . . He tried to defeat nature. . . . He believed he would be able to live with another person's organ. . . . That was daring. But if he had gone on living, he would have been the first human being of a new race—triumphant evidence of the greatness of mankind."

From a letter of Dr. Paul Benoist, March 14, 1953:

"Millions of people have enjoyed their drama. This was the first time, I think, that a wholly unknown patient became the hero of headlines. Who knows whether it was the spectacle of mother love or the longing of the human race for eternal life that made these millions hope for the miracle of a supply of spare parts for human organs? The experiment has failed. It has shown that even the close kinship of mother and son is not sufficient to prevent the rejection of an organ.

"The mystery remains unsolved. But anyone who knows human beings, knows their curiosity, their ambition, and their craving to live, must know that in spite of all the doctors' pledges the whole experiment will be tried again, perhaps even by those who have sworn to refrain."

5 / Edith Helm

Dr. John P. Merrill of Peter Bent Brigham Hospital, Boston,
in Great Adventures in Medicine:

"In 1954 we were confronted with a unique opportunity. . . . An alert physician in a nearby U. S. Public Health Service hospital was caring for a young veteran who was dying of severe kidney failure and high blood pressure. A daily visitor to his bedside was his apparently identical twin. Miller knew of our work on kidney transplantation. He also knew that biological incompatibility was the reason transplantation of tissues generally failed. He reasoned that if the two young men were identical twins, their tissues might not be incompatible. As is well known, identical twins develop from a single fertilized egg; they not only resemble each other in appearance but also have a high degree of biological identity."

The latest magazines arrived in Chandler on Tuesday or Wednesday of each week. Sometimes they came late, for Chandler is a country town thirty-odd miles from Oklahoma City. The issue of *Time* for the first week of January 1955 arrived on a Wednesday. There were no customers in the beauty parlor where Edith and Wanda Johnson both worked, and so they were free to read the magazine that Wednesday. The two girls were twins, daughters of Virgie and James H. Johnson. Their father had formerly run a dairy farm near Davenport, a few miles away, and was now working for the Chandler department of public works. The twins were twenty years old, pretty, slightly built, with brown hair and brown eyes. And they were so much alike that their teachers in Davenport had always confounded them. Even their mother occasionally could not tell them apart; their younger sister, Sandra, and their younger brothers, Kenneth and Jim, had equal difficulty.

On page 36 of *Time,* Wanda found a story headed "Twin Transplant." The story mentioned the fact that all kidney transplants hitherto had been failures. But recently, on December 23, 1954, a team of doctors at the Peter Bent Brigham Hospital in Boston had decided to venture still another transplant. A farm boy from Northboro, Massachusetts, who had come down with an incurable kidney disease while serving in the Coast Guard, had been sent to them from a veterans' hospital. His name was Richard Herrick; he was only twenty-three years old and had an identical twin brother named Ronald, who looked exactly like him. Since all their physical characteristics coincided so completely, there was the chance that Richard's body might not reject a kidney from his brother. Ronald, who intended to make a career of teaching, had been willing to give up one of his kidneys. Immediately after the operation Richard's new kidney had begun functioning, and both brothers were in good condition.

"Now look at that," Wanda said, handing the magazine to Edith. Neither of the girls could recall ever having been sick. And so Wanda laughed and added: "I guess we're safe. If you ever need a kidney you can have one of mine."

"And the same goes for you," Edith said.

Later they showed the magazine to their fiancés. Both young men were from the neighborhood, and Wanda's boyfriend, William Melvin Foster, whom they called "Buck," was virtually the only person who could tell the sisters apart. Buck worked as a mechanic and was preparing to go into the navy in San Diego.

"If Edith were sick and I wanted to give her a kidney, would you let me?" Wanda asked.

"Let you?" Buck replied. "It's your kidney. I guess you can do whatever you like with it."

Edith's fiancé was twenty-three; his name was Lee Helm. He had grown up on a dairy farm and was so tall and broad-shouldered that Edith looked like a doll when she stood beside him. He worked in nearby Sand Springs. He too laughed at the same question and said: "I guess the two of you don't have to worry about that sort of thing."

Wanda married Buck in October 1955, and Edith married Lee in November. When Buck went to San Diego, Wanda remained in Chandler. The Helms moved to Sand Springs, a little place consisting of a schoolhouse, a church, a store, and a great many cows. The R.F.D. mailboxes along the roads had no names on them, because the mail carrier knew everyone in town.

Lee's salary was small, and so Edith went on working in the beauty parlor. Every Sunday after church they drove out to the Johnson home in Chandler, where Virgie Johnson produced some especially delicious southern fried chicken. They were still a close-knit family who had a lot of fun together. But a few months after Edith's marriage they all stopped laughing abruptly.

It happened in February 1956. One morning at work Edith Helm felt ill, and suddenly she tumbled to the floor in a faint. A doctor thought she had a virus infection. Lee took Edith home to Sand Springs. But the virus proved stubborn. After a while Edith began vomiting frequently. Naturally, Edith thought she might be pregnant, and Lee took her to a doctor in town. The doctor also thought it was probably pregnancy. But since he discovered that her blood pressure was unusually high, he referred her to the hospital in Cushing, another small town farther north, where there were specialists.

The specialist in Cushing told Edith she seemed to be pregnant and gave her prescriptions for a number of drugs. But then he called Lee back into his office and told him that he did not want to worry his wife, but that if she were pregnant, she had also developed a kidney infection and her blood showed evidence of anemia. He recommended that Lee take Edith to Dr. Lewis in Tulsa. Lewis was a specialist in kidney and blood diseases.

Edith Helm in an interview in 1970:

"I didn't really think too much about it, but I guess my husband knew it was serious, because the doctors told him. But at first the baby specialist thought that I had anemia, and that's what he told him, lu—I can't even pronounce it, what I *did* have. They never did tell me."

By this time it was the end of March. The prescribed drugs did not help. Edith suffered from shortness of breath; her normally thin face swelled. And so Lee drove her to Tulsa.

Dr. Lewis quickly found out that Edith was not pregnant at all. The symptoms came from a chronic glomerulonephritis in its last stages; her illness must have begun years ago. He prescribed digitalis for Edith's heart, and then had a private talk with Lee.

In his short life, Lee had had so little to do with medicine that he could not believe his wife might be fatally ill. Yet that was what Dr. Lewis had to tell him. The doctor could not precisely predict how much longer she might live. In the end he added—and at the moment he said this it was intended merely as a parting flourish—that for sufferers from Edith's disease there was only one chance to prolong their lives. Doctors in Boston had discovered it. But the possibility existed only if such a patient had a twin, and there weren't all that many twins around.

Lee Helm was stunned for a moment. Then he recalled the article in *Time* that the sisters had jokingly showed him, and the girls' mutual promises.

"But she does have a twin sister, Doctor," he said. "And they're so much alike that nobody can tell them apart."

"She really has a twin sister?"

"Yes," Lee said. "Her name is Wanda Foster."

Lewis had the feeling that here was one of the most momentous events in his life in medicine. He briefly weighed the pros and cons. Then he asked Lee to wait for further word from him. And he telephoned Dr. John P. Merrill at the Peter Bent Brigham Hospital. Merrill was not a surgeon. He had not himself performed the operation described in *Time*, but had left the actual surgery to his associates Murray and Harrison. But he had been the kidney specialist in charge of the whole procedure.

Lewis asked Merrill about the condition of Richard Herrick, the twin patient who had received a kidney from his brother in December 1954. Was he still alive? A somewhat puzzled Merrill replied that Richard Herrick was indeed alive more than a year after the operation. Herrick's case was the first successful kidney transplant in history.

Then the prospects for a kidney transplant between twins were really good? Lewis asked.

If they were identical twins, Merrill replied. In the meantime he had carried out a second kidney transplant—the past February 6—between two brothers, Jesse and Louis Heilman of Washington. Louis would probably be discharged from the hospital shortly. But why was Dr. Lewis asking?

Lewis gave a brief summary of his case. Merrill wanted to know whether he was sure that the twins were identical and asked whether Edith and Wanda could come to Boston for examination.

Lewis replied that the matter was not so simple. They were not wealthy people, and the travel expenses to Boston alone would surely be a problem for them.

Merrill then asked whether certain tests could be carried out in Tulsa. Similarity of fingerprints, identity of blood groups, records indicating whether only a single placenta had been present at the birth of the twins. Finally, patches of skin should be grafted between the twins. If these were not rejected after several weeks, a kidney transplant could be considered.

Lewis promised to discuss these matters with local surgeons. Then he informd Lee. He explained the whole matter to him and emphasized that there was only one hope for his wife. Lee must talk with Wanda and find out whether she was really willing to give up a kidney if the tests proved that conditions were favorable.

Edith Helm in an interview in 1970:

"The doctor talked with Dr. Merrill. He said that it hadn't been done much and that it was risky, and they weren't even sure they'd do it when I got there. If we'd take the tests, they'd see if they could do it. I was there a month before they decided they'd do it. . . . I was too sick to care. I just didn't care. I was doing whatever people told me to. It got where I'd bleed out of my mouth and everywhere. It just became scary. My husband talked to my sister."

Wanda Foster did not hesitate. If a kidney of hers was needed, she would give it. Not just because she had promised.

Edith's mother had always been convinced that the girls were identical twins. But all she could remember was that Edith had been born first and had weighed 6 pounds, and Wanda fifteen minutes later, weighing 6¾ pounds. And so the tests were undertaken in Tulsa. Edith Helm was growing weaker from day to day, and the rides to Tulsa became more and more strenuous for her. During the early part of April surgeons took pieces of skin from each of the sisters and grafted these into the other twin.

In the meantime, people in Chandler and the vicinity had learned what was afoot, and were inquiring daily how matters developed. The first headlines appeared in the *Oklahoma City Times*. At last, on April 22, Lee once more drove to Tulsa with Edith and Wanda. The doctors found that the skin grafts had not been rejected. Dr. Lewis telephoned Dr. Merrill, who decided that the sisters should come to the Peter Bent Brigham Hospital. At once, if possible.

That was fine, Lewis said, but first he would have to talk over the matter of money with his patient and her husband. Merrill replied that because an experimental operation was involved, he would try to have a foundation pay for the treatment. Only the air fare from Oklahoma to Boston and $500 as a basic sum for the hospital would be needed; unfortunately the foundation could not assume these costs.

Lewis had another talk with Lee. Lee had no extra money, but he said with a kind of despairing resolve that he would raise it somehow. Throughout the drive home, he kept asking himself how he could raise such a sum immediately. But as soon as he arrived in Chandler, he was called to the telephone. It was Dr. Merrill's secretary. She said: "Lee, don't worry about the money. It's all taken care of. Dr. Lewis has a patient who was in the waiting room and heard about your problem. I'm not supposed to tell you his name. But we have the plane tickets, and we're sure to get the $500 for the hospital, too."

Edith Helm in an interview in 1970:

"There were some oil companies and businesses in Tulsa that put up the $500 for the hospital, and I know now who they all were. I believe the doctor's secretary called everybody to raise the money."

.   .   .

Enough money was raised for Lee and his mother-in-law to accompany Edith and Wanda to Boston. On April 24 they were ready to leave. The evening before, neighbors and friends brought them presents of suitcases and dressing gowns for the hospital. But Edith Helm was aware of all this only dimly. Later she could not recall the drive to the airport or the arrival in Boston on April 25, 1956.

Boston seemed like a foreign country to these people from Oklahoma. Lee and Edith's mother moved into a furnished apartment on Tremont Street. A few days later Buck Foster joined them; the navy had given him a furlough so that he could be with Wanda during the operation. Meanwhile, Edith and Wanda themselves vanished beyond the huge pillared gate of Peter Bent Brigham Hospital. Edith's strength had reached its limit; totally exhausted, she collapsed into her bed. But although the strange world and the narrow walls oppressed her, she felt no fear.

Edith Helm to Jerry LeBlanc, 1970:

"I think I was always sure it was going to be all right. I love God, put my faith in him. I think that helps a lot. I liked Dr. Merrill before I even met him. I liked the picture I'd seen of him. He had the bluest eyes, and he was just so friendly. He said he couldn't understand our Oklahoma talk. They talk so fast that I couldn't keep up with them, and they said we talk so slow they'd lose what we said first before we'd finish."

Although Edith Helm still did not realize how close to death she was, Merrill was quite well aware of it. The first unfortunate experiments in 1951 had not kept him from pursuing the possibilities of kidney transplantation in animals and then, in the case of Richard Herrick, once more venturing it upon a human being. There were some who claimed to see in Merrill's blue eyes and sharply chiseled, manly face the cold ambition of an experimenter. But there were also patients who saw in those same blue eyes something that inspired them with unquestioning trust.

Merrill's tests convinced him that at best Edith Helm had only a few months to live. She weighed just seventy pounds; she had become a pitiable little creature who, strictly speaking, was violating the laws of nature in staying alive. If she were to undergo the further extensive series of tests, her advanced state of uremia would have to be checked. On May 4, therefore, Merrill put her through the first of many hours of treatment with an artificial kidney.

Edith Helm:

"When they put me on the kidney machine I felt so good I wanted to go home, but they told me it wouldn't last. They said I could live only about three months, and they could just put me on the machine a few times. Then I wanted to go ahead and get it over with."

Nevertheless, for a short time she felt human again. And one day, after her second treatment with the artificial kidney, the door opened and a young man entered. He said that his name was Richard Herrick and he was the twin on whom Dr. Merrill had operated on December 23, 1954. Dr. Merrill had asked him to come over from Shrewsbury, where he was now working in a clothing store, to introduce himself to Edith. If she didn't mind, he wanted to tell her what had happened to him. Perhaps his story would encourage her to believe that she could get well again.

He drew a chair up to Edith's bed. He, too, had trouble understanding her "Oklahoma talk," and she had to listen very closely to understand his accent. But quickly they hit it off famously.

Before his operation, he told her, his blood pressure had been so high that he could only stagger about. Several times his doctors had changed all of his blood because there was no artificial kidney at the hospital he was in then. None of that had helped. They had sent him home "improved" all the same—because there was nothing else to do with him. There he had crawled around for a while, but in 1954 he was back in the hospital. When the doctors attempted to take X rays of his kidneys, they found the organs simply did not show up at all. Nevertheless, they had simply released him again after three days. For six weeks he had lain around home like a dying dog. Then an ambulance had to take him back to the hospital. He himself could scarcely remember that episode. At the time they had expected him to lose his mind. When they tried to put him in a bed, he fell into convulsions until he lost consciousness. Had Edith ever experienced that sort of thing? he asked.

No, she said, she hadn't had it that bad.

Then she had even more reason to trust that she would be well again, Richard said. He owed his life to a sympathetic doctor named Miller who had hit on the idea of transplantation between twins when his brother, Ronald, visited him. On October 26, 1954, Dr. Miller had sent him to Dr. Merrill. But Richard had only heard about that later. At the time he had not even been able to recognize his brother. On October 30 they had hooked him up to the artificial kidney. After that, he'd come to his senses for the first time in weeks. And on November 11, Herrick continued, he had felt so well that they had released him from the hospital for a while, because Dr. Merrill first wanted to make sure that he and Ronald were identical twins.

Edith said that it had been the same way with her. Since the treatment with the kidney machine, she had been feeling almost well again. But the doctors had told her the effect would not last.

They were right about that, Herrick said. Although they had given him machine treatments several times after that, he had only got worse more slowly. Finally they couldn't give him any more dialysis treatments, and he had begged them to operate on him because he could no longer stand it. The operation had been set for December 23. At the last moment he began feeling conscience-stricken about Ronald and had sent him a note: "Beat it, go home while you can." But Ronald had sent him a note back: "I'm here and I'm staying here." That was the way twins felt about each other. Anyhow, they'd operated on him for 3½ hours, leaving his old kidneys in for the time being and putting the new one into his pelvis. The kidney had started functioning at once. But of course that didn't mean much, because in previous cases rejection had come later. His brother had gone home after only two weeks, while the doctors still sweated it out with him. Then on the thirty-seventh day after the operation they'd released him, and he'd felt like a new man. He'd gained ten pounds.

All the same, they had tested him regularly, and were still testing him because he was the first person in the whole world who hadn't rejected his new kidney. Maybe they were still not quite willing to believe it. Finally, on May 23 last year they had removed the first of his diseased kidneys, and on June 21 the second. Meanwhile, Herrick concluded, he had been married and his wife, Claire, was expecting her first baby.

A baby! Edith Helm became animated. If she went home well, she said, she wanted to have children, too. And Herrick replied that she would undoubtedly get well and be able to have them.

After Herrick's visit Edith Helm felt definitely buoyed up. It did not occur to her that Merrill had the gravest qualms about the whole question of pregnancy in her case.

Merrill had abandoned the transplantation method that had proved so unsuccessful in 1951. Instead he had tried placing the transplanted kidney in the patient's pelvis and connecting it directly with the bladder. He had done this for Herrick. But in a woman this would mean that a transplanted kidney was situated in the immediate vicinity of the uterus. If he operated on Edith Helm and if the success he had had with Herrick were repeated, what would happen to the transplanted kidney if Edith ever became pregnant? Here were perils that might undo his whole experiment.

On May 17, after the tests had confirmed the identicalness of the twins and the road to a transplantation seemed clear, an incident occurred that thrust such problems as future pregnancy for Edith into the background, and brought the same problem to the fore in the case of Wanda. Overnight Wanda Foster fell ill with a severe infection of the ureter. It suddenly seemed that all thought of a kidney transplant between Wanda and Edith might have to be abandoned. For experience indicated that such infections of the ureter could flare up again unless they were completely cured, and were likely to do so particularly during a pregnancy. Wanda, too, was recently married and would probably be having children. If a latent infection of the ureter should then flare up and involve her single remaining kidney, Wanda herself would be in deadly peril. Given such a possibility, there could be no question of her donating one of her kidneys. The infection had to be overcome, and overcome completely.

For days this problem kept Merrill and the other doctors completely absorbed. Wanda was given antibiotics. But this treatment alone did not suffice. In order for the doctors to be completely sure that the infection was cured and would not become chronic, bacterial cultures were taken at regular intervals. Only after no more germs could be found was the crisis considered past. Shortly afterward, on May 23, the decision was made to undertake the third kidney transplantation between identical twins, and the first between two women.

At eight o'clock in the morning on May 24, Dr. J. Hartwell Harrison and Dr. Joseph E. Murray, assisted by Dr. David Hume, with Merrill standing by, began the now standard procedure in two adjacent operating rooms.

The date of the operation had become public knowledge in Boston after all this long prelude. That morning Protestant and Catholic churches opened earlier than usual so that people could pray for the sisters.

Edith Helm:

"When they decided to do it, they went right ahead. . . . They wheeled me in to where Wanda was just before the operation. I don't remember what we said to each other or if we talked. . . . We just looked at each other and could tell what we felt."

Lee, Buck, and the girls' mother waited in one of the hospital lobbies. At eleven o'clock they received their first word that the operations had gone well. Lawler with Ruth Tucker, Servelle with Jacqueline Cado, Hamburger's team with Marius Renard, and finally Murray and Harrison had successively developed the purely surgical techniques to the point that they were already a matter of routine. There was only one surprise. Although Edith Helm was just twenty-one years old, the illness had already caused traces of calcification in the blood vessels of her pelvis. These traces had to be removed. The infected kidneys were left in place, to be removed later.

After four hours, the two operations were completed.

Edith Helm:

"The doctors were so pleased with the operation, I didn't even have to ask them if it worked. The doctor that did the transplant, he came in and told me it was all working good. I had three kidneys then. . . . They said it would be a few days before they could be sure, in case I was going to reject it, but I think I was always sure it was going to be all right. Sister would come and visit me all the time after the operation. We'd talk about just everything. Home. There was never a 'thanks, sis'; we just didn't have to say things like that. She knew if it was the other way around I'd have done the same for her."

Between May 24 and June 7, 1956, Merrill once again (after the cases of Herrick and Heilman) discovered how easily a transplanted kidney would be accepted if the mysterious mechanism of the body's defenses did not begin to act. The new kidney worked so splendidly that within a few days the urea and electrolytic levels dropped to normal. Edith's visual disturbances ceased. Her blood pressure went down. She developed an almost unbelievable appetite. After a few days she was demanding her heavy home-town foods, above all southern fried chicken.

Edith Helm:

"They ruined me on potatoes, though. I just don't like 'em, mashed potatoes or anything. No other restrictions. I can eat whatever I want. . . . First thing I wanted when I got out was some fried chicken. Oh, they did have it in the hospital, but they just didn't know how to fix it southern style."

On June 7 she got out of bed for the first time and said good-bye to Buck, whose navy furlough was over. She also bade good-bye to her mother. A few days later, Wanda flew back to Oklahoma, less one kidney but in excellent health. From the next day on, Edith fell into a curious kind of depression, although her physical condition continued to improve from day to day. The entire family, once the suspense of the operation was over, had felt that they did not belong in Boston. Friendly as the people in the hospital were, it seemed like banishment to them. Letters and newspapers from Oklahoma had increased their homesickness; but as long as they were all together they had been able to bear it. Now only Lee was still there—and he felt just as forlorn as his wife. Moreover, his money was running out. Edith's low voice changed tone whenever she talked about farms, pastures, cows, and blue skies; finally she told the nurses and Merrill that she would fall sick again if they didn't let her go home.

Merrill, who wanted to keep his first successful case of transplantation in women under observation as long as possible, arranged for Lee to be given a job in the hospital, where he would be able to stay close to Edith. Finally, he also had Edith take on light tasks as a helper in the hospital, in order to distract her from her homesickness. Even so, by July she would not talk of anything but home. Merrill tried to explain to her that toward the end of the month he would have to remove the first of her two diseased kidneys, so that it was reasonable for her to stay in Boston at least until then. But Edith was recalcitrant. She told him she felt sure she would die if he didn't let her go home soon. At last Merrill yielded. Then, just before she left, Edith said she had one important question to ask him.

Edith Helm:

"I asked: 'Can I have children?' Because I wanted to have a big family. He told me I'd have to wait a while. . . . They told my husband I shouldn't have any children at all, but they didn't tell me."

In fact, Merrill had decided that in Edith's state of nervousness it would be better not to inflict such a disappointment. But he talked plainly to Lee, making the point that it would be dangerous to Edith to have children. He was fairly sure, moreover, that the aftereffects of the severe operation and of the operations to follow would prevent any pregnancy for a long time to come.

Back home in Chandler, Edith was received like a heroine. Reporters from Tulsa and Oklahoma City were waiting to greet her, along with half the population of the town. There were headlines and dinners of southern fried chicken. But since Lee, in spite of all this sudden fame, could not find a job, they moved in with Edith's parents until the end of July. Then they set out on the long auto trip to Boston.

Edith Helm:

"We stayed home a little over a month. I could do just anything I wanted. I didn't take anything. No medicine. No doctor's visits. The fact that I had three kidneys didn't bother me. I hated to go back, really. Every-thing was real nice and everything, but it wasn't like home."

Merrill found that all his tests showed normal values for Edith. Dr. Murray removed the first of the diseased kidneys, and on August 15, Lee and Edith went home to Chandler for the second time. They returned to Boston two months later, and on October 29, Murray extracted the second of the old kidneys. Two weeks later Lee and Edith were home for good.

So, at least, they thought. Lee found a job as a service station attend-ant in Chandler. They also found a home, and thought that now the long nightmare was behind them. They read the last newspaper stories about the "woman who made medical history," and Edith Helm thought rather wryly that there must be less painful ways of becoming famous.

But it was by no means all over yet.

Edith Helm:

"I told my husband I was pregnant, but he didn't believe me because he thought they had told him they were going to fix me so I couldn't, but they evidently didn't."

One and a half years had passed since the kidney transplantation when Edith Helm became aware of changes in her body. But this was different from 1956, when she had suddenly fallen ill and thought herself pregnant. This time there was nothing else wrong. She felt well and was certain that it could only be pregnancy. But Lee told her it was impossible. He had misunderstood Dr. Merrill and believed that after the operation Edith would never be able to have children. Thus he was all the more fearful that something was wrong with her kidney again, and he insisted that Edith write to Boston and that she at least consult a doctor in Tulsa.

But Edith was determined not to return to Boston under any circum-stances. Finally Lee talked to Wanda, who now lived in Cushing—after Buck Foster completed his service in the navy he had found a job working for a farm machinery dealer in Cushing. In the meantime Wanda had had her first child, Mike. Lee hoped that Wanda would persuade Edith to write to Boston. But Edith held her ground; at most she would go to see Dr. J. Douglas Green in Cushing, to find out whether she was right about being pregnant.

Green confirmed the pregnancy. But he had read enough about kidney transplants to know that no woman with a transplanted kidney had ever become pregnant before—simply because none had lived long enough. He informed Merrill at once—and the news of Edith Helm's pregnancy imme-diately alarmed the Boston team of kidney transplanters.

For Merrill there was only one possible recourse: he must bring Edith Helm to Boston at the expense of a medical foundation and keep her under constant observation. He was determined to interrupt the pregnancy if the new kidney was displaced by the expanding uterus, thus threatening its functioning and Edith Helm's life.

Merrill's alarm was not unjustified. In the first place, no physician had any experience with the effects of pregnancy in such a case. Moreover, other setbacks in recent months had undermined his initial optimism about the prospects of transplantation between twins. Since the operation on Edith Helm, Merrill and his team had transplanted more kidneys in twins. The first operation, in June, had been successful. But on September 1 he had operated on two fourteen-year-old twin girls, Dolores and Doris Huskey, whose parents had brought them to Boston.

Dolores had already been unconscious when they arrived in Boston. In spite of severe intestinal complications after the operation, the kidney had functioned for a while. But now, in December, the girl lay dying. Not because the kidney had been rejected. Something new and unpredictable had happened: the transplanted, completely healthy kidney had been attacked by the same disease of glomerulonephritis that destroyed Dolores's own kidneys. This experience had taught Merrill that transplantation between identical twins involved other mysterious problems, even though it did eliminate the problem of the rejection mechanism.

Merrill therefore asked Dr. Green to press Edith Helm to come to Boston at once. He would provide the funds for Lee to accompany his wife and would obtain a job for him in Boston for the next several months. And so Lee gave up his job in the gas station, and in January 1958, for the fourth time, he and Edith set out for Boston, in winter.

Edith Helm:

"I didn't want to go 'cause I felt good and I thought the doctor in Cushing could deliver me just as well. . . . But everybody said I had to go. I flew by myself. Lee came out later. . . . I could get up and go around the hospital. I never did have any trouble. I worried a little about the baby; I wanted him to be all right."

To his surprise, Merrill found that the pregnancy did not have the slightest effect upon the kidney. From January to the end of February 1958 he ran one test after the other. But the kidney was functioning perfectly. Nevertheless, he did not dare to let Edith Helm go back to Oklahoma—where the news media and the general population were taking as warm an interest in Edith's pregnancy as they had in the kidney transplant between Wanda and Edith.

From the Oklahoma City Press:

MOTHER TO BE IS HEROINE

"If a poll were taken of Boston's giant research center, Edith Helm of Chandler is a sure bet for the 'most valuable patient' title."

By March 1, as the time of the birth approached, Edith Helm was moved to the maternity ward. Dr. Duncan E. Reid, professor of obstetrics at Harvard University, took charge of her. On March 10, Merrill and Reid conferred once more and decided to deliver the child by Caesarean operation in order to prevent any possibility of damage to the transplanted kidney from protracted labor. The operation went smoothly and no complications followed. The baby was a healthy boy. In informing Merrill of the outcome, Reid remarked that, surprising though it might sound, in his opinion the baby would have been born easily without a Caesarean.

Edith Helm:

"Right after John was born they let me call my husband down in the lobby. . . . He was real pleased it was a boy and he said he'd have to call the folks. I had a name for a girl, but hadn't really picked one for a boy, so we ended up naming him after the doctor, John Merrill."

When Edith Helm was to leave Boston with her new baby, the hospital personnel made the occasion something of a family party. Helena Crocker, the nurse who had tended Edith at the time of the kidney transplant, carried the baby into the plane. In Tulsa swarms of reporters were again waiting, and the Helms' home was filled with presents for the child, enough to last for years.

But that was not the end of the story of Edith Helm. Late in 1959 she became pregnant for the second time. Again Dr. Green sent the pair to Boston, in April 1960. But when Merrill could detect not the slightest trace of kidney difficulty and observed that Edith was crying from homesickness, he agreed that she could have her baby at home this time. On August 5, 1960, again by a Caesarean operation, she gave birth to a six-pound daughter, whom they named Vicki.

In 1963 she read in a newspaper that Richard Herrick, who had given her such encouragement seven years before in Boston, had died. She wrote to Richard's wife in Shrewsbury, Massachusetts, and learned that Richard had died not of a kidney ailment, but because his heart had given out under the strain of severe pneumonia.

That was not the whole truth—possibly Claire Herrick herself did not know the truth. Merrill knew, however, for his autopsy showed that Ronald Herrick's kidney, with which Richard Herrick had lived some nine years, had been attacked by the same glomerulonephritis that had destroyed his own kidneys earlier. Thus the mysterious case of Dolores Huskey was repeated.

In April 1964, Edith Helm was expecting her third baby. This time she lost it—it was born dead. A few years later Lee took over a small dairy farm. Edith and the children moved into a one-story white farmhouse north of Chandler, where they could look over the endless succession of green hills and survey their herd of grazing cows. For a while Edith even resumed the farm work she had done in her childhood. To a reporter who visited her in 1970 she said: "I feel so good they even sold me health insurance last year. I'm lucky to be living at all, and every day is just something extra I wouldn't have had. So I don't worry about dying."

6 / Georges Siméon

United Press International, Boston, April 12, 1959:

"Massive doses of X rays all over the body of a Wisconsin man saved his life in a kidney transplant operation, the first such successful surgery between *nonidentical* twins in medical history. The operation, generally regarded as a medical break-through, was announced yesterday by Peter Bent Brigham Hospital doctors. John M. Riteris, 23, of Milwaukee, who was discharged yesterday, received a normal kidney from his brother, Andrew, on January 24. . . . Prior to transplantation a large dose of total body X-irradiation was administered in the hope of suppressing the rejection response in the sick twin which might fight off the new kidney."

Georges Siméon, a Parisian postal clerk, entered Necker Hospital on April 28, 1959. On the arm of his wife, Armande, he passed through the gate and went on to the ward where Marius Renard had come to his sad end. By nature Siméon was a stocky fellow, of sturdy constitution. Now he was emaciated, although he was only thirty-seven years old, and he walked unsteadily. For the past eight years he had been slowly dying—but as yet he did not know it. Armande, however, knew that Georges was suffering from glomerulonephritis and that he had reached the last, fatal stage of the disease.

Previously, Georges had never been seriously ill. On the contrary. As a young man he had been a considerable athlete, and when in the war year of 1942 he and his brother, André, had been sent to forced labor in Germany—like tens of thousands of other Frenchmen—he had borne up well through it all and come out of that difficult time in good health. In 1945 both brothers were home again. Georges had returned to his job in the post office and that same year married Armande. In 1946 they had their first child, Danielle, and in 1948 a second daughter, Michèle, came along. Theirs was a peaceful house and a peaceful family.

Possibly the disease had begun with a throat abscess from which Georges suffered in 1949. At any rate, that was his family doctor's opinion after an examination in 1951, when Georges complained of being tired all the time. This doctor had subsequently told him: it's nothing serious. But in the future he must keep to a salt-free diet, avoid proteins as much as possible, and come in for a checkup every few months. What the doctor told Armande, however, had a very different sound: chronic nephritis, and incurable.

Armande had resolved to keep Georges ignorant of his condition as long as possible. She had desperately kept to this resolution, although the strain exhausted her. Her brother-in-law, André, had helped in the deception and in keeping up Georges's hopes. For the story of Georges and André resembled that of Edith Helm and Wanda Foster in this respect: they were an inseparable pair.

Armande had arranged for a double set of medical reports: a genuine version for herself and a false and favorable version that she could show to Georges. In 1952 she had given birth to a son, Patrick, and in 1956 to a daughter, Ghislaine. And through the years she had continued her deceptions and consolations—until in 1958 she read an article about kidney transplants between identical twins. André had commented: "If Georges ever reaches that point and he can be helped in such a way, fine. I'm healthy and Juliette would understand." (Juliette was his wife and the mother of his four children.)

Georges and André were twins, but that they were identical twins seemed hardly likely. Georges was stocky, André slightly built; Georges deliberate, André lively. Armande nevertheless began to cherish hope—simply because she wanted to hope.

On the other hand, to talk with Georges about kidney transplants would have meant telling him that he was fatally ill. Once, when Armande and André noticed an article about kidney transplants on Georges's table, André said, as if joking: "Have you read that? If those funny kidneys of yours ever go on strike in thirty years or so, you can have one of mine."

Georges waved that aside with his usual composed air. They never knew for certain whether or not he believed their deceptions.

Then, at the beginning of the year, he had begun going downhill so rapidly that he could no longer perform his post-office job. More sinister still, Armande observed that he was reading everything he could find on kidney diseases. She could not very well take the books away from him. And although she had sometimes wondered earlier how well she was really fooling him, now she trembled daily that he would discover the whole truth. Then, in the spring of 1959, she suddenly dared to hope again. *France-Soir* and other newspapers were publishing sensational reports from Boston. A Professor Merrill and several other doctors had once again transplanted a kidney from one twin to another, and the patient was still living—although the twins had not been identical. Their names were

John and Andrew Riteris, and they were ordinary twins, as Georges and André probably were.

André advised Armande to write to Professor Merrill and describe Georges's situation. After some hesitation, she did so. She scarcely dared to hope for a reply. But Merrill did answer—and had even attempted to write in French. She kept his letter carefully, even though it seemed like a very uncertain draft on the future. For Merrill had explained to her that he could not undertake another operation between nonidentical twins for a considerable time. The transplant of the Riteris brothers had been done only a few weeks ago, and he must wait to see whether it was successful.

A considerable time did not mean forever, Armande told herself. However, during the past few weeks Georges's decline had accelerated to such a point that something had to be done.

Armande had heard about a Dr. de Beaufond. He was well along in years, but was supposed to have helped many people suffering from kidney diseases. Armande had therefore applied to him—a rather difficult matter, for Beaufond had already more or less retired from active practice. She had asked him to examine Georges personally and do whatever could be done, but not to say anything that might deprive him of hope—not even if his case was really hopeless.

Beaufond, a kindly old gentleman, had granted her request and gone along with the game of deception. But to Armande he said bluntly: "To my knowledge there is nothing that can help your husband. If there is some new development, there is just one Paris doctor who would know: Professor Hamburger at Necker Hospital. I'll write to his assistant, Dr. Crosnier. If you take the letter to the hospital, I'm certain Professor Hamburger will look into your husband's case."

At Necker Hospital, Armande had to wait for a long time. But at last Professor Hamburger gave Georges an appointment for April 28. On that day Armande conducted Georges through the labyrinth of ancient courtyards and corridors to Hamburger's ward.

Professor Jean Hamburger in a report on the case of G.S., October 17, 1959:

"His general condition was fair. Face sallow. Percentage of urea in the blood was 3.45 grams per liter. . . . The condition corresponded to the last stage of a protracted, chronic nephritis. Consideration of all prognostic aspects led to the conclusion that the patient . . . had only a few months to live."

Armande Siméon's recollections:

"Professor Hamburger listened to the whole story. Then he said: 'You have four children. . . . At home your husband might be taken suddenly by an attack and die right there. Therefore it would be better for him to stay with us.' And so I left him there."

As she hesitantly stepped through the gate and out onto the rue de Sèvres that afternoon of April 28, 1959, she suddenly realized that Hamburger had said not a word to her about any chance of saving Georges. Instead, he had plainly implied that his one concern was to make the slow process of dying easier for the sick man. Armande decided not to go home. Instead, she set out for Roissy-en-Brie, where André had built a house in 1958 and where he now lived with Juliette and their four children, Annie, Silvie, Jean-Thierry, and Philippe. André worked nights in a print shop and therefore often slept by day. He was already up when Armande arrived and sorrowfully told him that she had left Georges in the hospital. Undoubtedly the staff would do their best for him there, but she also knew that they would let him die. The only thing that could help him, she said, was a new kidney. Why couldn't the doctors at Necker do what had been done in Boston? After all, they were French doctors, and among the best in Paris. If she and André wanted to help Georges, they had to do something right now. And she asked André to come with her to see Dr. de Beaufond.

It was evening. The children went to bed. Juliette Siméon sat listening in silence.

André Siméon's recollections:

"My sister-in-law begged me to give my brother a kidney. And I was determined to. . . . Still, I couldn't help thinking: what will happen if the new kidney doesn't take—or if the surgeon who operates on me has a bad day? Then I'll also be leaving behind a widow and four children."

Armande Siméon's recollections:

"André and I talked over the whole thing with Dr. de Beaufond, and he answered: 'Only Hamburger can decide that.' So we went to see Hamburger with Dr. de Beaufond—my brother-in-law and I."

Georges Siméon's recollections:

"That was it. When my brother talked with Professor Hamburger, the doctor told him: 'No, no kidney transplant in human beings has ever succeeded except with identical twins. You must know that I had that unfortunate experience with little Marius. I cannot take the responsibility for another human transplant. People would say that I am experimenting on human beings.'"

Armande Siméon's recollections:

"Dr. de Beaufond helped us in those decisive days . . . because he understood all the medical language better than we did. Hamburger said it was all very complicated. But later, when we went on pressing him, he promised to get in touch with Professor Merrill in Boston. . . . So then he telephoned Professor Merrill. . . . I still remember because I was sitting in another room while he was on the telephone."

André Siméon's recollections:

"I think the case of young Marius Renard must have hit Professor Hamburger particularly hard. It was only after we kept telling him, backed by Dr. de Beaufond, that Georges's case was altogether different and just like the last case in Boston, and that we were twins and I wanted to give one of my kidneys, that he finally consented."

Georges Siméon's recollections:

"I suppose the doctors should have told me they wanted to do a transplant. But Hamburger thought that if he told me, then I'd know how desperate my state was. But in secret I knew a lot more about it than they thought. I'd read that with a urea level of 2 grams to a liter of blood a person might have six months to live. In the hospital I found out that I had 3.5 grams per liter. So I knew I really didn't have much time. . . . But I kept cheering myself up with new hopes. That's the way we human beings are. I'd seen . . . other patients who had to come to the hospital only once every few months. And I thought maybe the professor could do something to fix up my blood again. . . .

"Finally Armande asked my brother to talk to me."

André Siméon's recollections:

"I went . . . over to Georges and told him everything. . . . At first he wouldn't hear of it. . . . And I said: 'What's the matter, my kidney isn't good enough for you?' And he said: 'This is nothing to joke about. Suppose something goes wrong with the operation.' So I asked what else he wanted to do. 'Do you just want to wait for death?' Well, in the end he finally said yes, and I told him: 'Don't worry.' "

Memory is always a merciful filtering of the past. Unfiltered, the reality of those two months from the end of April into June 1959 had been pretty horrible for Georges Siméon and his family.

Georges, Armande, and André had read that in the case of John Riteris, X-radiation had prevented rejection of the kidney. But they had no real idea of what was involved in bombarding the human body with X rays. Hamburger, on the other hand, did know. Ever since he had been engaged in the transatlantic exchange of experiences, he had known the price for a success like Merrill's recent one. And that explained his hesitation.

He and his associates had also tried to approach closer to the puzzle of rejection after the death of Marius Renard. They had, moreover, studied the efforts of other scientists, principally in England and America. It had long been known that a very large number of substances, when they enter the bodies of men or higher animals, cause the formation of defensive substances which combat the intruding foreign material. Even before the turn of the century, these substances had been given the name "antigens," and the body's defensive substances were called "antibodies."

It had furthermore been demonstrated that the body tissues of every human being contain antigen characteristics that are typical of the particular individual. This means that when a foreign organ is grafted into a body in a case of transplantation, the host reacts by the formation of antibodies that ultimately cause rejection of the transplanted organ. The alarm reaction, which begins as soon as foreign substances or tissues intrude, depends principally on the lymphocytes, white blood corpuscles that, like scouts, report the entrance of the foreign elements to certain centers of the body, such as the bone marrow and the spleen. In some still largely unclarified manner, so-called immunocytes are then formed; hordes of these fall upon the foreign tissue and within a relatively brief time destroy it by the formation of antibodies.

These processes explain why there is no such activating of the defensive apparatus between identical twins. Since the twins have developed from a single egg cell, the tissue of neither is foreign to the other. One identical twin's tissue does not act as an antigen to the other twin's tissue. And thus the strategy for preventing rejection reactions was becoming clearer. Obviously, the aim must be to cancel out the mobilization of the lymphocytes, the immunocytes, and the whole apparatus connected with them, chiefly in the bone marrow and the spleen.

At about the same time that the operations on Richard Herrick and Edith Helm had taken place, American experimenters had shown by animal experiments that the whole alarm and defense system could be paralyzed by a massive dose of X rays. Skin grafts between unrelated animals healed when the recipients were exposed to such a dose of radiation beforehand. Unfortunately, the radiation had to be so massive that it had a terrible side effect: it destroyed the entire blood-forming system in the bone marrow. Without the formation of blood, every living organism perished; and so, in spite of the successful transplantations, the host animals eventually died. The radiation was like a tremendous club that smashed the animal's ability to survive in order to make possible the grafting of a patch of skin.

In 1957 the British scientists Voss and Bekham attempted to keep a dog alive by implanting into it healthy bone marrow from another dog, thus making up for the destruction by radiation of the first dog's own marrow. The recipient remained alive for some time; moreover, a skin transplant grafted at the same time as the bone marrow healed with unusual rapidity. An "adjustment" had been achieved between the host's organism and the transplant from the donor.

The results of these experiments were by now familiar to those doctors and surgeons who were investigating the problems of transplantation. But who could or would risk applying them to human beings? Who would expose a nephritic patient—even if he were on the brink of death—to such an enormous dose of X rays that he would virtually be condemned to death twice over, both from his kidney disease and from the radiation? Who, moreover, would risk implanting in this twice-condemned patient bone marrow from another person, either a corpse, a living person, or even the kidney donor, in order to save him from the destruction of his blood? And who, finally, would implant a kidney into this violently changed body in the hope of keeping this twice-dying patient "alive"? The thought seemed monstrous. Perhaps Hamburger, too, had considered and rejected this course. At any rate, he had not attempted it. Yet by the time he was becoming involved with Georges Siméon's fate, he must have learned that this seemingly monstrous experiment had been undertaken by John P. Merrill a year earlier—in May and July 1958.

Merrill had risked the experiment on two patients, a woman (G.L.;

these initials alone were revealed) and a twelve-year-old girl (known only as W.N.). Both patients had been born with a single kidney and had suffered accidents in which their only kidney was destroyed. Both were condemned to death because neither had a twin who might have given her a kidney. And so Merrill had exposed them to 600 roentgen units of radiation in the one case, and 700 in the other, and then had implanted into Mrs. G.L. the bone marrow and kidney of a dead child. But the kidney had never functioned. The patient had not accepted the bone marrow and died from the consequences of the radiation.

The twelve-year-old child, on the other hand, had received bone marrow from her own mother and had resisted death for twenty-five days. Then she had died of hemorrhages, so that Merrill, Murray, and Harrison had been unable to implant a kidney that they had also planned to take from her mother.

From Dr. John P. Merrill's scientific report:

"In human beings, however, in spite of numerous attempts, whole body irradiation, with permanent survival of homologous bone marrow, has not been successful. In two cases we have attempted this in patients as a preliminary to renal homotransplantations. Both patients died primarily of the effects of radiation depression of hematopoiesis [blood cell formation]. The technical problems . . . made this approach seem unfruitful."

Diary notes of a Boston doctor:

" 'What monstrous acts! What cruel gambling with human lives!' I can just see those headlines when our failures (and admittedly our sometimes cruel failures) are subjected to the 'light' of publicity. And yet anyone who refuses to see that every genuine or even presumptive advance in medicine must be associated with mistakes, sacrifices, grief, or cruelty—anyone who will not see that is a romantic fool.

"If it had not been for the two patients who died after seemingly useless exposure to fatal radiation, no newspapers would have been able to print banner headlines about John Riteris half a year later. They wouldn't have been able to serve up for their readers another of those popular stories about the latest miracles of medicine.

"The death of those two patients prompted Merrill and his associates to abandon transplantation of bone marrow. Instead, they hit on the idea of reducing the fatal radiation to the nearly lethal dose of 450 roentgens; such radiation did not completely destroy the bone marrow and the lymphatic defensive system, but did put both out of action for several weeks.

After such a period these systems generally recover. Merrill's hope was that the period of inaction would suffice to give the kidney recipient's body an opportunity to adjust to the antigens from the foreign kidney."

When Merrill first heard about John Riteris on December 13, 1958, he decided to try out the new idea on him. Riteris, twenty-four years old and Lithuanian by birth, had come to America as a child with his parents and his twin brother, Andrew. While serving in the U. S. Navy, he had learned that he was suffering from chronic nephritis. Thereafter he began dying "inch by inch" in the usual way. In December he had been admitted to the veterans' hospital in Wood, Wisconsin, where his entire supply of blood was changed. The process had to be repeated several times. Finally he had been sent to Merrill in the hope that Merrill could save him, as he had Richard Herrick and Edith Helm, by transplanting a kidney from his brother, Andrew. But Merrill discovered that John and Andrew were not identical twins; they had no more in common than ordinary brothers. It was then that he decided to try transplantation after "nearly lethal" radiation on Riteris. On January 16, 1959, John Riteris received whole-body radiation with 250 roentgen units, and on January 23 he was exposed to another 200 units. The kidney was transplanted on January 24, 1959.

A few weeks after Georges Siméon entered Necker Hospital, he was still lying in his bed and waiting. He now knew that the doctors intended to transplant one of André's kidneys into him, and he experienced hours of terror in which he wished that they would never take him to the operating room. But immediately afterward thirst and pain made him hope that they would get to it as soon as possible. From what was going on around him, he could deduce that preparations for the "great adventure" were in progress. His fingerprints were taken. A tiny patch of André's skin was grafted into his skin. And he heard that all the studies had proved that he and André were, in fact, not identical twins.

André was now coming to the hospital frequently. His kidneys were X-rayed, and he informed Georges that it was going to be his left kidney. But otherwise there were no signs of an impending operation. Georges learned only that some rebuilding was going on in the women's ward, and that it was being undertaken because of his operation. Many special technicians came and went.

Recollections of a former technician at Necker Hospital:

"The rebuilding occupied much of our attention. We found out that radiation before a kidney transplant was no simple matter. The idea was to repress the rejection process, the defensive reaction to the new kidney. For that purpose Siméon had to be irradiated from head to foot, with radiation far more intense than anyone had ever been subjected to. There was a fine line to be drawn; he had to receive just enough radiation, but not so much that he would die of it. For if the radiation eliminated Georges's defenses against André's kidney, it also did the same for his defenses against all infections. Professor Merrill in Boston had had to learn that the hard way. One infection after another had arisen, and Professor Hamburger did not want to take such a risk. He therefore had a special room set up for Siméon, which would be completely sterile and would be entered only by doctors and nurses in sterilized outfits."

Armande and Georges Siméon learned little about such medical problems, and they surely knew nothing about the ordeal of John Riteris, who had been operated on five months previously. To be sure, his new kidney had functioned well from the very day it was implanted. But shortly afterward he was seized by such shivers that his entire bed rocked, while his temperature rose to 104 degrees. Day after day the fever persisted. His intestinal system failed. He was stricken by jaundice. His white blood corpuscle count was 50 per cubic millimeter, instead of the normal count of 5,000 to 7,000. In a short while the count fell to zero. He no longer had any antibodies whatsoever. The radiation had done its work all too thoroughly, and Merrill had the patient put on the critical list.

Throughout all this the new kidney continued to function. But there was suddenly an invasion of coli bacteria in the blood, and dangerous microorganisms appeared in the urine. Septicemia was developing. To cap it off, Riteris was suffering agonies of pain in the right side of his body. Merrill's surgeons conducted a second operation. They discovered a severe infection of one of Riteris's diseased kidneys, which had been allowed to remain as in the cases of Herrick and Edith Helm. There was nothing to do but to excise both the old kidneys. After this the patient's temperature went down. Blood tests also revealed that the white blood corpuscles with their lymphocytes and antibodies were again present. The body's resistance mechanism was once more mobilized. For Merrill this meant new fears that the patient's body would reject the foreign organ.

Riteris was subjected to another radiation treatment of 100 roentgen units, and then to still another. What followed were new fever spells and oral complications that made it impossible for the patient to eat. New microorganisms infected his urinary system. He was given massive doses of antibiotics, but this led to all kinds of side effects. It was not until March that the fever slowly receded. Once more the white blood count rose, indicating a return of the body's resistance mechanism. This time, though, Merrill would not put the patient through another, and fifth, bout of radiation. He could only hope that the body had meanwhile "accepted" the new organ. And apparently this hope had some grounds, because by the beginning of April, Riteris had made enough of a recovery to be able to go home. He was back at the Peter Bent Brigham Hospital on the first of May because of an unhealed fistula from the second of his operations. The new kidney, however, except for a slight albumin excretion, was serving him well.

Once more John Riteris was sent home. But Merrill was still very cautious about calling the experiment a success. Meanwhile, Hamburger was being kept minutely informed about each new phase of the case.

Professor Jean Hamburger in an interview in January 1970:

"By 1959 we had ample evidence that massive radiation would destroy the body's power to create antibodies. It was only logical to make use of this method in order to overcome the rejection process in organ transplant."

But he was highly conscious of the other consequences of radiation, and knew that these were more or less inevitable. The most he could do for Georges Siméon was to fend off all sources of infection during the time that the patient would be without any defenses of his own.

It was by no means easy to set aside such an isolation room in the overcrowded, ancient hospital. Siméon would be kept there from the time of the first radiation. The room was equipped with air conditioning and atmospheric filters, as well as with ultraviolet lamps, which bathed the room with germ-killing rays both day and night. The air was pressurized, in order to repel the entrance of unfiltered air when the door was opened. A glass panel was installed through which the patient could be observed, and a speaker system by which conversation could be carried on.

An adjacent room was made into a sterilizing chamber where the doctors and nurses would don sterile robes, gloves, and masks before approaching Siméon's bed. Any article being brought into Siméon's room, as well as his food and drink, would first be made germ-free here.

By the sixteenth of June both rooms were ready. Five days more were devoted to experiments with the sterilizing techniques. By June 21, Hamburger was convinced that the bacteria count could be kept to a minimum.

Only then was the decision made to go ahead with the great adventure and administer the first, well-nigh lethal, radiation treatments.

Necker Hospital did not have sufficient apparatus for this. There was only one place in Paris that had—the Gustave Roissy radiation institute in Villejuif. Early one morning two orderlies carried Georges Siméon through the gray corridors to a waiting ambulance. One of Hamburger's assistants, Dr. Antoine, who had also looked after Marius Renard, told the patient where he was being taken. From this moment on Georges Siméon knew that the hour of decision had come.

They carried Georges Siméon through the halls of the bleak-looking concrete building. A heavy door opened and he was in the presence of two doctors and a young woman: Dr. Tubiana, Dr. Lalanne, and Madame Dutreix.

He was carried through still another door into a large concrete-walled room where he was laid on a table between two panels of glass. He was shown the strange machine that would administer the radiation. It was about ten yards distant, a mysterious thing which reminded him of science-fiction stories. The doctors were speaking to him, instructing him to double up as he lay on the table, with his knees drawn up to his chest. The machine had only a narrow radius, although it stood so far away, and the rays had to penetrate his whole body. This was possible only if he rolled himself up. So he obeyed their orders, although he had the feeling that he was too weak to stand very much of this.

Georges Siméon's recollections:

"They left me there, in the big room all by myself.

"There were mirrors set into the concrete walls, and small windows through which the doctors could watch what was happening. I was also given a speaker, so that I could let them know when I couldn't stand it any more. They also told me what to do when I couldn't keep that position any longer, so that the rays would go on reaching my whole body evenly.

"It is simply indescribable to lie that way, all alone, with only a voice now and then coming in over the speaker. And then I was aware that there were these rays striking me, and that at a certain point they would be deadly.

"Of course, the doctors had gone into it all very deeply. They must have run many experiments, with animals or what have you. But I kept wondering if they actually knew just how much one could take without dying. I lay there for about six hours on that table between the concrete walls and the machine. No, I can't describe it. . . ."

On that morning of June 22, Georges Siméon received a total radiation of 260 roentgen units. Madame Dutreix made certain tests to make sure that the rays had penetrated evenly throughout his body. Then the ambulance took him back to Necker Hospital.

And now he found himself in bed as totally cut off from the world as he had been on the radiation table in Villejuif. There were four walls covered with antiseptic paint, a table, two chairs, one window, and a door to the anteroom from which he could be observed by the nurses—all bathed in an uncanny blue light from the ultraviolet lamps.

The one familiar "human" thing there was the TV set, which Armande had brought from home so that he would not be absolutely cut off from the world. The set, too, had been sterilized. When the doctors came in to see Georges, he could recognize them only by their height, their eyes, or their voices, for their faces were hidden behind surgical masks. Even their feet were shod in clumsy sterile boots.

He felt enormous relief when he saw Armande's familiar face with her anxious brown eyes through the window. André's thin face was also there, nerved up to look encouraging. "Well, old boy," André said, "we've come a long way. The thing is practically behind us now."

In fact, it was only the beginning. After Georges Siméon had spent several days in his "prison" cell and had got used to touching nothing that had not previously been sterilized, not even a newspaper or a pencil, two male nurses entered the anteroom. That was on June 28.

The two scrubbed themselves like surgeons, and then opened the door and brought in a box that rather alarmed Siméon for a moment, for at first glance it looked like a coffin. It might be called a plexiglass casket. The male nurses explained that the glass box was sterile, and that they had to use it to transport Georges to Villejuif for a second dose of radiation. He had to be moved in a sterile container; otherwise he might encounter germs of infection on the way, and then all the measures of the past week would have been in vain.

They bedded him down in the "coffin." Beside him was a flask of oxygen so that he would not suffocate when the airtight glass lid was closed over him. For a while Georges felt frightened as he was carried to the ambulance in the yard. It was weird being driven through the city in a glass coffin and watching life in the streets through walls of glass.

Georges Siméon's recollections:

"And in Villejuif they lifted my box onto a cart and rolled me into the cellar. There they opened the 'coffin.' They laid me on the table and made me double up again. And the cobalt bomb began firing at me for the second time. Again it went on for five or six hours. Then I was put back in the box and breathed oxygen, and they drove me back. I can't describe it. . . . I could never explain it to somebody who wasn't there."

That June 28, Georges Siméon received 200 roentgen units. Once more the distribution of the radiation in Siméon's body was measured carefully, as if he were a creature in some strange, inhuman technological world.

And then Hamburger set the date for the transplant: the evening of June 29.

André Siméon bade good-bye to his wife and children and came to Necker Hospital. For the thirtieth or fortieth time he walked in through the ancient portal. He was assigned a bed in a room one story higher than Georges's prison cell, and waited for the doctors to remove one of his kidneys.

Georges Siméon's recollections:

"In the afternoon a doctor came—I no longer remember which one, but it wasn't the professor—and told me they were going to operate that evening. He gave me a form to fill out—I had to state that I agreed to all their procedures. And I said I did, though all of a sudden I didn't feel the least bit sure I agreed. But I knew . . . there wasn't any other way out for me. . . . The doctor wanted to say something comforting to me. So he said: 'If it doesn't work, you'll still have your own kidneys. We're not taking them away from you.' I answered that he knew himself what was wrong with my kidneys and that I couldn't keep going long on them. He got the message and didn't say anything more, just went quietlike out of the room."

André Siméon's recollections:

"Around five o'clock in the afternoon the professor came and told me: 'Now's the time.' I said I'd like to go over to see my brother first and have a few words with him, because after all nobody could be sure and all that. . . . I waved to Georges through the window and said the kind of thing we always used to say to each other when we were kids: 'We'll pull it off, don't you worry. You'll go to sleep and when you wake up it will all be over.' Then I returned to my room. After that I had to go up to the top story. There they put me into a cold bath until my body temperature dropped to 85 degrees. There was some delay . . . before they were able to take me down into the operating room. By then my temperature had shot up again, higher than it should have been . . . and one of the doctors asked me—I suppose he thought he was going to relieve my tension that way: 'Well, which kidney do you want us to take?' I tried to answer him in the same tone: 'The best one, of course.' . . . Then they gave me an injection and that was the last I knew."

From Professor Jean Hamburger's report on the operation:

"The surgical procedure took place on June 29, 1959. . . . In one operating room the kidney was removed, and implanted in an adjacent room. . . . The kidney was removed by J. Auvert. The donor's body had been reduced to a temperature of 85 degrees by a cold bath, in order to lower the kidney's oxygen requirement and to increase its resistance during the period in which it would be without blood supply. . . .

"The left kidney was removed. . . . Its implantation was carried out by J. Vaysse, M. Chevrier, and Mademoiselle Lenègre. Blood circulation of the transplanted kidney was interrupted for a total of forty minutes. . . . The ureter was sutured to the right side of the bladder. The operation on the donor lasted two and a half hours, on the recipient four and a half hours."

Armande Siméon's recollections:

"Dr. de Beaufond was present throughout the whole five hours of the operation, in spite of his age. I waited in André's room because I wasn't allowed into Georges's room on account of the sterilization. . . . But in the middle of the night, right after the operation, Dr. de Beaufond came to me and said the operation had gone well . . . and that now we would have to wait to see how the radiation worked and whether Georges had been saved."

Georges Siméon's recollections:

"I think it was two days after the operation before I really woke up. All I know is I was horribly thirsty but wasn't allowed to drink anything. . . . It was awfully hot—awfully hot at the end of June or the beginning of July. . . . I was allowed to rinse out my mouth but had to spit the water out again. The whole thing is a horrible memory that I'll never forget."

Certainly he would never forget that. But he would also never forget that the real hell began the day after the operation.

Hamburger and his associates were prepared for the fierce reaction that the massive dose of radiation would produce in Siméon's organism. Siméon was not prepared.

When the reaction began, he had just been told (and had also felt) that the new kidney was working as if it were his own. In the first twenty-four hours it produced 1,800 cubic centimeters of urine. The urea content of his blood dropped rapidly.

André, who lay in bed waiting for every scrap of news that Armande or one of the nurses could bring him, heard about this and sent a note to Georges: "Well, you ought to be damn proud of my spare kidney that piddles so nice." Armande brought the note to Georges, and for the first time he smiled at her through the window. But that was his last genuine smile for a good while. A few hours later the fever commenced.

His temperature rose precipitately. It reached 102 and shortly afterward 104. Georges's entire body burned. Then he would be racked by shivers. The world melted away around him; he was only dimly conscious of the figures moving about him, taking his blood pressure, doing electrocardiograms, removing blood samples from him, or taking smears. He was scarcely aware that all the while the kidney continued to function regularly. Nor did he learn that so far all the bacteriological studies showed not the slightest trace of an infection. That proved that the sterile "prison" was serving its function well. The fever and chills that racked him were entirely the consequence of the radiation he had undergone in Villejuif.

The effects of the radiation remained within tolerable limits as far as his red blood cell count was concerned—further deterioration was kept in check by transfusions. On the other hand, the white blood cell count dropped to virtually nothing. First the leucocytes vanished, then the granulocytes, then the lymphocytes.

The ability of the blood to coagulate had been disturbed. Within a week red spots from epidermal hemorrhages covered Georges Siméon's body. Meanwhile the fever continued to rage. When Georges at last recognized Armande's face behind the window, he was so weak that he could barely lift his arm or talk to her. Terrified, Armande demanded that the doctors tell her what was the matter with Georges. But the sole comfort they could give her was to explain that the fever was natural and would pass as soon as his bone marrow recovered—and that the kidney was functioning. It was filtering Georges's blood so efficiently that the urea level had dropped to 1 gram.

On July 8 there were signs of slight improvement. The fever dropped, and André, who was not feeling too well himself, left his room for the first time and went to the window of the sterile room. He saw how depleted Georges was—too weak to eat, too weak to talk. Desperately, André tried to rally him. He called through the speaker system: "What's all this fuss about? Do you want us to have gone to all this trouble for nothing? If you don't eat, you won't get back on your feet, and I'll have lost one of my kidneys for nothing."

He succeeded in coaxing a tremulous smile out of Georges.

Georges Siméon's recollections:

"I'd read more about kidney transplants than they knew. . . . I'd read that the sewed-up blood vessels heal well at first, but that between the fifteenth and twentieth day complications set in and that the foreign body is rejected. There was a lot of uncertainty about the whole thing, and all I could do was wait."

On July 13 the brief spell of improvement came to an end. A new wave of fever ensued. Once again the nurses, the doctors, the laboratory assistants came rushing through the corridors with their test tubes. But even on the day that Georges's temperature rose above 104 and he was again shaken by violent chills, there was no sign of any infection. Once again these symptoms were the consequences of the radiation.

The experience accumulated in Villejuif had taught the doctors that several such "waves" of radiation effects were not unusual, and that the attacks of chills and fever would continue until the bone marrow recovered and the lymphatic system resumed its functions. Since the urea level had reached its lowest value so far on July 13—0.32 grams—Hamburger was not excessively disturbed. But he knew only too well that he was working in an area between unknowns and uncertainties. Along with the bouts of fever came attacks of diarrhea which lasted for days. A human being, Georges Siméon, lay in his bed with an operation wound, a catheter into his bladder, burning with fever, dependent for his simplest bodily functions upon the aid of "sterile phantoms." . . . Was he still a human being?

To Armande he undoubtedly was. He was her husband, the father of her children, no matter how humiliatingly he was deprived of control over his own body. But was he in other respects still a human being, or was he merely a laboratory animal, racked by his own illness and the cruelties of medical technology, merely an organism that was being measured, checked, and observed?

On July 14 the radiation crisis suddenly and without warning took a disastrous turn. The doctors were truly alarmed. Abruptly, the quantity of urine diminished. The capacity of the kidney to excrete urine, which had increased to 45 cubic centimeters per minute, dropped to 25 cubic centimeters, then to 9. At the same time the urea level in the blood rose once more. Hamburger had never forgotten that January day when Marius Renard's transplanted kidney had suddenly begun to fail. Was he again to be confronted with the same phenomenon? Had the hopes he had placed in radiation been an illusion? On July 18 the kidney's ability to excrete urine dropped to only 6 cubic centimeters per minute, and at the same time the urea level in the blood reached 1.27 grams per liter. By July 19, Hamburger could only think that the great new experiment had failed and he was facing another defeat, Siméon a painful death.

Siméon himself, burning with fever, his kidney failing, once again was only dimly aware of what was happening to him and around him. He may have vaguely noticed several unfamiliar faces, but he did not know that among them was Dr. John P. Merrill, who had flown from Boston bringing the meager consolation that he had observed a similar crisis in the case of John Riteris. Dr. Merrill conjectured that this was the moment when under ordinary circumstances the transplanted kidney would have been rejected. Presumably a struggle was taking place in the tormented body between forces seeking adjustment to the foreign tissues and forces opposing that adjustment. It would soon be seen whether the effect of the radiation had been strong enough to make adjustment possible.

Armande and André suspected that things had reached a crucial point in Georges's struggle for life, but fortunately they had only vague intimations. They did not know that Hamburger had almost given up hope. When Armande learned that Merrill had come from Boston, and when she actually met the American doctor in the corridor and he shook her hand, she decided that he had flown to Paris especially to save her husband and that now Georges was under the best of care.

July 20 was a day of ferocious Parisian summer heat. The doctors were ready to give up. Suddenly, in the morning, one of the nurses reported that the patient's excretion of urine was increasing again. And that increase continued. On July 21 the fever began to fall, slowly at first, then rapidly. At the same time growing numbers of white blood corpuscles reappeared in the samples of Georges's blood. The count rose from 50 to 100, from 100 to 1,000. The bone marrow was once more coming into play. The paralyzing effects of the radiation were being overcome. Had Merrill's theory been correct? Had the radiation repressed the defense mechanisms long enough for the new kidney to adjust?

From July 23 to 26, the kidney function improved steadily with each passing day. The blood pressure, which at times had reached heights of 190/110, dropped. The last ripples of the waves of fever passed. On August 10 the urea level reached completely normal values.

The operation wound healed without complications. All that remained was general physical weakness. This was the inevitable result of

Georges's subjection to the inferno of radiation. But by the last days of July, Georges was sitting up in bed. When Armande appeared at the window of his "cell," he talked at length with her about the children, their schooling, and finally about a house of their own in Montgeron, which he had been meaning to build for a long time. Such plans had had to be put aside when his health failed.

Georges Siméon's recollections:

"On the twenty-third and twenty-fourth day I began to tell myself for the first time: It's working. I'm going to make it."

By August 10 all his blood values were so normal that the doctors for the first time appeared in his room without their ghostly wrappings. Shortly afterward, Siméon was allowed to leave his sterile cage, in which he had spent nearly fifty days. He was transferred to an ordinary sickroom. There Hamburger observed him for another five days, and Armande and André led him around the ancient corridors for brief walks.

This time Hamburger had so effectively kept the operation secret that no reporters bothered Georges Siméon when, on August 15, he left Necker Hospital and went home—pale and thin, but confident.

André Siméon's recollections:

"Before he went home I went to see Professor Hamburger and asked him: 'What's going to happen now? How long will he be all right?' But the doctor didn't know. He said: 'It may be a year or two, or three, maybe even longer.' . . . So there was nothing for us to do but hope, and we hoped."

Hamburger himself did not dare to be overly optimistic. He had seen too many things go wrong, and was fully aware of how little he knew, to entertain any false hopes. If Georges Siméon survived for a long time, his survival, like that of John Riteris in Boston, would signify that the rejection of transplanted organs could be prevented by the use of radiation. On the other hand, radiation was undoubtedly a frightful, a "heroic" method. But if it did prove effective, would it not mean a turning point in the history of organ transplantation? After several weeks Hamburger requested Georges and André to return to the hospital for a postoperative examination. André was already leading a normal life once more. And Georges, too, was making an amazing recovery. He was obviously developing into the stocky, sturdy man he had been in his healthy days. His new kidney was performing at only 80 per cent of normal kidney function. But all other test values were normal. And he was preparing to return to his job at the post office.

Georges Siméon's recollections (recorded in December 1969 in his new house in Montgeron, on a slope above the valley of the Seine):

"Hamburger told me that someday, when I had recovered further, he would have to remove my useless old kidneys. Maybe next year. . . . Then, a few days before Christmas, my wife had to go through another period of worry. I suddenly had violent abdominal pains and high fever. . . . I myself felt perfectly sure that it had nothing to do with the kidney. I'd often had irritations of the appendix. But Armande called Necker Hospital, and Professor Hamburger said for me to be taken there at once. They thought that now the rejection was beginning."

Georges Siméon did not know, and was never told, that in the meantime (on October 17) John Riteris had been rushed to Peter Bent Brigham Hospital because he was showing all the symptoms of kidney rejection. Merrill and his team of surgeons exposed the new kidney and found their fears confirmed. . . . Consequently, on October 19 and on November 16 and 21, Merrill subjected Riteris to more radiation. Fortunately, the rejection crisis was thus overcome, and Riteris returned home on November 28.

Aware of these developments, Hamburger and his associates were understandably concerned when Armande Siméon reported the sudden deterioration in Georges's condition. To their relief they discovered that there had been no disturbance of the kidney's functioning at all. Georges Siméon was right. He was suffering from an acute phase of his chronic appendicitis.

Georges Siméon's recollections:

"They operated on my appendix, and by New Year's Eve I was back home. André, Juliette, Armande, and the children, we were all together, and after all those years I drank a glass of champagne—to the toast that we would all stay together. . . .

"On January 31, I went to the hospital for the third time and they removed one of my old kidneys, and on February 17 the other one. Both were useless by now. They'd lasted just long enough, until I received André's kidney. . . . And now it's been ten years. . . . And believe me, that kidney works normally and there haven't been any complications in all these years."

Dr. Anatol Coudahei in a letter dated October 1, 1962:

"Let us recall that the triumph in Georges Siméon's case was regarded as a great break-through. It appeared that science was overcoming the rejection mechanism. Today, two years later, we know that we succumbed to a cruel error.

"Let us sum up what happened. After Georges Siméon, Hamburger made five attempts to transplant kidneys after combating the defense mechanisms with whole-body radiation. He tried transplants from mothers to children and from sisters to brothers. The results have been crushing.

"Patient D.M. of December 14, 1959. Donor: the mother. Radiation: 450 roentgen units. Death after 25 hours.

"Patient C.G., thirty-eight, December 31, 1959. Donor: sister. 450 roentgen units. Death after 10 days.

"Patient A.M., twelve years old, May 6, 1960. Donor: a sister. Radiation: 430 roentgen units. Death after 21 days.

"Another patient, Panayotis Yannopoulos, who came to Paris from Greece after reading reports on the Siméon case, and who received his mother's kidney on December 19, 1960, seemed to be the only one who promised some success. Yannopoulos recovered sufficiently to return home to Athens, but there he died.

"The balance sheet for the experiences of John Merrill in Boston with transplants under 'nearly lethal' radiation seems to me equally devastating. From July 16, 1959, to May 1962, he tried the same operation nine more times: between father and son, mother and daughter, brother and sister. All nine patients died; maximum survival was 18 days. Up to the present no one has been able to explain why John Riteris and Georges Siméon survived, thus arousing such deceptive hopes. Perhaps the reason was that they were twins, even if not identical twins, and that the rejection reactions between twins of any kind are somewhat milder; or that their tissues were more compatible for other unknown reasons. In any case, what saved these two seems not to have been the whole-body radiation."

Joseph E. Murray, John P. Merrill, and J. Hartwell Harrison
in Annals of Surgery:

"Of the twelve patients conditioned with total body irradiation, only one has survived."

Francis D. Moore, Surgeon-in-Chief, Peter Bent Brigham Hospital in Boston, May 1962:

"Irradiation given in one or two doses has to do its whole job in one sledge-hammer blow. Each cell is hit hard—how hard, we never know —and recovery is slow or may never occur."

Professor Jean Hamburger in an interview in January 1970:

"Every advance in medicine also involves a certain risk. We try one thing or another, and very often we do not know how it will turn out. . . . Altogether, we irradiated nearly forty cases before operation, including a . . . case on February 2, 1962, in which the first kidney transplant in the world between nontwins succeeded. The young man, who received a kidney from a first cousin, still enjoys the best of health. Soon afterward, however, we abandoned the radiation method because it was harder to carry out and more dangerous in its immediate reactions than other procedures."

Dr. Anatol Coudahei in his letter of October 1, 1962:

"Had we been forced back to the place where we started before the irradiation method was developed? We would have to answer this question affirmatively were it not for certain recent evidence that the idea of knocking out the body's defensive mechanism has some prospects of success. New transplantation experiments with animals undertaken by the Boston team have shown that various chemicals developed since 1951, particularly 6-mercaptopurine and azathioprine (Imuran), distinctly inhibit the rejection mechanism. Although these drugs were originally developed for use against cancer, they seem to possess the ability to inhibit the defenses against alien organs. They prove to be particularly effective when used in conjunction with cortisone.

"Unfortunately, Imuran is extremely toxic. Merrill has since tried it in six transplant operations, and in November 1960 and May 1961 he lost two of his patients from Imuran poisoning, although in both cases the transplanted kidneys functioned until the patients died. Moreover, the combination of Imuran and cortisone—like radiation—weakens resistance to infection. This led to the deaths of other patients.

"After five such tragic deaths, in April of this year Merrill shifted to a triad of drugs, the third being the new drug actinomycin. Possibly he has discovered a new approach to preventing rejection. But this method is extraordinarily difficult, for it involves a balancing act between re-pression of rejection, defense against infection, and poisoning by drugs. . . . Consequently, the tendency at the moment is to turn away from the whole question of transplants and continue to develop the artificial kidney to the point that permanent treatment of patients with chronic kidney diseases may be possible."

7 / Clyde Shields

"Are you getting up to go to work?" Emma Shields asked from bed.

"No, I can't do it," Clyde Shields answered.

His voice was hardly recognizable, though ordinarily it was so vigorous and sonorous that those who knew him would have said it was his most prominent characteristic.

That was on a December morning in 1959. The sky above Seattle was still dark, and a cold morning mist hung over the city. The Shieldses' house, 132 Southwest 119th Street, was about half a mile from the city line, in the southwestern part of the city. Most of the houses in this area were small, with flat roofs, modest yards, and carports. Clyde and Emma Shields had bought their house in 1943, two years after their marriage. In 1953 they had added on to it after a third son, Tom, came along; by then they already had two boys, Eddie and Jimmy. That year, incidentally, marked the time that Clyde Shields's health had gradually begun to go downhill.

"I'll call Dr. Clausing," Emma Shields said as she got up.

"You and the doctor," Clyde Shields said. "How long do the pair of you think you can kid me? I know I'm done for."

"The doctor knows more about that than you do," Emma Shields retorted. She was aware, of course, that Clyde was right, and she had long been girding herself for the day when he would wake up and tell her, "I can't do it." To be precise, they had both girded themselves for that, she and Dr. Vernon Dale Clausing, ever since that day in 1953 when Clausing had discovered albumin in Clyde Shields's urine. After a careful examination he had explained to Emma Shields that her husband had a chronic disease. There was nothing that could be done for him except recommend a salt-free and protein-poor diet and hope that during the years Clyde Shields still had left some cure for the disease would be discovered.

Thereafter, Emma Shields had done everything in her power. But how could you forbid a strong man like Clyde, who was only thirty-nine years old, to eat meat and salt? Nobody looking at him would

168

suspect he was suffering from a disease that was inwardly consuming him, and that this disease would take another four or five years to kill him. By this December morning in 1959, six years had passed, and the moment of truth had arrived.

"I'd better call Johnson's too, and tell them you can't come," Emma Shields said.

Johnson Manufacturing Company was a machine shop where Clyde Shields had a responsible job.

"Tell them I may be back on my feet tomorrow," Clyde said, but he himself did not believe it. For the past week his illness had been getting him down. He felt "like a dog," he said; it was as if someone were pulling the rug from under his feet.

Dr. Clausing found him thoroughly depressed. "Well, Clyde," he said, "I could see something was wrong with you for a good long time. But there was no sense bothering you about it. You would only have had needless worries. But now it really is getting serious. You have a kidney disease, and we have to do something about it."

Clyde Shields in an interview with Henry Marx:

"The doctor did not tell me, he told my wife, and she did not tell anybody. They were the only ones who knew what situation I was in, at least up to 1959. . . . The kind of physician he was, being the kind of family doctor he was, he probably felt inclined to do more than he might have done with some other patient. In fact, he showed how it bothered him that I was going downhill the way I was. He had me hospitalized and told me, and told my wife, he would not let me out until he knew that there was something that could be done for me."

At the time he spoke in such high and mighty terms, Dr. Clausing did not know for certain whether anything could be done for Clyde Shields. All he could fall back on was having blood transfusions and other supportive measures administered to his patient. These produced only a temporary effect. Clyde Shields returned home, but by the end of January his blood pressure had risen to 230/140. He vomited almost everything he ate and had difficulty walking. He lost his job at Johnson's, so that his family had to live on his disability insurance.

In the meantime Dr. Clausing read everything he could find in medical literature about the most recent developments in the treatment of kidney disease. He studied all the reports on kidney transplants and queried the Boston kidney transplant team. It was not encouraging to hear that following the few successes with twins and the Riteris brothers, all the patients had died after X-radiation. Clyde Shields had no twin brother, and a man of Clausing's temperament would not for a moment consider subjecting his patient to the tortures of radiation with such dubious prospects of success.

From the problems of transplantation, Clausing turned to the latest developments in artificial kidneys. All such artificial kidneys were by now far superior to the machine with which Kolff had started in Kampen. Just like Kolff's first machine, however, they were suitable only for short-term treatment of acute kidney failure. They had saved many patients by tiding them over the interval their own kidneys needed in order to recover. But it was still impossible to carry out more than ten or twelve treatments, or to keep a sufferer from chronic kidney disease alive for any significant length of time.

During the first weeks of February, Clyde Shields's condition deteriorated from day to day. Then, in the middle of the month, Clausing received news of a new "experimental program for renal patients" that was being undertaken, oddly enough, not in Boston but in Seattle itself. The program had been initiated by the University of Washington Hospital there.

In the big, yellowish building in the northwestern part of Seattle a Clinical Research Center had been established to give doctors the opportunity to try out new methods in medicine. This center was now engaged on a promising program involving the artificial kidney. According to the reports Clausing read, the secret lay in a specially constructed connection to the blood vessels, made of Teflon; it had been discovered that the human body displayed a high degree of tolerance for this newly developed plastic, so that it could be used for repeated treatments.

The man responsible for the basic idea was a young doctor named Belding H. Scribner. Dr. Clausing at once got in touch with Scribner, who readily explained the apparatus that he and several other doctors and technicians had invented. It consisted of a pair of Teflon cannulae that were to be inserted more or less parallel into a vein and an artery of the patient's forearm. During treatment with the artificial kidney, the cannulae would be connected with the tubes running to and from the machine. When the treatment was over, the tubes were removed, but the cannulae remained in place until the next treatment, their open ends linked with a U-shaped Teflon tube, thus completing the circulation of the blood. This arrangement was called a "shunt." It had been shown that animals could carry the shunt, covered only with a light bandage, on their legs without being hampered in their movements.

Clausing had the feeling that he had found the solution he had been so desperately looking for to save Clyde Shields. Unfortunately, Scribner had not finished his explanations. So far, so good, he said—but the shunt was still in the stage of animal experimentation. He could not yet think of trying it on a human being.

How long would it be before he was willing to risk that? Clausing asked. And he described his patient Clyde Shields, an otherwise strong, healthy man who was slowly dying from kidney failure. Shields was in a hopeless state, he said, and the whole thing was tragic; the man's life expectancy now amounted to a few weeks at most. Clausing begged Scribner at least to take a look at Clyde Shields. He was convinced, he said, that Clyde and his wife would be willing to take any risk, if only it involved a real chance, no matter how small.

Scribner demurred, but at last said he would go so far as to study a written report on Clausing's patient.

Clausing drew up the report at once. To his enormous relief, he was soon asked to send Shields to the Clinical Research Center so that Scribner could examine him personally. The following day Emma Shields helped her husband into their station wagon and drove him to the hospital, on the university campus between Lake Union and Portage Bay. As she led him down the corridors to Scribner's wing, she felt as if she were entering a courthouse where a trial for life was about to take place.

Clyde Shields in an interview with Henry Marx:

"They did not decide immediately. They weren't ready yet, and I believe they were still thinking it over. Dr. Scribner was a frank young man, and the first time he talked with my wife and me, he said I would have to try to hold out for a while, that they were working day and night on the shunt but were still having problems. I went there as an outpatient for about a month. But my condition kept getting worse, and by the beginning of March they apparently made the decision to use the artificial kidney. After they decided, they told my wife they were rushing it because I was running out of time. So they rushed into something for which they normally would have taken a little more time. They also told my wife they didn't know what was going to happen. When you get so sick that you would gladly accept anything to have a chance, you are eager to get on with it and at least try it. I think that was the case with us. I said to my wife: 'Regardless of what, you give those people permission to do anything they want.' I did not want any deterrent in their progress as far as I was concerned."

Dr. Belding H. Scribner in a report:

"On admission to the hospital early in March, he was barely able to walk to the bathroom. His speech was thick and his sensorium clouded. . . . His cannulae and arm plate were inserted on March 9, 1960, and dialysis begun immediately. (We would not dialyze immediately any more because of the danger of hemorrhage. . . .)"

Dr. Scribner was well aware that he was venturing into totally unexplored territory. He was a sports-loving young man whose every free hour was spent sailing or swimming in the waters around Seattle—despite the fact that he had undergone a corneal transplant and owed his sight to a dead man's eyes. He was a person prepared to take risks, but he was also keenly conscious of the problems involved. The mountain of medical books and technical journals surrounding him in his small office even in later years testified to the thoroughness of his research—as the Impressionist paintings on the walls did to his wider interests.

He knew that there was no saying how the plastic would behave in the long run. Scribner could not tell precisely how long the human body would tolerate the cannulae in blood vessels, in spite of the material's compatibility with tissue. Nor did he know how often the shunt would have to be moved to other parts of the body. It had cost him and his team much labor to develop connectors that could be attached to the open ends of the artery and vein cannulae. These had to be so made that both the plastic tubes of the artificial kidney and the U-shaped shunt could be attached securely and quickly. They also had to be firm enough so that between treatments, when the patient's blood was circulating through the shunt, no end would come loose, for that might mean the patient would bleed to death.

There was also the problem of providing the arterial cannula with an "injection system" through which the blood, enriched with heparin, could flow for much longer periods than had hitherto been customary in the use of artificial kidneys. Heparin was essential to prevent coagulation in the plastic tubes of the machine. Even the thinnest of injection needles protruding into the cannula had caused the formation of blood clots before the heparin could take effect. Finally, good results were achieved with finely sharpened silver needles that were not allowed to protrude through the wall of the cannula.

The dialysis solution constituted another problem. Large quantities were needed, so that long treatments could be carried out without having to change the solution too often. Scribner wanted a solution that would suffice for at least twenty-four hours. The solution had to be cooled to discourage the growth of bacteria during such a prolonged treatment. But whether that would be enough to keep the dialysis solution sterile had not yet been proved; perhaps there would still be danger of infections. In any case, blood cooled by contact with the dialysis solution could not be returned to the patient's veins at that temperature. Consequently, the tube carrying the dialyzed blood back from the artificial kidney to the patient's body had to be warmed by passing through a bath of hot water. To add to these complications, another injection system was required in the vein cannula, this time to inject protamine sulfate, which counteracted the effect of the heparin and restored the blood's ability to coagulate.

On the morning of March 9, 1960, Shields's subclavian artery was shut off with a tourniquet and two Teflon cannulae inserted into an artery and a vein of his forearm. These tubes, thin as spaghetti, were stitched firmly into place. By the time the minor operation was done, Shields was scarcely conscious. His vitality was ebbing fast.

The machine with the tubes, the large, chilled dialysis tank, and the warming bath was standing in readiness. The tubes were filled with an antiseptic solution. Before Scribner's team fastened the outflow tube to Shields's arterial cannula and released the clamp on the subclavian artery, five liters of sterile saline solution were run into the opening of the tube. The blood that came pulsing into the tube immediately afterward propelled this solution before it into the artificial kidney. After the solution had emptied out of the end of the return tube, the tube was attached to the vein cannula. This procedure was necessary to prevent air bubbles from entering the blood stream.

Everyone breathed a sigh of relief when this first step went off without a hitch and Shields's blood began pouring steadily through the tubes of the artificial kidney.

Scribner had no idea how long the first treatment would have to last in order to ward off the fatal coma into which Shields would otherwise be slipping. Perhaps a whole day, perhaps two, perhaps more. A tourniquet to compress the subclavian artery lay ready to hand in case one of the plastic tubes slipped off the cannula in spite of all precautions. That did not happen, but another complication soon ensued. Suddenly the unconscious Shields was shaken by violent chills. The reason was quickly discovered. In its short path back into the patient's body, the blood was not being sufficiently warmed by the hot bath. Shields was quickly wrapped in an electric blanket, and the chills ceased. Then another danger arose. Bacteriological tests showed that hundreds of thousands of bacteria per cubic centimeter were developing in the dialysis solution. Their number rose from hour to hour. The solution had to be changed, and all the apparatus that had come in contact with the old solution was disinfected once more.

Anxious hours passed, until it became clear that Shields had suffered no harm. It seemed miraculous.

During the first twenty-four hours of treatment, checks showed that the artificial kidney had removed considerable quantities of urea from the patient's blood, but not yet enough to relieve his desperate condition. Another twenty-four hours passed before Shields showed the first signs of improvement. He awoke. His mind cleared. Finally, after fifty uninterrupted hours, the dramatic change occurred: he spoke clearly. Thereafter, from hour to hour he declared that he was feeling better and better. After seventy consecutive hours he was still very weak, but for the first time said that he was feeling "human" again.

After a total of seventy-six hours, the connection to the machine was removed and the arterial and venous cannulae joined with the shunt. The shunt, on the outside of the arm, was sprayed with hexachlorophene and covered with a light bandage. Shortly afterward, Shields was able to sit up, even to stand up.

Clyde Shields in an interview:

"The marvelous thing about the first dialysis I had was like changing from darkness to daylight. . . . But they told me that it was only the beginning, and we would have to see."

It was indeed only the beginning. Aside from the unusual length of the treatment, what had been done did not differ essentially from previous short-term experiences with the artificial kidney. The real test of the shunt as a long-term device was still to come. For a day, Clyde continued to feel well, but the following night he was awakened by violent headaches. He felt intense pressure on his chest. Alarmed, Scribner found that Shields's blood pressure had again risen to 240/130. At the same time his weight had increased by nearly nine pounds. Within a short time Shields's heart had enormously enlarged, and his lungs were filled with fluid which made it hard for him to breathe. Obviously the dialysis, though successfully removing large quantities of metabolic wastes, had for some unknown reason thrown the saline content of the body completely out of balance. The result was a large accumulation of body fluids that burdened the heart and raised the blood pressure to dangerous heights.

Clyde Shields was hooked up to the artificial kidney for the second time. The crucial question—whether the shunt would function; whether attachment to the machine at the same spot would work twice—was answered immediately. The U-shaped tube was removed without difficulty and the tubes from the machine slipped effortlessly over the cannulae. Once more Shields's blood poured through the dialysis solution.

This time Scribner employed a solution with a lower hydrostatic pressure, so that Shields's blood released large quantities of fluid into the solution. But it was a long time before the blood pressure slowly dropped down to 130/100. Shields was again disconnected from the machine. But he did not feel well; his sight was disturbed, and he felt giddy as soon as he tried to sit up. Had too much body fluid been removed this time? Was the blood pressure now too low? Tests confirmed this conjecture—and foreshadowed the enormous number of problems Scribner would have to overcome before he found the proper equilibrium.

For the third time Shields was connected to the artificial kidney. In the midst of this new crisis it was some consolation to Scribner that the shunt again functioned faithfully. At least Shields did not have to suffer the repeated puncturing of veins and arteries that had been the bane of all patients who had previously undergone dialysis. But this did not mean that the crisis was over. If Shields's fluid and electrolytic equilibrium could not be restored, if he died under treatment with the artificial kidney— what a price to pay for the first successful use of the shunt.

The machine ran. Once again the dialysis solution was changed. Hours passed without any essential change in Shields's condition. Then at last the blood pressure began to show a rise. When it reached 150/80, Shields suddenly declared that he was feeling well again. Shortly afterward, he was taken back to his room. He was now wide awake. The enlargement of his heart reduced within a short time. Only the retinas of his eyes showed fresh hemorrhages from the violent alternations in blood pressure.

Scribner carefully observed his patient for several days. No new crisis ensued. Soon Clyde Shields got out of bed and began walking, stooped and weak, but without aid. He was extremely tired, yet he kept repeating that he felt human again, that it was like returning from darkness to broad daylight.

During the period of observation, Scribner pondered the possibilities that underlay the idea of prolonged treatment with the artificial kidney. What was the point of keeping chronic nephritics alive perhaps for years if "life" meant no more to them than dragging out a helpless existence in a hospital room? The patients must be enabled to live a life worth living, interrupted by semimonthly or perhaps weekly (he simply did not know how frequent) trips to the life-preserving machine in the hospital. Such treatment made sense only if the patients could return to their jobs, or at least could take up some new and fulfilling occupation.

When the seventh day passed without a relapse, Scribner surprised

Clyde Shields by asking whether he did not want to return home to his wife and children.

Shields showed signs of fright. Scribner had saved his life. He felt safe under his care and was afraid of being banished from the doctor's presence. "No, please not. I don't think I ought to go home. . . ."

But after another day had passed without a crisis and without the need of any further treatment, there seemed reason to think that sizable intervals of normal life could be interposed between treatments. When Emma Shields visited, Scribner had a talk with her. This time he asked whether she wanted to take Clyde home.

"Of course," she replied unhesitatingly. Then she, too, seemed struck by a touch of fear, for she asked whether Clyde could really be well so soon. And what would happen if he had a sudden relapse?

He could understand her anxiety, Scribner said. Nevertheless, she must try taking Clyde home. If she were prepared to act as Clyde's nurse, it would be an enormous help both to Clyde himself and to the medical team who were trying a unique experiment. The routine would not be difficult—she would have to spray the shunt daily, put antiseptic salve on the junctures, and apply a fresh bandage—that was all. In addition she would have to know how to make a tourniquet on Clyde's arm, in case the shunt should somehow loosen and a hemorrhage begin. But, Scribner said, he believed that this would never happen; still, if it did, she must be able to give Clyde first aid. Otherwise, she must watch out for the moment when Clyde began to complain about tiredness or nausea. Then she would have to drive him to the hospital for his next treatment. Did she think she could handle that?

Emma Shields promptly said yes. Of course they would all do what they could. The boys would be happy to have Clyde back home, and they would be on hand to help him if she had to take a job and so couldn't be at home all the time. They were living on Clyde's unemployment payments now, and she had no idea how she was going to pay the medical bills. They'd already considered selling the house. But—that wasn't Scribner's concern. They'd do as he said.

Scribner replied that she need not worry about the cost of the treatment. There was the John A. Hartford Foundation, which sponsored research into kidney diseases. The foundation would certainly assume the costs of this case. "Clyde," Scribner said, "is the first person who will be living permanently on the artificial kidney. The experiences we have with Clyde will determine whether thousands of other patients with kidney disease can be kept alive. If you and Clyde co-operate in this experiment, your help is worth more than the most whopping bill a hospital could present to you."

And so Emma Shields learned to deal with the shunt. A few days later she drove her husband home.

Clyde Shields:

"My wife was not only my driver, but also my nurse. She took wonderful care of me. And the kids—well, they all knew what was the matter with me all along. . . . In the beginning there were so many crises that my wife would sometimes drive me to the hospital five times in a day."

On March 20, 1960, Clyde Shields's second life began, as the first of all renal patients who would spend the rest of their lives dependent on the artificial kidney. On the very day that he was sent home, Scribner decided to enlist a second patient in his pioneering program. This was a twenty-two-year-old shoe salesman named Harvey Gentry. On March 23, Scribner's team inserted a shunt into Harvey Gentry's forearm and next day connected the young patient to the "kidney."

Once again there were difficulties. The treatment had to be interrupted after twenty-four hours because too much heparin entered Gentry's blood. The incisions into which the shunt cannulae had been inserted began to bleed, and two blood transfusions were needed before the hemorrhages could be stopped.

Nevertheless, the dialysis treatment helped sufficiently for Harvey Gentry to return home on March 26. Scribner waited until Gentry's family reported that he was once again bothered by nausea and vomiting. Then he was attached to the kidney for the second time. This treatment, too, went off without a hitch. Gentry's condition continued to improve—fortunately for him, for otherwise he would scarcely have had the strength to survive the crisis that came during the next treatment, early in April. During that dialysis, he suddenly went into convulsions. It turned out that through a mechanical error the dialysis solution had been not cooled to the freezing point, but warmed. A tremendous multiplication of bacteria took place—the bacteria count far exceeded that in the case of Clyde Shields. Gentry's blood swarmed with bacteria that again brought him to the brink of the grave.

This shocking incident made Scribner initiate even more stringent precautions. But it was days before Gentry recovered. Still, that was not the last of the crises. On April 7, Gentry underwent his third treatment, and there was no trouble. Once more he was fortunate, for he was strong enough to survive the next relapse, which came on April 9. It showed what potentialities for mischief there were in the shunt.

Gentry was young. After the third treatment, he went out with some friends to gather mussels in the waters around Seattle. He was not particularly careful about the shunt in his arm. He began running a high fever, and soon afterward pus appeared along the sides of the cannulae. Scribner prescribed erythromycin in the hope that this drug would knock out the infection. But on April 15, Gentry had to be hospitalized and treated with more antibiotics. Time was pressing now, for no one knew how long he could manage until his next dialysis. After several tense days Scribner saw no alternative but to remove the shunt. Any day might bring a return of the symptoms of uremia. And soon they came. It now became imperative to hook the patient up to the artificial kidney. In this desperate situation, Scribner tried to insert the cannulae at the same spot once more. But this effort failed, and he had to use Gentry's other arm in order to attach the young man to the life-saving mechanism.

Probably it was only Gentry's youthful strength that helped him through this third crisis. But after several dialyses in the course of the next two weeks, he recovered to such an extent that for the first time he was able to return to his job, although not full time.

During those dramatic April days, Clyde Shields as yet knew nothing about his fellow sufferer. Shields himself was much too taken up struggling through the early stages of a new life that, as he realized during those first weeks at home, would chain him forever to a machine.

Dr. Belding H. Scribner in his report on Clyde Shields and Harvey Gentry:

"C.S., while he is able to live at home and carry on some activity, has not been rehabilitated to the point of being able to return to full-time work. He simply lacks the stamina. . . . During March and April, C.S. felt well most of the time between dialyses and even on the last day before the next dialysis. Toward the end of April, however, one to two days before his weekly dialysis, he began to feel weak and vomited, especially in the early morning. . . . A program of shorter dialysis twice a week will now be instituted to try to improve the situation. . . . C.S. seems to require one or two units of packed cells per week to maintain his hematocrit in the mid-20's. Red cell survival studies before the initial dialysis and after the first dialysis revealed a cell life of about one-half normal, which was not changed by dialysis. . . . As of this writing, C.S. is now in his tenth week, and H.G. in his eighth week, of dialysis therapy. The preliminary experience suggests that the useful life of patients dying of chronic uremia can be prolonged and that the cannulation technique provides access for repeated hemodialysis. In addition, these patients provide an unusual opportunity for investigation of the many problems encountered in patients with chronic renal failure. . . . The research opportunities seem limitless and involve many fields of interest to both the clinician and the basic scientist."

The first chapter in Clyde Shields's life as Exhibit 1 lasted until December 1963. During this period he experienced virtually everything that a guinea pig could possibly undergo. In the effort to determine what lengths of time were most favorable for treatment with the artificial kidney, Shields was subjected to dialyses of widely varying duration. Emma Shields repeatedly drove her husband to the hospital for his treatments. Sometimes he felt well; at other times he was again prone to vomiting, weakness, itching, and trembling. At last Scribner found that two treatments weekly, each lasting from fifteen to seventeen hours, produced the most favorable results. But this did not mean that he could establish a firm rule. The renal metabolism of every human being depends upon so many reciprocal chemical influences that the duration of treatment must vary widely. Harvey Gentry and a third patient named Rolin Heming, whom Scribner accepted for his experimental program during this time, required altogether different periods of treatment.

Clyde Shields's case also showed that it was necessary to keep constant check on salt and fluid intake, in order to avoid blood pressure crises. Clyde had to weigh himself daily to determine what quantity of fluids he could drink. Once he tried to escape his "life in chains" and go for a drive with Emma and the children into the mountains around Seattle. The consequence was so wild a fluctuation in blood pressure that he nearly died.

Shields had to battle a series of psychological crises as well. After the initial relief had subsided, he was hard hit by the realization that he was at the mercy of a machine. This led to profound depressions. Emma found him "hard to get along with." Many patients after him were to have similar reactions. His was the state of mind of the prisoner with a life sentence who realizes more and more inescapably that freedom is something he will never know again.

When Scribner took Clyde Shields to Chicago to present him to a medical convention, the incident proved something of a narrow escape. As yet there were no jet planes from Seattle to Chicago. Prop planes required more than six hours' flying time. Scribner and Shields left Seattle on a Saturday and returned on a Monday, just in time for Shields to be rushed directly from the airport to the artificial kidney. Such experiences intensified his sense of being a prisoner, and it was a long while before he became accustomed to his chains.

Thanks to Emma Shields's care, the shunt itself functioned perfectly from week to week, and subsequently from month to month. But after a while signs of intolerance appeared in the arteries and veins. The shunt had to be moved to the other arm, and later implanted in the legs. Large scars developed at the old shunt sites. Shields's example showed that the shunt could not be left longer than half a year at one spot in the body, and often not as long as that. As the years passed, the search for new places to implant it would necessarily become more difficult.

The years 1960 and 1961 passed, and Clyde Shields was still alive. He could not, however, return to his job. In 1962, though, he felt strong enough to work "a little" around the house. He had a lathe and a 1915 Ford in the shed attached to his garage—he had bought the old car in 1956, meaning someday to turn it into a plaything for his children. Now he began spending many hours in his workshop—between drives to the hospital and the many hours at the artificial kidney. These hours troubled him less and less as the machine was continually improved. During most of the treatment he slept, or played his accordion on and off. But the period of surprises had not yet ended. Slowly, his body began to show unfamiliar symptoms. He suffered severe attacks of gout. He had spells of burning pain in his feet. These were the first symptoms of a nervous disease that could lead to paralysis. Scribner suspected that they were consequences of the prolonged treatment with the artificial kidney. Dialysis might well produce changes in the metabolism of the nerves; no one knew anything about this yet.

When all other measures failed, Scribner began lengthening the time of Shields's dialyses—and to his joy the neuropathic symptoms gradually disappeared. He had not yet discovered that they were, in fact, a side effect of the treatment and later appeared in a large number of his patients.

Meanwhile, however, new symptoms developed. Clyde Shields's joints swelled. Later there were pains in his bones. At times he had to use a cane to walk. High doses of vitamins brought some improvement. But Shields did not recover completely; he continued to be hampered in walking. Scribner was learning that damage to the bone substance appeared to be a side effect of prolonged dialysis; later he was to see the same phenomenon in one out of every five of his patients.

Nevertheless, Clyde Shields lived. In 1963 he was fitted with his fifth or sixth shunt. More and more he became aware of his role as Exhibit 1, and he began to live for that role. Formerly, he had not been much of a reader. Now he read everything in the medical journals about artificial kidneys. He obtained one of the pioneer models, which was no longer in use, and mulled over possible improvements to the machine.

Meanwhile, news of Scribner's method of permanent treatment by dialysis was spreading throughout the United States. Patients began coming to Seattle from everywhere. The artificial kidneys Scribner had at his disposal did not suffice to treat even a small part of these patients. Responding to necessity, Scribner founded a committee of doctors, clergymen, and judges to decide which patients were to have priority. At the hospital Clyde Shields witnessed the press of patients and saw the despair, the disappointment, and the fear of death that overwhelmed the rejected.

In 1963, Shields was one of the first patients to be connected to a new, larger "kidney" that was nicknamed "the monster." It was capable of taking care of fifteen patients simultaneously. The experience of lying beside the machine along with many other patients, telling them about his own experiences and inspiring them with confidence in the treatment, heightened Clyde Shields's sense of his importance.

Clyde Shields:

"The first years were tough. Lots of the equipment looked like a Rube Goldberg machine. . . . Actually I have enjoyed being part of this program, although it has been a disturbing part as far as my health is concerned. The participation in it has been a rewarding thing to me, and I feel I have contributed something to the end result."

In December 1963, Scribner witnessed the fulfillment of a dream he had cherished for a long time. In spite of all the setbacks, Clyde Shields recovered to such an extent that he could consider returning to his work. He found a job as a machinist at the Elliot Bay Plywood factory fairly near his home. The company allowed him to leave early twice a week, on Tuesdays and Fridays. On these days Emma called for him around noon and drove him to the hospital. At one o'clock he was attached to "the monster" and underwent dialysis until five o'clock the following morning. Then Emma took him back to the factory.

This was the beginning of the second chapter in Shields's story, which lasted from December 1963 to March 19, 1969. During this period Shields had to undergo the insertion of twenty more shunts. Scars covered his arms and legs. He also regularly needed transfusions of red blood cells to combat his anemia. Finally it became necessary to treat him on the machine not two or three but four times a week, for nine hours at a stretch. Only then did he feel strong enough to continue his work. His greatest treat was going on picnics with Emma and the children; once they even drove as far as the wooded country along the Spokane River in the eastern part of Washington State.

The file on Clyde Shields in Scribner's department had swollen enormously; it had become the bulkiest case history in the University Hospital. In addition, it proved to be an invaluable medical chronicle, because Shields, reading constantly and learning more and more about the problems, observed himself closely and was able to report every new development to Scribner.

At this time a second center for dialysis was set up in Seattle's Swedish Hospital. The number of patients who could be treated thereby increased, but a great many still had to be turned away. Only the well-to-do could afford to come to Seattle from other states, or even from distant parts of the state of Washington, and settle there for permanent treatment. For those who lived too far away or had only average means, there was no chance for treatment. To Scribner's mind, there were only two possible solutions to this problem. Either numerous kidney treatment centers would have to be set up throughout the country or the artificial kidney must be made so safe and simple that it could be installed in a patient's home and the patient or his family taught to run it.

The second solution involved serious financial problems, for even this simple an artificial kidney would cost up to $7,000. Moreover, there were many medical risks to be considered. Home treatment involved an increased danger of infection, of hemorrhage, or even of death from carelessness in the preparation of the dialysis solution. And human as well as medical problems must be reckoned with. There were not many women like Emma Shields. Many people might be able to nurse their spouses during a short illness. But how many would be prepared to share their lives for years with a sick person and a machine?

Nevertheless, Scribner decided on the second course. Henceforth he gave priority to patients whose relatives pledged to attempt machine treatment in their homes. The hospital facilities could be reserved for patients who had no relatives or no funds.

The day Emma Shields for the first time connected her husband to an artificial kidney at home was March 19, 1969. The next chapter in Clyde Shields's role as Exhibit 1 had begun. Just as Emma had learned to care for the shunt conscientiously, she now learned to handle all the details of working the artificial kidney. Scribner had a machine, a hospital bed, and all the necessary appliances installed in Clyde's basement. Clyde himself fixed up his basement as much as he was able to. He began putting up wood paneling, to brighten the place where he would spend many hours four times a week. Alongside the bed stood a telephone, so that he could call Emma and the children or Scribner for help. He took a new job with the Lawrence Manufacturing Company in Seattle; the plant was only a fifteen-minute ride from his home, and he could work the night shift. That shift began at midnight and ended at seven o'clock in the morning. At 7:15 A.M. he was back home.

On Mondays, Wednesdays, Fridays, and Saturdays, Emma connected him to the machine immediately after he reached home. She had developed great skill in handling the shunt, filling the dialysis tank, and checking Clyde's blood pressure. For each treatment she mixed approximately 150 liters of water with 16 liters of dialysis concentrate, which a truck brought regularly from Denver. Then Emma set the machine in operation. In a short while Clyde fell asleep. About four o'clock in the afternoon, when the treatment was coming to an end, he awoke. He then had eight hours before he went off to his job on the night shift. On days when he did not need treatment, he slept from seven to twelve in the morning, and in the evening from seven to eleven. In the intervals he tinkered with the old Ford, sat in the back yard, watched television, or read. He was now forty-nine years old, and over the years had lost considerable weight. He looked older than he was. His bones still ached. In 1970 he received his fortieth shunt—this time on one of his thighs. But—he was alive.

Rolin Heming also survived. He, however, was never able to work. Harvey Gentry could not make the psychological adjustment involved in living with the artificial kidney. He was too young to live as a prisoner. In 1968 he pleaded so hard to have a kidney transplant that his mother gave him one of her kidneys. But the kidney did not function and he was forced to return to his fetters, to the machine.

Thus Clyde Shields remained, for Scribner, the best and decisive proof that a human being could stay alive on dialysis and in addition could work—if he learned self-discipline and renunciation, and if he had a family prepared to care for him day and night.

Clyde Shields in 1971:

"Looking back at the progress over the years, I would say it was marvelous. . . . Even the grandchildren already know what's the matter with Grandpa, and sometimes I take them down to the basement, show them the machine, and we make jokes about it."

8 / Melbourne Doucette

Pawlow Bronsky, June 1969:

"Henceforth the artificial kidney will present more and more patients with a makeshift life. But what monstrous machines, what an expenditure of technological skills, chemistry, and money is necessary to create a substitute, and moreover still an imperfect one, for an organ that nature has made the size of a small clenched fist! Permanent treatment with the artificial kidney must be counted among the bizarre excesses of man in the stage of technocratic civilization. Civilized man, surrounded by tubes, plastics, glass, and pumps, drowns in a deluge of chemicals, is condemned to slavish dependence on a machine. The question is whether he will not after all—in spite of all the science-fiction propagandists of medicine—one day regard the eternal sleep of death as more tolerable than this kind of artificial existence."

New York Times, May 13, 1970:

"Suicide among chronically ill kidney dialysis patients is 400 times more prevalent than suicide in the general population. . . . The data were based on a study of 3,400 patients who were hooked up to blood filtering machines at 125 dialysis centers across the country. . . . The patients sometimes gorged themselves with food they should not have eaten. . . . The greatest number of deaths, 117, came from not following the regimen required of a patient undergoing hemodialysis. Twenty-two patients withdrew from dialysis, which means certain death."

Dr. Belding H. Scribner to Henry Marx,
March 25, 1970:

"Younger people do better on transplants, because they find it difficult to adjust to dialysis life."

Pawlow Bronsky, September 1970:

"So long as medical science is not able to discover the cause of fatal kidney disease and overcome it, only one humane solution remains to us: to solve at last the problems of kidney transplantation, in other words, the ingrafting of natural organs. And it seems as if Merrill's team in Boston succeeded, from 1961 to 1964, in achieving the first effective suppression of rejection by the use of drugs. We are witnessing the fruits of that work today."

Anna Doucette came from the tiny Italian village of Beffi, fairly close to Aquila in the Abruzzi. Her maiden name was Anna Berardinangelo. Her father had been the village constable in Beffi until he emigrated to the United States in May 1954, taking with him his wife, Giovanna, and his children, Alderio, Anna, Valia, and Bruna. They settled in the vicinity of Boston. Anna was fifteen when she arrived in the New World. Her memories of Beffi included a cluster of houses under a glaring sun, a dusty village street on which the chickens scattered when an occasional automobile passed, and a boyfriend named Giuseppe whom she was sure she loved and to whom she had promised marriage the day before she and her family sailed from Naples.

Anna was different from her mother, Giovanna, who went on being an Italian woman in Boston, as subservient to her husband as any woman of Beffi. Anna was as self-willed as she was pretty; after a few weeks in America she became convinced that all American women must be happy because they seemed to lead such a free life—a life inconceivable to a woman of Beffi. Pretty soon she had picked up some English and found a job as a seamstress in Wakefield, a Boston suburb. Moreover, she was becoming so enthusiastic about the life of American women that her parents decided to send her back to Beffi so that she could keep her promise to Giuseppe, as custom required.

One more time Anna obeyed her father. In the summer of 1955 she sailed back to Naples, accompanied by an aunt. But when she saw Giuseppe waiting on the dock, she realized that her love must have been mistaken, that Giuseppe would never fit into the new world she had discovered, the world she now wanted to belong to. After several appalling weeks in Beffi, during which Giuseppe bombarded Antonio Berardinangelo with vehement letters complaining about his daughter, Anna made use of her return ticket without her father's authorization and went back to Boston without Giuseppe. For weeks afterward her parents refused to speak to her. Possibly they would have been even more obdurate if Alderio, her brother, had not at this time married an American girl named Evelyne Doucette—and thus broken out of "the walls of Beffi."

Soon afterward Anna met Evelyne's brother. Melbourne, or Mel, as his family and friends called him, was eighteen. He was attending Bentley College in Boston, studying accountancy. Anna fell in love with him, and when they decided to marry, had no doubt that she would be a good wife to him. Still, she wanted to be a "free American girl" also. Only years later, when she was already swept up in the drama of Melbourne's life, did it become apparent that he had fallen in love with her precisely because she was not what she was so determined to become: a cliché American girl. She had really changed much less than she knew. What she had brought with her from Beffi still remained—in particular a patient, honest, loving, courageous spirit.

First signs of the nemesis that struck Melbourne and Anna appeared in November 1961, three and a half years after the June day on which they were married in 1958. To Anna, that day had been the symbol of her final liberation. Before her marriage she had been permitted to meet Melbourne only on Sundays. And even then her father had insisted that she be home by nine o'clock at the latest. On their wedding day Melbourne and Anna set out in a four-year-old Chevrolet for a honeymoon trip through Massachusetts and Vermont. Then they moved into an apartment in Wakefield. Mel had a job with the Wakefield Daily Item Company by day and continued his college studies evenings. Anna kept on working so that they would soon be able to realize their dream of a house of their own. On May 2, 1959, Anna gave birth to her first child, David Joseph. A few months later Melbourne finished college and got his first real job, at Schroeder Industries. By 1960 they had saved enough to buy a lot on Spruce Street for $2,500, and in the spring of 1961 they obtained a long-term mortgage and built a small $25,000 house on their land, close to the edge of the woods. A few months later, on August 28, their second son, Dean John, was born. Anna had hoped for a girl, but she was happy about this second boy. She had given up her job and now devoted her full time to caring for Melbourne, the children, and the house.

Melbourne was twenty-three. He was highly capable; in a few years he expected to be able to open an independent accountancy bureau. Anna was twenty-one. A peaceful and serene life lay before her, she thought—worlds removed from the constraints of Beffi, from its grinding poverty and prayers for rain.

Three months later, within the span of a few weeks, her life was totally changed.

Anna Doucette's recollections:

"That morning in November Mel did not feel well. He threw up. That went on for several days. We thought that maybe he was allergic to something in the new house. I called our doctor, and when we went to his office on November 15, Mel's hands were so white that I was scared stiff. The doctor thought it wasn't anything serious. But shortly after Thanksgiving, Mel felt so miserable that I drove him to Melrose Hospital in Wakefield. On account of the vomiting they thought that he might have a stomach ulcer. But they had a kidney specialist from Mass General [Massachusetts General Hospital] there and he asked Mel about his earlier illnesses. Then Mel remembered that at sixteen he'd had a sore throat and his urine had turned red. The color disappeared again, and so he paid no attention to it. But the red color always came back whenever he had a sore throat. After that hint, the specialist found that one of Mel's kidneys was completely gone and the other almost. He didn't tell us right off that it was hopeless. But they kept Mel at the hospital. And somehow I knew. I can't describe what it feels like when you realize that a young man you thought completely healthy is suddenly going to die. I didn't want to believe it—our whole lives lay before us, as they say."

Melbourne Doucette stayed at Melrose Hospital several weeks. Although he received frequent blood transfusions, he changed from a healthy-looking young man to a pallid invalid. Much as Anna fought against the sudden annihilation of her hopes, she realized that Mel could no longer work and would lose his job. Perhaps she became aware for the first time that the country she so admired could be just as merciless as the Abruzzi where employment and survival were concerned. She did not dare to think of what the hospital would cost or how she would pay the bills. And she knew she would have to sell the house if she could not meet the mortgage payments. But her people had a tradition of hard work. She went back to the shop where she used to work. She sat at the sewing machine all day, drove to the hospital to see Melbourne in the evening, and at night took care of the household tasks.

Shortly before Christmas, Melbourne came home. But he was no longer the man who in November had been building kitchen cabinets for the new house. By New Year's Day he was again so weak that Anna had to take him back to the Melrose Hospital emergency room. Once again he came home after a blood transfusion. But on January 9, after Anna had gone to work, he collapsed, and was saved only because an old friend, John Welsh, happened to be visiting and rushed him to the hospital. Anna did not hear about it until she returned home that evening, just in time to answer a telephone call from their family doctor.

Anna Doucette's recollections:

"He told me right out on the telephone: 'He doesn't have long to live.' I didn't know what to say. Right after that, the hospital called and said that Mel was very bad. I said desperately that I'd come at once, but first I had to find somebody to take care of the children. Then they told me in that case to wait, he's asleep now, and we'll call you again if there's any change."

Melbourne's steadily worsening kidney failure had led to an accumulation of fluid in the lungs that threatened to suffocate him. Melrose Hospital had no artificial kidney, and so the doctors at the hospital tried to do what they could with oxygen, heart stimulants, and transfusions. Toward four o'clock in the morning it appeared that Doucette's heart was giving out. Anna left her children asleep and drove through the darkness to the hospital with the feeling that Melbourne was already dead and she would never be able to speak to him again. She felt enormously relieved when she entered the ward and saw he was still alive. He spoke with difficulty, but said: "Calm down. I'm not going to die." It was clear that he did not realize how serious his situation was.

Anna Doucette's recollections:

"I asked the doctor desperately whether there was any chance to keep Mel alive. He shrugged. But I kept thinking how young Mel was, and about the children. I kept after the doctor. Finally he said they might try to transfer Mel to the Peter Bent Brigham Hospital where they had artificial kidneys and could prolong his life for a while. He telephoned them. But the answer was: 'We won't have a bed free for two weeks at the earliest.' "

Anna drove home, woke the children, took them to her sister Bruna, and then rushed to work. For, ghastly as she felt, she could think of only one thing: she must not lose her job. She inquired about Melbourne's health insurance and learned that it would not pay more than a part of the hospital bill. She was advised, however—this was some small consolation—to apply to a foundation for help. She also inquired at Peter Bent Brigham how much the bill would be for a stay of several weeks, and learned that it would amount to thousands of dollars. Anna knew she would never be able to raise such a sum unless she sold the house—and even that would be far from sufficient. She tried to forget money and the future. Her mind was filled with a single thought: Mel must go to Peter Bent Brigham.

Anna Doucette's recollections:

"Mel survived the waiting period and was taken to Peter Bent Brigham on January 21, 1962. . . . They placed him in the section for kidney research on the ground floor, pretty close to the main entrance. Doctor Merrill was in charge there."

Francis D. Moore, Surgeon-in-Chief, Peter Bent Brigham Hospital, in his book Give and Take, 1964:

"Mr. M.D. (PBBH 1–19–87) was 24 years old at the time of his admission to the hospital on January 21, 1962. . . . In the 12 years since the artificial kidney was first used, many procedures had changed. Besides the use of dialysis on the artificial kidney, it was possible to wash the surface of the peritoneal cavity and remove waste products in this way, called 'peritoneal dialysis.' . . . This procedure was much easier and less expensive than the artificial kidney. . . . [But] the danger of infection was ever present. . . . Mr. M.D. was treated initially by peritoneal dialysis. . . . A plastic button was placed in the abdominal wall so that the small tube for peritoneal dialysis could be inserted without pain or inconvenience."

Joseph E. Murray, John P. Merrill, et al., in the New England Journal of Medicine, *June 13, 1963:*

"Six hospitalizations were required during the next month. Dialyses became less effective, and congestive heart failure reappeared. Peritonitis developed, with ileus, vomiting, and abdominal distention."

Anna Doucette's recollections:

"The dialyses became more and more horrible and painful for him. I knew he wouldn't be able to stand them much longer. In February, when they kept him in the hospital again, I went to see Dr. Merrill. I got up all my nerve and asked him: 'Couldn't you do a kidney trans-

2THE KIDNEY PATIENTS

plant on Mel?' To my surprise Dr. Merrill didn't say no right off. Instead he said: 'We might try if a brother or some other relative would donate a kidney.'

"Mel had four brothers, and so I felt some hope. But I would have had to ask them for a kidney myself. Mel couldn't ask them. He still didn't know how bad off he was, and I didn't want to agitate him by telling him I was looking for a kidney for him. I didn't know how I could ask his brothers, Joe, Paul, Thomas, and Norman, so I went to Mel's mother and told her the whole story. She promised she would think the whole thing over. But I sensed that she didn't like the idea. All the same I waited desperately to hear something, but there wasn't another word from her about the matter. My brother, Alderio, offered a kidney, but they couldn't use it any more than they could my own. Then Dr. Merrill saw me in the hospital and asked what I had accomplished, and I told him: 'Forget it.' But he asked then whether Mel would object if he tried a kidney from a dead person. I was surprised, because in all I'd heard about transplants before it was always twins or relatives. But I so much wanted Mel to live that I would have agreed to anything. I made up my mind to tell Mel the whole story, even if it meant his finding out how deathly sick he was."

Anna knew nothing of Merrill's bitter experiences with the application of X rays. Nor did she know of his first experiments with Imuran, or of the deaths that had followed the efforts to prevent rejection by administering large quantities of this highly toxic drug. In the interval he had undertaken animal experiments using a combination of Imuran, steroids, and actinomycin, and he was now waiting to try this combination on a human being, in the hope that it would prevent the rejection of kidneys from nonrelated persons.

Anna Doucette's recollections:

"I asked Mel: 'Do you want to go on with this dialysis torture, or would you consent if Dr. Merrill grafted a foreign kidney into you?' Mel was too weak to be surprised or even to think it over. He whispered: 'I wouldn't care what happens if I didn't have to endure this dialysis any more.' He'd also never heard about kidney transplants between unrelated people. I didn't say anything to him about a kidney from a dead body. He just whispered once more: 'If you think it's possible, okay.' "

So the decision was left to Anna. And when she saw Melbourne lying in his bed, helpless and hopeless, she decided to risk anything.

The burden seemed to lift when Merrill explained his intentions. He would be taking a kidney from some person who had just died. The operation would be part of a research program supported by the Hartford Foundation, the U.S. Public Health Service, the Atomic Energy Commission, and other public bodies. So Anna would not have to worry about the costs.

Anna Doucette's recollections:

"After the first few weeks in Peter Bent Brigham, Mel was treated free. . . . The insurance paid only a part of the $3,500 hospital bill for the first weeks. . . . Otherwise we would have been financially ruined."

Francis D. Moore in Give and Take, *1964:*

"The assumption of clinical success [with a combination of drugs] was based wholly on animal work in the laboratory."

The decision was made. Merrill had his first patient, and since transplantation itself had become a routine operation, it only remained to find a donor. During the last week of March, Dr. Murray, Dr. Couch, or Dr. Wilson slept at the hospital, in order to be right on hand in case a sudden death provided a kidney donor. There were three false alarms before a suitable donor was found on the night of April 5.

Anna Doucette's recollections:

"I was at the hospital after work on April 5. At nine o'clock I went home, so I didn't hear about what happened until later on. . . . They said they tried to telephone me, but I didn't answer. Maybe I really didn't hear the bell."

Joseph E. Murray, John P. Merrill, et al., in the New England Journal of Medicine, *June 13, 1963:*

"On April 5 a kidney from a 30-year-old . . . man who had been maintained at 20° C. before death during an operation became available. . . . The transplant was performed in the usual fashion."

Anna Doucette's recollections:

"Anyhow, I went to the hospital Friday as usual. I went into his room and saw him asleep in his bed. So I tiptoed out to the ward nurse.

She said: 'He was operated on last night.' And then she gave me a sterile gown and a mask for my mouth and eyes—I wasn't supposed to visit Mel without these for the time being."

The fact that Anna found her husband in an ordinary sickroom without sterile precautions was part of Merrill's approach. Through daily checks on Melbourne's defensive reactions to the new kidney and constant surveillance of his entire defensive system, the doctor hoped that he would be able to recognize the first signs of either rejection or infection. By sensitive use of Imuran, steroids, actinomycin, and other antibiotics, he planned to repress the first indications and thus avoid the necessity for the monstrous "sterile apparatus" connected with radiation repression.

All available methods were employed to keep a close watch on the situation. Among these methods were kidney biopsy and bone marrow puncture. In the first, a fine hollow probe was inserted through the skin, subcutaneous tissue, and fatty tissue into the kidney in order to punch out bits of kidney tissue for microscopic examination. In the second, bone marrow was removed, usually from the sternum, in order to determine the condition of the blood-forming system. Both procedures were controversial, involving some risk and causing a great deal of pain. Moreover, there was suspicion that the procedures themselves, if frequently repeated, might lead to kidney and other damage. Merrill also did not know to what extent Imuran or actinomycin damaged and slowly poisoned the very kidney they were supposed to protect against rejection. He began his experiment by giving Doucette 200 milligrams of Imuran per day. This was only one-third of the dose employed in Merrill's ill-fated experiments in 1960 and 1961. Thus began his advance into the unknown. An account of the bare facts would read as follows:

1st–6th day after operation: 200 milligrams of Imuran administered daily with sodium carbonate to prevent damage to the stomach. Alarmingly little functioning of the new kidney: 427 cubic centimeters of urine produced the first day, dropping down to 165 cubic centimeters. Accumulations of fluid throughout the body, including the face. Edema forced resumption of peritoneal dialysis; 4 liters of fluid removed. Continued albumin excretion, high blood pressure.

7th day: First kidney biopsy through operation incision. Evidences of distinct damage to the kidney tubules. Unclear whether this is a consequence of transplantation or beginning of a rejection crisis. 200 milligrams Imuran.

8th day: Again 200 milligrams Imuran. Rise in temperature. Fever of 103 degrees. Pussy discharge. Infection.

9th–13th day: Immediate increase in Imuran dose to 300 milligrams to combat rejection. Increase in kidney excretion to 3,000 cubic centimeters and more. Distinct improvement in spite of high blood pressure and high urea concentration.

20th–25th day: Decrease of white blood corpuscles to 900. Indication of new damage to body's defenses against infection caused by Imuran. Confirmation of this diagnosis by bone marrow puncture. Temporary halt to Imuran dosing.

26th–31st day: Improvement in white blood corpuscle count and immune responses. Consequently resumption of Imuran, dose reduced to 100 milligrams. Third kidney biopsy shows numerous cellular changes. Albumin excretion. Signs of continued efforts to reject transplant.

32nd–42nd day: High fever, intense feeling of illness. Excretion of albumin. Increase in urea level. Fourth kidney biopsy. New evidences of rejection. Increase of Imuran dosage appears justified. 200 gamma (millionth of a gram) intravenous actinomycin for three days. Fever drops.

43rd–48th day: Slow improvement in kidney function. Second bone marrow puncture. Sufficient resistance to infection. Increase in Imuran dosage to 150 milligrams. In addition, 200 gamma actinomycin.

49th–53rd day: Despite continuing high blood pressure and excretion of albumin, erythrocytes, and leucocytes, indications that rejection is being overcome. Decision to remove first of diseased kidneys in hope of lowering blood pressure. Nephrectomy without complications. Fifth biopsy of the new kidney. Renewed suspicion of rejection.

54th–60th day: In addition to Imuran, increased doses of actinomycin, up to 250 gamma. Disappearance of albumin in the urine.

62nd day: In view of persistent high blood pressure, decision to remove diseased right kidney also. Blood pressure drops after operation.

63rd–72nd day: Diminution of excretion; suspicion of a new acute rejection crisis. Increase of actinomycin dosage to highest value so far, 500 gamma. Return to normal kidney excretion with continued high albumin and urea levels.

73rd day: Diminution of white blood corpuscles; evidently renewed weakening of defenses to infection. Therefore reduction of Imuran to 100 milligrams. Improvement in defensive reactions, but reduction of kidney activity and increase of blood pressure. Reserpine and 200 gamma actinomycin. Diminution of albumin excretion and improvement in kidney function.

The seventy-third day was June 17, 1962. After work Anna drove for the 148th time from Wakefield along the Fells Way, from there by way of the McGrath Highway to Memorial Drive, and finally down Massachusetts Avenue to the gates of Peter Bent Brigham. She drove during the rush hour, when the streets were jammed with cars and "Mass Ave" became a nightmare. But she had not missed a single day, despite the snowstorms and icy roads of winter, the heavy fogs of spring, or now, when the first summer heat wave was coming on. Anna knew nothing about Imuran and actinomycin, but she knew when Melbourne suffered, when he thought he was going to die, and when he felt better. She had seen him with his face so swollen with fluids that he could scarcely talk. She had seen him thrashing in bouts of fever, or exhausted by the two new operations, which the doctors had described as proceeding "without complications." She had known that the kidney biopsies were an agony, and that the drugs he received day after day made his intestines rebel.

But after the thirtieth or fortieth day she had slowly begun to think that his course was now upward. Melbourne had begun to sit up and even to walk about a bit—emaciated one day, suddenly weighing a few pounds more next day because the new kidney was not doing well. By early June he seemed sufficiently improved so that she would have liked to take him home to the children. Yet she did not dare express such wishes, for she knew that only the doctors could prolong his life, that they were asking no money, and that they had the right to keep him in the hospital as long as seemed necessary to them.

Anna Doucette's recollections:

"Merrill didn't say much, but all the doctors looked more relaxed. They could have discharged Mel in June. But they kept him there, maybe because they wanted to show him off."

When the seventy-ninth day of Melbourne Doucette's survival began on June 23, he was the first human being to have lived for nearly three months with a kidney from a nonrelative that had been treated for rejection solely by drugs. Merrill continued to be on his guard against premature optimism. How dreadfully he had been deceived, in the end, by the case of Riteris. Yet there was no denying that for seventy-nine days he had successfully fought down the invisible foes for which Melbourne Doucette was a battlefield. He still had no idea whether he would annihilate the enemy or was only temporarily holding it at bay. Nor could he say whether the enemy would not outlast the "battlefield" itself, which was being daily bombarded by poisons.

From the eightieth day on, Merrill allowed Anna to take Melbourne home for several hours a day; the rest of the time he remained under supervision at the hospital. From June 24 to July 3, Anna drove that familiar road four times a day. But she did it gladly; at least Melbourne could be home for a few hours. While she sewed, he sat quietly watching; or else he played with David Joseph and Dean John, who were now three and one years old.

On July 3, Merrill decided to release Melbourne, on condition that he be brought to the hospital for an hour or two every day. Anna took her long overdue vacation. For the first time she visited friends with Melbourne or drove to the seashore. On July 14 they celebrated the hundredth day of his survival.

Anna Doucette's recollections:

"A hundred days—who ever thinks of what a hundred days of life can mean? And they meant a great deal, because the day after he had edema again and we were frightened."

They had good reasons for fear. A sixth kidney biopsy suggested that another rejection crisis was beginning. In addition to the usual Imuran, Merrill several times prescribed 300 gamma of actinomycin. But this time both drugs proved insufficient. On August 11, Merrill stepped up medication with 80 milligrams of the cortisone preparation prednisone. A seventh kidney biopsy showed that this new combination was effective within a few days and had stopped the incipient rejection process. But at the same time the prednisone—for unknown reasons—drove the urea levels to dangerous heights. Merrill began wrestling again with the enigma of his drugs—and Melbourne recovered to such a point that he was able to drive himself to the hospital while Anna was at work.

Anna Doucette's recollections:

"For a while we were happy. When you've felt death so close, you can be modest. I usually finished work at three-thirty in the afternoon, because I did piecework and I was a fast worker. Then we drove to the shore. By the end of September it was already 170 days since the operation. But around this time Mel had a dangerous relapse."

On September 22, Melbourne suddenly developed pulmonary edema. Once more there were indications of rejection. The crisis was combated with Imuran, prednisone, and actinomycin. But the prednisone had such a bad effect on Melbourne's resistance to infection that, on October 4, Anna brought him to the hospital running a high fever. He had developed pneumonia. After many fearful hours, he responded to penicillin. In order to encourage his immunity responses, however, Merrill had to cut back on the Imuran and prednisone. The result was, on November 12, another attempt to reject the kidney. Once more Merrill had to resort to the cortisone and actinomycin.

Merrill's patient seemed to be endlessly rocking on a seesaw. In December the violence of the rejection crisis apparently diminished. On December 4, 1962, after the 242nd day, Merrill thought he might be able to achieve some sort of "armistice" if Melbourne were kept on 100 milligrams of Imuran daily and 25 milligrams of prednisone (in addition to a number of other drugs). Because of constant anemia he also needed regular transfusions of red blood cells. Yet all these measures did not suffice to keep his kidney functioning in a normal manner. Albumin excretion and high urea values continued—but he lived. And at Christmas 1962 he at last returned home. He was pale and had the round "moonface" of all those who are treated for a long period of time with high doses of cortisone.

But he was home.

Anna Doucette's recollections:

"We drove to the hospital several times a week, but now he wanted to work and make himself useful. So he built a wooden partition in the children's room. At Christmas our children had presents again for the first time, and in February 1963 we bought an electric typewriter and Mel dug up a few clients whose bookkeeping he could do at home in our basement. We couldn't fly very high, but occasionally we'd forget for a while that he was really living on borrowed time."

Boston Herald, *March 16, 1963:*

DEAD MAN'S KIDNEY SAVES LIFE

"Doctors at Peter Bent Brigham Hospital identified a Wakefield accountant yesterday as the subject of a kidney surgical procedure which made medical history last April. . . . Melbourne Doucette, Jr., 25, of Spruce Street, the father of two boys, is leading an active, happy, near-normal life a year, less three weeks, after the surgery, which the doctors now classify as successful. . . . The doctors watch him like hawks on the hunt."

Anna Doucette's recollections:

"It really looked as though we'd come through. . . . In the summer of 1963, Mel even helped my brother, Alderio, build his house. He climbed up on the ladder. But then on November 18, Mel suddenly doubled over in pain. We'd got to be so optimistic that we thought it was because he'd eaten hot dogs. . . . He wasn't supposed to eat anything spicy. So we thought that was probably the reason for his attack. But on November 22, the day President Kennedy was assassinated, he had to go back to the hospital."

Francis D. Moore in Give and Take, 1964:

"Then, as if to put the entire procedure to its severest test, Mr. M.D. developed acute appendicitis 18 months after his transplant. The appendix lay right next to the transplanted kidney. It was badly infected and partially perforated. It was removed. The patient's course was stormy for a while. . . . But this was not all. This kidney, the first to show long-term function after transplantation on drugs, displayed a continuous . . . reduction in function. Although Mr. M.D. was home and at work, his condition was not quite perfect."

Anna Doucette's recollections:

"After he came home from the operation, Mel again had to go to the hospital every day. Finally Dr. Edward Hager admitted to me that they were looking for a donor for a second new kidney for him. When Mel heard about that, he knew he was going to die. By then he knew enough about transplants so they couldn't fool him. . . . But still he wanted to live. 'Ma. I need a kidney,' he said to his mother, and this time she answered: 'I'll give you one of mine.' But her kidney wasn't suitable.

"Finally the doctors said they'd look for another kidney from a dead person. Then they found out that in the children's hospital a child was going to be operated on for hydrocephalus—they remove a kidney to help the condition. So they could take the kidney from this child."

Francis D. Moore in Give and Take, 1964:

"On January 22, 1964, 21 months after his transplant, a second kidney was placed in the patient. . . . The kidney was placed in the other side of the pelvis."

Anna Doucette's recollections:

"After everything had gone well for so long, we almost believed that anything was possible and it would be possible to start all over again from the beginning. But when Mel was allowed to get up, he felt pain in his left leg, on the side of the new kidney. He was in a ward, and a patient discovered a bloodstain on Mel's sheet and shouted: 'Jesus, he's bleeding.' The artery in Mel's leg had burst open. It was sewed up. But a few days later the same thing happened. Again Mel was operated on. On the way back to the ward the artery opened up again. Then they tried a kind of plastic shunt. Mel was in terrible pain and was given Demerol. Before long he started looking longingly at the clock, because he was waiting for the Demerol. He'd become addicted."

John A. Welsh, Melbourne's friend:

"After the second transplant, the doctors had left the left side of the pelvis open where the second kidney was. You could see the kidney lying there. The ureter of the new kidney had been too short and they hadn't been able to attach it to the bladder. So the urine ran outside and they couldn't close up the incision."

Anna Doucette's recollections:

"Besides the old drugs, Mel was getting more and more new ones. They brought on an attack of jaundice. Mel's liver and bone marrow stopped functioning. Finally he was transferred to the intensive-care unit on the first floor. In May . . . on Mother's Day, I took the children with me. Ordinarily, I didn't want them to see their father in the condition he was in. . . . They had an exercise room there, with steps for practicing climbing."

John A. Welsh:

"During the time he was practicing climbing steps with that open incision and the kidney, Dr. Wilson once happened to be standing near him. Mel asked Wilson anxiously: 'Doctor, what can I do if the kidney falls out?' Wilson answered jokingly: 'Why, we'll pick it up again, that's all.' At first Mel was shocked, but I comforted him and kidded him till we both laughed."

Anna Doucette's recollections:

"The kidney functioned somewhat. But all his other organs had been ruined by the drugs. Mel . . . could no longer get up. On July 2 I telephoned him from my job and he told me he no longer had any pain. I thought that was a good sign. But at one o'clock they called me and said:

'Anna, he's in a coma.' I never drove so wildly as I did that day. But all I could think of was that I wanted to talk to him once more. When I got to his room, there were so many doctors standing around his bed that I couldn't see him. And when they noticed me and let me go to him, he didn't wake up, and I never talked to him again."

So Melbourne Doucette's life ended on July 2, 1964, about two years and three months after he had received his first kidney and Merrill's experiment had begun.

Anna had to learn, like millions before her, that life goes on. She worked to provide for her children and keep the house. A few years later, in October 1966, she married John A. Welsh, Melbourne's friend, and in time had two more children. Slowly, the memory of those years of tragedy was blunted by the passage of time. Nevertheless, her thoughts kept returning to Mel's painful death, and she began to ask herself whether she had acted rightly when she asked Mel to risk a transplant. "I can only hope it was right," she says. "But I didn't know any other way. I couldn't go on watching the way he was suffering then. He was so weak that he had to crawl up the stairs in our house on all fours. It wasn't a life, there was no human dignity in it."

She did not say whether she had ever asked Dr. Merrill if her action was right. If she had, he would undoubtedly have answered yes. For Doucette's fate had given him many of the answers he was seeking.

Francis D. Moore in Give and Take, 1964:

"Looking back over the development of immunosuppression, it appears that the drugs have provided the most practical and safest means of achieving transplant acceptance. . . . They are toxic and far from perfect. New and better drugs will be developed; the use of multiple drugs is fully justified by both theory and practice."

Michael E. DeBakey in the Journal of the American Medical Association, February 19, 1968:

"Had research in transplantation never moved from the experimental laboratory to the operating room, problems peculiar to human subjects would have to remain unknown and therefore unsolved, and persons living today with transplanted kidneys would surely have died."

9 / Jefferson Davis

From a letter of Philippe Biset to his mother, Paris, April 4, 1963:

"Yesterday, at Foch Hospital, Genevieve and I were able to have another talk with Professor René Küss. He again assured us that the invention of the new drugs provided the best chances for success if Papa is to have a kidney transplant, and that he is continuing to look for a donor kidney for him. He's a very frank and natural person, and knows we have been waiting for almost four months and that Papa's sight is almost gone because of his high blood pressure. But a hundred other people are waiting besides Papa, he said, and in the last month there have been no more than six kidneys available. We asked again whether he couldn't take a kidney from me. But he says it's out of the question because I have kidney stones. We feel nearly desperate. Now Papa could be helped by a kidney transplant but there's no kidney for him."

Joseph E. Murray, John P. Merrill, et al., in the New England Journal of Medicine, *June 13, 1963:*

"The selection of donors has been a changing problem. The legal restrictions make the logistics of obtaining cadaver donors difficult. Although many potential recipients are resident in the hospital at all times, awaiting a traumatic or unexpected hospital death, only a few suitable cadaveric kidneys become available in the course of the calendar year."

Gerald Leach in The Biocrats: Ethics and the New Medicine:

"The annual demand for kidneys in the United Kingdom is between 2,000 and 3,000 . . . in the United States between 8,000 and 12,000. In 1967 there were about 100 kidney transplants in Britain, but the National Health Service plans to increase this figure to 600 in the next few years. The remaining candidates for kidney transplants will die or go on kidney machines."

New Orleans Times-Picayune, *October 11, 1963:*

"Tulane University physicians have made the first recorded transplant of monkey kidneys to a human being. . . . Dr. Keith Reemtsma, spokesman for the Tulane team, said the implanted kidneys have been functioning so far, but he would not speculate about future developments."

In the autumn of 1963, New Orleans' Charity Hospital had been in existence for twenty-four years. In all that time the hospital had not added a single new stick of furniture. Day after day lines of impoverished patients moved past the doorman for whites, the doorman for blacks, and past a guard with a pistol in his holster. Sometimes there were 1,000 or 2,000, sometimes as many as 5,000 in a single day, who waited hour after hour for advice or aid. Sixty thousand or more might be treated in a year. They came on foot, by bicycle, by jalopy, or, if they had no vehicles at all, in cabs or ambulances. Some days and nights, an ambulance roared up with howling siren nearly once a minute, and the attendants unloaded the dying, the suicides, the victims of accidents and poisonings, the sufferers from acute asthma. The patients lay or sat in narrow corridors that served for waiting rooms, the contagious and the noncontagious side by side, and had to prove they were really indigent before they were sent on—whites and blacks separately—to doctors and nurses. The medical staff, few in number, overworked and exhausted, quickly and curtly treated the ambulatory cases and had the severe cases assigned to the wards.

In a single year 48,000 patients passed through the wards, were healed or died. This tremendous horde of sick also constituted a tremendous body of material for medical study—for only a passage separated them from the skyscraper that housed the Tulane School of Medicine. Tulane doctors and students could study every common or uncommon disease by going no farther than the Charity Hospital.

Among the thousands who came to the hospital in October 1963 was a forty-three-year-old black who bore the distinguished name of Jefferson Davis. From the time he was sixteen Jefferson had worked as a banana carrier on the water front, handling the cargoes of bananas that freighters brought into the mouth of the Mississippi from Central America. He came originally from Georgia, had hardly known his parents, both now dead, and had seen little of his brothers and sisters for the past thirty years. Word had reached him that one of his brothers had been killed in a fight sometime after being released from a Chicago jail. He spoke a Louisiana dialect and belonged to that generation of blacks who were faithful churchgoers and regarded their hard life as the will of Providence.

Brought to the hospital by ambulance, Jefferson was in the last stage of glomerulonephritis. Aside from the normal hard lot of a black family in the South, life had treated him pretty roughly. His first wife, Ruby, the mother of his four children, was long since dead, either of a stomach ulcer or cancer of the stomach. His second wife, Dolores, was religious to an extreme. She decorated the walls of their house in the black slum around North Claiborne Avenue with pictures of Jesus and hoped for heavenly release from the earthly vale of tears. Dolores had bravely taken over the care of Jefferson and his four children, Morris, Richard, Alvin, and Julia. Then she herself had taken sick and had had to apply to Charity Hospital. After a serious operation she had returned to their thirty-dollar-a-month house but in the meantime the children had vanished. Jefferson had had to give them into the care of an aunt, who had registered them with the welfare department; now she was unwilling to return them because if she did she would lose the welfare payments. Perhaps that was just as well, for shortly afterward Jefferson had collapsed on the pier under a load of bananas. Since he had been a soldier during the war, he was taken to the Veterans Administration hospital, just across from Charity Hospital. But he had not recovered.

He had no very clear notion of what was wrong with him; all he knew was that it had something to do with the kidneys. The doctors had given him pills and attached him to tubes, through which they pumped water into him—that is, he had been treated by peritoneal dialysis. Then they had sent him home. But his legs were swollen; he could not work, and had to live on welfare and what little Dolores earned as a cleaning woman for the United Parcel Company. For the past year he had been so weak that he had spent most of his time sitting on the porch, breathing the damp air with increasing difficulty.

By June, Jefferson could scarcely move from his bed to the porch. Dolores had taken him back to the veterans' hospital. But nothing could be done for him there, and he had been transferred to Charity Hospital. Possibly, he was told, the doctors from Tulane would know some way to help him. When two attendants carried him into a ward for blacks jam-packed with beds, only a foot or two of floor space between them, Jefferson's face was more gray than black, and the lips under his mustache were blue. Clearly, if he were to be helped, he would have to be helped soon.

Keith Reemtsma in the Journal of the American Medical Association, *March 7, 1964:*

"Our decision to re-explore renal heterotransplantation [transplantation of kidneys between members of different species] was prompted in part by a certain clinical urgency. The patients awaiting transplantation could not be maintained indefinitely on dialysis and we were unable to obtain, in some instances, suitable human kidneys from either cadavers or volunteer donors. . . . Early in this century renal heterotransplantation in man was attempted. . . . In 1905 Princeteau inserted two pieces of rabbit kidney into a nephrotomy incision in a child with anuria. . . . Jaboulay reported, in 1906, transplantation of pig and goat kidneys into humans with no success. Unger, in 1910, used kidneys from nonhuman primates but these grafts did not function in man. . . . The recent development of effective immunosuppressive agents has prompted a resurgence of a clinical effort in transplantation."

Keith Reemtsma was a thirty-seven-year-old surgeon, a Californian by birth, the son of a Presbyterian minister who had worked for many years among the Indians of the Southwest. As a child, Keith lived in various places in Arizona, Oklahoma, and Utah. He attended medical schools in Idaho, Pennsylvania, and New York, and in 1957, full of energy, ambition, and enterprise, came to the Tulane University School of Medicine in New Orleans.

Soon he turned his attention to the new field of kidney transplants. He managed to convince the Public Health Service and the U.S. Navy that it was time to proceed systematically with a program of research in the transplantation of animal kidneys to human beings, using immunosuppressive drugs, and was given research grants from these institutions. He planned to experiment secondarily with kidneys from rhesus monkeys, primarily with kidneys from chimpanzees, as these were the primates most closely related to man.

With the co-operation of Dr. Kenneth Burns of the department of animal biology at Tulane, he obtained a number of research animals. Burns had in his cages no fewer than fifteen chimpanzees, who bore such names as Adam, Vicki, Peanut, Tony, and Sarge—most of them unmanageable animals formerly in zoos or circuses, and sold to the laboratory for from $500 to $1,000. Reemtsma and his associates, Brian McCracken, Prentice E. Smith, Robert L. Hewitt, Charles Pearce, the microbiologist Charles W. DeWitt, and several others, had initially undertaken organ transplants between various species of animals—monkeys, dogs, and cats. But in spite of the experience they had gained, they fully realized that they would never find out how animal organs behaved in human beings without operating on human beings. They had begun developing a surgical method for the transplantation of monkey or ape kidneys to men. Since it could be foreseen that a single kidney from even a ninety-pound chimp (let alone from a much smaller rhesus monkey) would scarcely suffice to assume the work required of a human kidney, they had set up a program involving the implantation of both of the monkey's or ape's kidneys into the human pelvis.

When bulletins from Boston continued to report favorable results with transplants under the influence of Imuran, Reemtsma speeded up his own program. Nevertheless, another surgeon, Claude Hitchcock in Minneapolis, nearly forestalled him. Hitchcock had implanted a human kidney into a patient, and when this kidney failed after only three days, on February 16, 1963, he made a desperate attempt with a baboon kidney. The experiment failed; the patient died a few days later. But Reemtsma was not going to let this failure discourage him; he continued his preparations for an initial experiment with a human being.

He had, however, no illusions concerning the difficulties of finding patients who would be prepared to accept implantation of a primate kidney. It was October, in fact, before he found a willing patient, a thirty-two-year-old black woman named Mildred Heard. She had had seven children, and her seventh confinement had left her with an inflammation of the kidney which had gone unattended. In March 1963 she was taken to Charity Hospital, already unconscious. Twice she was sent home, somewhat improved. But in August she was back in the hospital for the third time, dropsical, her heart failing under the burden, near death. In vain she had been treated with peritoneal dialysis. Because there was no human kidney available for transplant, Mildred Heard was finally told that the only chance of help for her would be the transplantation of several monkey kidneys. Since the doctors had to count on the possibility that they might be accused—"in the North"—of misusing a black as a guinea pig, they went through every nicety prescribed by medical ethics, prudence, and the law. They warned Mildred Heard that she would be "the first" and that they as doctors could not predict how the operation would turn out. But no one could tell how much Mildred Heard understood of these explanations. In any case, she gave her consent. Reemtsma and his colleagues began treating her with Imuran, and on October 8 implanted in her both kidneys from a rhesus monkey. To their satisfaction, the kidneys began functioning after ten minutes. All went well for five days. But on the seventh day the kidneys abruptly stopped functioning, and on October 16, Mildred Heard's condition forced the doctors to resort to peritoneal dialysis again.

On the same afternoon that Jefferson Davis received his first peritoneal dialysis at Charity Hospital, Reemtsma reluctantly decided that the monkey kidneys must be removed from Mildred's body. This operation was performed on October 18; both kidneys showed extensive cell degeneration. Mildred Heard suffered severe internal hemorrhages—and on the night of October 20 she took her last breath through a tracheal incision.

Reemtsma and McCracken had already studied Jefferson Davis's case history and had selected him as the next possible candidate. A few days later they went to his bedside to give him the same careful explanations they had given Mildred Heard, and to ask him the same questions.

Keith Reemtsma in the Journal of the American Medical Association, *March 7, 1964:*

"The use of a transplant from a nonhuman primate was discussed with the patient and he consented to this procedure."

Dr. Brian McCracken to Jerry LeBlanc, *1970:*

"He knew all along and he accepted it from the first."

Transcript of a conversation among Jefferson Davis, Keith Reemtsma, and Brian McCracken, from a tape recording:

QUESTION BY DOCTORS: Didn't you agree to the operation after having all the details explained to you?

JEFFERSON DAVIS (*slowly, with frequent pauses*): You told me that's one chance out of a thousand. I said I didn't have no choice. I said I couldn't live with my own [kidneys]. I'm very sick and I'm tired of suffering. That's why I got no choice. That's why my mind is made up, going on through. After all, I knew that woman had hers done—well, I got scared there. Well, the doctors told me no two patients alike. Well . . .

QUESTION: You remember talking about the operation before we did it?

DAVIS: Yes, I does. You told me it gonna be animal kidneys. Well, I ain't had no choice.

Dolores Davis to Jerry LeBlanc, *1970:*

"I didn't know myself anything about those monkey kidneys, I tell you. They never told me about that and I never signed no consent to do that. I don't know if he did, but if he did he never told me. They said, the doctors, that they'd do a transplant, but they never said it'd be a monkey, a chimp, you know. I didn't know that until they did it. When it came out in the papers . . . that's the first I knew about it. I didn't know what to say, but he said, he told me: 'I didn't have no choice.' But he made medical history, the doctors told me that much."

. . .

On the ninth floor of the Tulane medical school building, on November 5, 1963, the ninety-pound chimpanzee Adam, whose blood group corresponded most closely to that of Jefferson Davis, was anesthetized and his body temperature cooled to 30 degrees centrigrade. Surgeons Prentice E. Smith and Robert L. Hewitt removed both his kidneys, and while Adam died the surgeons carried the kidneys into a small operating room paved with aquamarine tile in Charity Hospital. Here Reemtsma and McCracken had prepared Jefferson Davis for the implantation. The operation proceeded in an atmosphere of calm, for the case of Mildred Heard had taught Reemtsma and his colleagues that the transplant itself involved no great problems and that nonhuman primate kidneys would actually function in their new environment. The great questions concerned the period after the operation.

It took only thirty-nine minutes for Adam's kidneys to be attached to Davis's blood circulation. Barely ten minutes later the kidneys began functioning more vigorously than had the kidneys from the rhesus monkey. Within the first twenty-four hours they excreted no less than 7,300 cubic centimeters of urine. During those first days Davis—who to his astonishment and confusion awoke to find himself in a private room—recovered amazingly. On the fourth day, however, his temperature suddenly rose to 103, and at the same time the quantity of excreted urine dropped drastically. Reemtsma, fearing a first rejection crisis, increased the amount of Imuran and actinomycin Davis was receiving. In order to be sure he was doing everything possible, he also had the implanted kidneys irradiated three times with high X-ray dosage. To his relief, Davis responded to this treatment within a few days. The fever dropped. The kidneys resumed their full activity.

Reemtsma regarded this as confirmation that the Boston immunosuppressive treatment would, as he had hoped, also be effective against the rejection of animal organs. Within a short time Davis was able to sit up, and soon to stand up, walk, eat, and sit in a chair to watch television—as an experimental subject who daily grew more interesting and more important, he had been given his own television set.

From the transcript of the tape-recorded conversation between Jefferson Davis and his doctors:

QUESTION: How do you feel now?
DAVIS: I feel just like a person never been sick a day in their life. . . . I can eat things I never ate before since I got sick. . . . My strength started coming back in three days after the operation. . . . I'm not short of breath, no. Before the operation I couldn't walk from here to this door-

knob. . . . The dinner I really enjoy was the other day, they gave me pot roast and sweet potatoes.

QUESTION: Do you have any pain? . . . You didn't find the operation too tiring?

DAVIS: No, I didn't. . . . My only pain is some from urinating. I know that going to pass. I get a little, blood clots, blood clots come. Well, I expect that 'cause monkeys they eat sand and things like that, 'cause I seen sand the other day.

QUESTION: Do you have any regrets?

DAVIS: I don't have no regrets about the monkeys.

Jefferson Davis continued to improve. He felt comfortable in his room and several times exclaimed: "God bless the monkeys." His only wish was to have Dolores with him. Reemtsma therefore arranged for Dolores Davis to be provided with a bed in Davis's room. When she finished her work at the United Parcel Company in the evenings, she came directly to Charity Hospital, a small woman with close-cropped curly hair and gold-capped teeth that flashed when she smiled.

Dolores Davis to Jerry LeBlanc, 1970:

"When Jefferson was in the hospital I was there with him all the time. I stayed there, and they even fed me at the hospital. They figured, I think, that he did better when I was there. . . . The hospital was separated then, the blacks in one place and the whites in another. They never came together. But they was good to me. They let me give him his orange juice in the morning—it had to be unsweetened—because they figured he took it better from me, the things I give him. The kids, they didn't know much 'cept that he was sick. They didn't come around much, 'cause kids always something to do their own. . . . I stayed there every night, and he'd say to me: 'Aren't you tired? Why don't you go home?' But I'd stay. I'd say: 'Never mind, I'm staying.' "

Davis survived the second, the third, the fourth week as well. During that fourth week, however, he began running a high fever for the second time. Reemtsma suspected that this was a sign of a second rejection crisis. But with the aid of actinomycin and X rays it, too, was quelled. When the fifth week began, Reemtsma's faith in the success of the experiment began growing from day to day. The chimpanzee kidneys seemed to be functioning so remarkably well that the urea content in Davis's blood dropped to completely normal levels. On December 12 the sixth week of his survival began. On December 15 he felt so well that he began talking about spending Christmas at home. A day later Reemtsma decided to announce the happy outcome of the operation. Reporters from the newspapers, the news agencies, and television were invited to a press conference set for December 17. Reemtsma was prepared to introduce his patient and at the same time—as the climax of the conference and proof of success—to give Davis permission to go home on December 18, so that he could spend Christmas there.

Jefferson Davis was alarmed when he was told that he was going to be introduced to reporters and photographed. His impulse was to lock the door of the room and barricade himself behind his television set. But he was persuaded by the promise that he would be allowed to go home next day, and that Reemtsma would sit beside him at the press conference. Dolores brought him his only blue suit, and on December 17 he was shown into a room filled not only with waiting reporters and photographers, but also with doctors he had never seen before. He realized that he was something of a celebrity. And in fact, even though Reemtsma explained to the reporters that the operation was an experiment whose future developments could not be predicted, the case of Jefferson Davis promptly became a medical sensation.

New Orleans Times-Picayune, *December 18, 1963:*

CHIMPANZEE DONOR: PATIENT OUT OF HOSPITAL

MEDICAL HISTORY WAS MADE IN NEW ORLEANS TUESDAY

"For the first time on record a human being was well enough to leave the hospital after his own failing kidneys were replaced by chimpanzee kidneys.

"The 43-year-old Negro patient, whose name is Jefferson Davis, could hardly believe his own good luck. To be snatched from almost certain death—

"'Doctors told me I couldn't live unless I had this operation,' said Davis. . . . 'Now I feel fine—practically good as new.'"

National Observer, *December 23, 1963:*

ORLEANS MAN SURVIVES WITH CHIMP KIDNEYS

"Mr. Davis is the only living survivor of what may someday become a routine medical procedure—the use of animal organs as spare parts for ailing humans.

"Tulane University Medical School doctors held back the news about Mr. Davis until he was well enough to leave the hospital for Christmas at home with his wife and four children. Before leaving Mr. Davis faced reporters and declared: 'I will outlive you all.'

". . . 'The most significant finding in the present case,' Dr. Reemtsma said, 'is in the demonstration that rejection can be reversed in heterotransplants.' Heterotransplant is the transplant of tissues and organs from one species to another."

The day after the conference was a Wednesday. Clouds hung above New Orleans, darkening Jefferson Davis's room when the nurse brought him a morning newspaper. He studied his own picture and read about what an important man he was. He also read what he was supposed to have said, including things he did not recall having put that way. But maybe he was wrong; everything had been so confusing.

Outside, a sleety rain was falling; the air was damp and cold. Still, no one advised against his going home as planned. A nurse drove him in her own car down the long, dreary, slippery stretch of Claiborne Avenue. On the sidewalks outside the houses, where the newsboys had tossed them, lay more newspapers with his picture, soaking up the damp. When the car stopped in front of his own small house with its sagging veranda and peeling green paint, the neighbors stuck their heads out of windows or pressed their noses against the windowpanes, for they had seen Jefferson on their TV screens.

The nurse accompanied Jefferson into the house. She explained to Dolores that she must give him only soup and fruit juices for the present, and his medicine from three different bottles three times a day. If Jefferson did not feel well, she must telephone the hospital at once. Then the nurse vanished into the bleakness.

Dolores Davis's recollections:

"I wondered why they'd let someone as sick as him out of the hospital when it was so cold, but he said he wanted to be home for Christmas, so they let him. . . . He just walked out, like anybody. No wheel chair, no nothing. And he had these monkey kidneys in him right then. Well, the kids weren't home right then. . . . I made him green pea soup, which was his favorite, and he liked that. . . . A lot of our friends and people came by the house, just to look at him, because he was on television and in the newspapers, and I guess they thought they'd see something different, maybe he'd start to become a monkey or act like one, but they could all see he was just like anybody else, no different you could see."

There was, in fact, a difference between Jefferson and the visitors; he seemed very gray-faced again and suddenly began to feel much weaker than he had been at the hospital. He had never been one to talk much anyhow, and now he sat silently in the tiny living room watching television. Dolores had only a small Christmas tree, because money was short and she was three months behind on the rent. But the members of the Baptist Church had brought the family a carton of Christmas gifts. And Jefferson was glad to be back home. The first day, he thought that he might be able to stay home for good. He kept looking out at the veranda and saying: "When they let me go, all I'm going to do is sit out there and wait for the mailman." He knew he'd never have the strength to go back to work and thought the mailman would be bringing him his veteran's pension.

They went to bed early because it was cold in the house. Jefferson slept at the head of the bed while Dolores lay at the other end, so that she could get up quickly if necessary to bring him water or medicine. Next morning he felt still weaker, although Dolores made sure he was taking his capsules and pills on time. He had great difficulty getting up, and suddenly said: "If I don't come home again, I hope you can buy your own house. Then you wouldn't have rent to pay. All these years we've been paying and we don't get no thanks for it, they throw you out in the street if you can't pay for a while." He talked about his union life insurance; if he died Dolores would receive a fortune—$6,000—which would surely be enough for a house. His train of thought worried Dolores; he must be feeling a lot worse than the day before.

Dolores Davis to Jerry LeBlanc, 1970:

"He'd walk around slow, like any sick person you'd see. . . . That last day he said he was feeling weak. . . . He barely had strength to walk into the kitchen, which was just the next room. He sat at the kitchen table and he told me he didn't feel very good. I asked him could I get him something to eat, but he says: 'What you got?' and I say: 'I got some of that green pea soup you like,' and he say: 'But I done had that yesterday!' . . . I says: 'Would you like to lay down?' So he lays down. . . . But after a while he said: 'I want to go back to the hospital,' so I call them and they came for him. In an ambulance."

Jefferson Davis's Christmas at home had lasted only two days. When, on December 20, he was carried through the corridors of Charity Hospital back to his room, he was running a high fever. Reemtsma assumed at first that this was a third rejection crisis. But that was not the case. In the two days at home a horde of pneumococci and other bacteria had invaded his drug-weakened bronchia and lungs. Although Reemtsma immediately reduced the dosage of Imuran and cortisone, a case of pneumonia developed that would not respond to antibiotics. For sixteen days Jefferson

Davis, suffering greatly, hovered in a no man's land between life and death. Now and then he returned to consciousness; then he would talk about the banana carriers' union, the insurance, and Dolores buying a house. During the last thirty-six hours he fell into a state of shock. On January 6, 1964, he died.

Dolores Davis to Jerry LeBlanc:

"On Monday they told me he'd died. And they said again that he'd made medical history. But he was dead, and, well, there was a check in the mail first of January, but he died and there was no more checks. They don't make mistakes about that. . . . And the house, nothing came of that. He got $6,000 insurance, and it went $1,000 to each of the children and $2,000 to me, and maybe that sounds like a lot, but I can show you the bills and Louisiana Undertaking Company got most of it, more than half, 'cause I'm the widow and I gotta pay for his burial, but the kids don't. . . . The funeral cost more than a thousand. . . . He had his picture in the paper and people wanted to see him. They said he made history. . . . He lay in the funeral home and you never seen so many curious people. They had to get in line to see the body. I was standing up there at the head of the casket and people would come up to me and say they was sad, and I cried. . . . And Reverend Zach Banks, he got up in the pulpit and said Jefferson Davis was a nice man, and he attended his church, and he said: 'He was a good man,' and everybody said: 'Yeah,' and they repeat this: 'He was a *good* man, yeah, he was a good *man*,' and everybody sang 'Amazing Grace.' . . . They were sad, and I was the saddest because a good man, when you lose a good man, well, they said, a good man is hard to find."

Weeks after the earth of Rest Haven Cemetery in New Orleans had closed above Jefferson Davis, his name continued to appear in newspapers and magazines all over the world—the name of the first human being who had lived for a while with chimpanzee kidneys. Reports stemming from the press conference of December 17 spread rapidly because they sounded the note of victory, of triumph over death. The news of Jefferson Davis's death made its way slowly, never reaching many newspapers. Months later some periodicals were still expressing the hope, based on Davis's supposed survival, that his case would usher in a new era in which unlimited numbers of transplant kidneys for nephritic patients would be raised on chimpanzee farms.

But even if the true story had been broadcast, the hopes that had been aroused would not have subsided quickly. Reemtsma himself refused to be discouraged. Studying the autopsy report on Jefferson Davis, he noted that the cells of the transplanted kidneys had shown no "infiltrates" and his blood vessels had been "unchanged." The report did mention "degeneration of the kidney tubuli," but attributed that to the prolonged state of shock Davis had undergone before his death. Reemtsma and McCracken decided that Jefferson Davis's death was a result of his having returned home too soon, under unfavorable conditions, so that his death in itself did not provide an argument against the feasibility of kidney transplantation between chimpanzees and human beings.

A week after Davis's death, on January 13, 1964, they undertook their next operation, on Edith Parker, a black schoolteacher of twenty-three. And up to February 4 they made three more transplants of chimpanzee kidneys to patients in Charity Hospital. Their hopes suffered a severe blow when the last three patients in succession died of infections. The doctors now concentrated their efforts on Edith Parker. She recovered swiftly, although she passed through several rejection crises and constantly ran high fevers for which they could find no explanation.

In her case Reemtsma did not commit the error he thought he had made with Jefferson Davis of letting him return home during those cold December days. He kept Edith Parker in the hospital two, three, and finally four months. Day after day her condition was checked and her drug dosages adjusted.

In the summer of 1964 more and more doctors came to New Orleans from all over the country to see for themselves what Reemtsma had accomplished with this young black girl. They came even from Europe—among them Paride Stefanini, director of the Second Surgical University Clinic in Rome. He arrived in New Orleans at the beginning of the eighth month after Edith Parker's operation. She was now working as a teacher at Charity Hospital's nursing school. Like other visitors, Stefanini had the impression that Edith Parker was doing "brilliantly"; he regarded her as a persuasive example of medical progress. Stefanini returned to Rome determined to follow Reemtsma's example.

But a few weeks later, on October 14, 1964, Edith Parker died—despite all the supervision, all the checkups, the careful watch for the slightest signs of rejection reaction or infection. This time the explanation could not be failure to fend off infections. There was only the terrible question of whether there were not, after all, rejection reactions between man and ape that had not been controlled by the painfully developed procedures for fighting rejection in transplants between human beings. The shock of Edith Parker's death, after all the hopes that had been placed in her, was so great that Keith Reemtsma gave up the idea of continuing such experiments on human beings.

Nevertheless, he remained convinced of the necessity of animal transplants; he was not yet prepared to abandon entirely the underlying concept. He returned, however, to working with animals alone, and continuing his laboratory tests. It must have struck him as a sad, painful echo of his own experiences when he learned, in June 1966, that Paride Stefanini, his enthusiastic visitor from Rome, had implanted a chimpanzee kidney in a seventeen-year-old shepherd from Orune, Sardinia, and that the boy had died within a few weeks—just as had Mildred Heard, Jefferson Davis, Edith Parker, and the others.

Francis D. Moore in Give and Take, *1964:*

"Despite ultimate failure, the study of heterotransplantation will never be the same again. Prior to this study . . . most students in this field would have predicted that the chimpanzee kidneys never would have functioned and would have been rejected immediately and permanently. . . . A seemingly impractical and visionary operation . . . had opened up an old field for renewed study in this matter of obtaining healthy tissues."

Keith Reemtsma (at this time chairman of the department of surgery at the University of Utah):

"All efforts to date in transplanting animal hearts or kidneys to man have failed, but more recent laboratory experience indicates we are further ahead toward breaking the cross-species barrier than we thought possible. It won't happen next week or next month, but in the long run I foresee the use of nonhuman organs to supply the demand."

Transplanted Lungs and Hearts

1 / John Richard Russell
Boyd Rush

From a Rivista Scientifica *interview, June 1968;*
questions by Robert Hall, answers by Dr. Seibert:

QUESTION: From medical literature it appears that the first human being whose own failing heart was replaced by another heart was not Louis Washkansky in Cape Town, but an unnamed patient at the University of Mississippi Medical Center Hospital in Jackson. It seems the transplant was carried out by James D. Hardy, chief of the surgical department of the Medical Center, on January 23, 1964.

ANSWER: Correct. Today there is no longer any reason to withhold the name of this first patient. In connection with preparations for a scientific publication, Hardy recently asked the patient's relatives for permission to release his identity. This permission was granted. The first heart transplant patient was a man named Boyd Rush of Hattiesburg, Mississippi. He was brought to Jackson, unconscious, on January 22, 1964.

QUESTION: Are you in a position to tell us about Boyd Rush and this little-known operation?

ANSWER: Certainly. However, you must permit me to go a bit far afield, for the background of this first attempt at a heart transplant goes back many years. During those years all the technical problems as well as all the moral doubts involved in heart transplantation were thoroughly examined for the first time. Above all, the fate of another little-known patient played an important part in the story. His name was John Richard Russell. Hardy operated on him in Jackson on June 11, 1963, six months before the operation on Boyd Rush. He was the first person to receive a transplanted lung, and this lung transplant was the experience that encouraged Hardy as he moved on toward risking the first heart transplant.

The ambulance that drove up to the University of Mississippi Medical Center in the northern part of Jackson on April 15, 1963, came from Parchman, Mississippi's principal prison. It brought to the hospital John

Richard Russell—fifty-eight years old and a "lifer." For the past six years he had been an inmate at the institution, which includes eighteen different prison camps in the northern part of the Mississippi delta. There between 2,000 and 2,500 prisoners work in the sultry heat on endless stretches of cotton and soybean fields.

Parchman was not noted for being an especially humane institution. Each of its camps held from 100 to 150 convicts. There were no cells and no bars, but each camp was surrounded by fences and towers with heavily armed guards, and the Mississippi delta in this region was so flat and empty that it would be hard for anyone to escape undetected.

The prison files had John Richard Russell down as a murderer. On September 9, 1957, a court in Kosciusko, a small, dreary cotton town northeast of Jackson, had found him guilty of the murder of fourteen-year-old Clarence Woodston. But people in Kosciusko had other ideas about the verdict, which was based largely on Russell's confession. Even Johnny Poole, the sheriff who arrested Russell, had been surprised by the harshness of the verdict and sentence. He felt sure that Russell, in a fit of jealousy, had fired wildly around him and had hit the boy by an unlucky accident.

Russell in general was an unlucky fellow. At the death of his father, a Mississippi poor white, his mother had moved the family to Kosciusko. There John began working, though he was only ten, to help provide for them all. He never finished school. At sixteen he married; his wife, Louise, bore him two daughters, Fay and Mary Ellis, and a son, James. They lived in an old frame house on Elm Street. At the time of the crime he was a short but brawny man with dark hair, a big nose, prominent cheekbones, and a firm chin. People said that he looked like Broderick Crawford, the movie and television actor who specialized in tough-guy roles. He had always been a hard worker, who allowed himself a Saturday-night bender in the Kosciusko bars, like most of the men in the neighborhood. Sheriff Poole said many of these men carried guns, called "Saturday-night specials" because they were used in shootings mostly on that one night, after heavy drinking.

Russell had allegedly been pursuing his brother Grady's wife. One day he approached her at her home on the edge of town, where several boisterous card players had gathered, and Russell began firing his pistol wildly. While the card players fled, the boy was struck by one of the bullets—no one even knew how the boy happened to be present. In any case, the boy lay on the porch with a bullet through his heart. Sobered up by what had happened, Russell handed the sheriff his gun and confessed.

Now, as he was carried into the hospital six years later, he was no longer the Broderick Crawford type he had once been. He was a wreck spewed out by the infirmary at Parchman because the prison doctor did not know what to do with him and the University of Mississippi Medical Center was responsible for severely ill or dying inmates. Since the previous December, Russell had suffered six or seven attacks of pneumonia. The antibiotics given him in Parchman had proved ineffective. Moreover, his legs had been swollen and dropsical for a long time and he was excreting albumin. Before he was loaded aboard the ambulance for Jackson, he had been placed in a special camp where invalids were put to making brooms or tending bees. But this light work had scarcely helped. At the slightest movement he became acutely short of breath. He coughed until his face and fingers turned blue, and brought up bloody mucus from his lungs.

The armed guards who accompanied him to Jackson were aware of the symbolic nature of their assignment; they drove back with the conviction that John Richard Russell was finished. The torrid soybean fields of Parchman had done him in—the guards were certain they would never see him again.

Russell was brought to a medical center that was not yet one of the show places of medical progress. As Russell was carried through the spartan hospital corridors into a room reserved for sick white prisoners, black and white freedom marchers from the North, with some southern blacks, were moving down the roads of Mississippi. Less than a year had passed since James Meredith registered at the University of Mississippi as the first black student in its history. In this troubled world, halfway between the past and the future, it was difficult to practice science. Race questions distorted every aspect of Mississippi medicine. Perhaps nobody knew that better than James D. Hardy, chief of the surgical department at the University Medical Center.

Hardy had been born in Alabama. Tall, limber, with slightly graying hair, he appeared casual and easygoing, with an underlay of incisiveness. He lived with his wife and pretty daughters five miles northeast of Jackson, in a large white plantation-style house filled with books, works of art, old furniture, and fine rugs.

When Hardy took charge of the small surgical department of the hospital in 1955, he was not yet thirty-seven. He had taught surgery at the University of Pennsylvania for a time and then had headed the department of surgical research at the University of Tennessee. He was a member of that remarkable generation of surgeons who could operate on any part of the human body; and his all-round abilities had proved a bitter necessity during his early years in Jackson. But he was not interested in routine work alone; his was a youthful spirit that called for bold innovations in surgery. And, among other things, that meant transplant surgery.

James D. Hardy in retrospect:

"Our first transplant experience, and I think everybody else's, was with the kidney. . . . I was interested in the kidney from the standpoint of people who were coming here. We didn't have a chronic dialysis unit, and you could help them to a certain extent with peritoneal dialysis, but of course you never could seem to get them off it. And so we got interested in kidney transplants about the same time they did in Boston, following their lead, of course. . . . And to me, being a thoracic surgeon, the idea of going on to the lung was natural.

"One particular patient catapulted me into being interested in lung transplants. . . . We had this man who had an intestinal obstruction and he had been sucked out. He went to the operating room, and the tube used to suck out the fluid was clamped off just for the time when he went from the floor to the operating room, and then it was opened again. But somehow during that time he vomited and sucked material into his lungs. And here we had a man, a young man, clearly able to live a long life if he could live a few days—the fact is, if a person can live a few days he will get over that condition all right. But he didn't live those few days. There is no way known to tide a man over for this period and let his lungs recover from this acid material from his stomach. He died, and it was at that precise starting point that we set out to try to do with lungs what we had done with the kidney."

Compared to the prison buildings of Parchman, the hospital was a comfortable world to John Richard Russell. He did not know that James D. Hardy, seven years after he had taken charge of his department, was still fighting to get replacements for outmoded and inadequate equipment. Russell, from the moment he came to in a bare white room and found himself in bed beside other prisoners, felt enormous relief.

His difficulty in breathing tormented him, although he was a man inured to pain. In Parchman he had discovered that it was possible to endure an enormous amount of physical abuse and psychological cruelty, but that one thing was worse than all the rest: the craving for air and the fear of suffocation. Often he had had the frightful feeling that the winter mists above the Parchman flatlands were crawling into the buildings, filling his lungs and blocking off the air passages. Sometimes he wanted to jump to his feet and run and run until one of the guards shot him and relieved him for good of his sufferings. He was such a simple fellow that he could not really imagine what was wrong with his lungs. He had no idea how a lung functioned, did not realize that it consisted of hundreds of tiny vesicles. He could not imagine these vesicles filling with air at each inhalation, passing the oxygen of the air on to the circulating blood, removing carbon dioxide from the blood, and giving it up to the outside with each exhalation. All Russell knew was that he could no longer breathe properly and that the left side of his chest felt like a piece of lifeless cement.

It had been particularly bad in the leaden heat of the dormitory, when on summer nights he would sit up in bed drenched with sweat, coughing incessantly while the other prisoners railed at him to be quiet. One of the attendants at the infirmary, who had previously worked in a hospital, told him that in Jackson they had oxygen in bottles. The bottles would be placed by the bed, and once you had oxygen you were safe—you couldn't suffocate. This information consoled Russell greatly as he was being moved to Jackson. Once there he said little, but he did ask whether there was oxygen and whether he would be given any. The male nurse looked at him in astonishment and then assured him that of course he would be given oxygen as soon as it was needed.

Russell had long since stopped fearing death. He was over his remorse about the dead boy, and also over his regret that he had confessed to being guilty without understanding that there were different kinds of guilt, and that once he had declared himself a murderer nobody could help him. He had long passed the period of hoping that someday he would be free again and able to go home. If he still hoped for anything, it was that here in the hospital he would be able to see not only his wife, Louise, and his daughters, Fay and Mary Ellis, but also his son, James. His wife and one daughter were back home in Kosciusko; Fay was working in Carthage. But James was in the army; he had been sent far away, to Germany, and Russell's grave illness offered the only chance that the army might fly James home, to let him see his father once more. Otherwise, Russell hoped only that he would be able to breathe easier and that if he had to die, he would not die of suffocation.

James D. Hardy in retrospect:

"Between 1956 and 1963 we undertook about a thousand experimental lung transplants in animals, mostly dogs, but including some apes and pigs. Many of my associates, such as Dr. Watts R. Webb, Dr. Martin L. Dalton, and Dr. Fikri Alican, participated. Of course, there was already a long history of such experiments on animals. It began as early as 1907, when Charles Guthrie in Pittsburgh connected a kitten's lung to the blood vessels in the neck of a grown cat. But truly decisive experiments did not begin until around 1950—those undertaken, for example, by Juvenelle in our country or Metras in France. On the whole, all experiments began with removing one lobe of a lung from a dog and then reimplanting the same lung in the same animal. The idea was to avoid rejection and first find out what the technical problems of such transplants were and whether the transplanted lung would function at all. We took the same course; only later did we switch to transplanting from animal to animal.

"In this work we were trying to solve three fundamental questions. First, we had to develop a safe surgical method for the transplantation. It turned out that this was not too difficult. It was easiest if we removed the left lobe of the lung, leaving behind the stump of its junction with the bronchial stem as well as the two pulmonary veins and the pulmonary artery, and connecting the new lung to these stumps. In order to facilitate the connection with the pulmonary veins, both veins together with a part of the left atrium of the heart, into which they flowed, could be removed. In removing the donor lung, this same part of the atrium was taken and then sutured to the recipient's heart.

"The answer to another question was more difficult. Lung respiration, as is well known, is directed by brain centers through nerve channels. If a complete lung, with both lobes, is removed, these nerve connections are destroyed and the new lung is without any regulation from the brain center. Ultimately we discovered that we always had to leave behind a part of the old lung in order to preserve the regulatory function.

"The third problem was the most complicated. How long, we asked ourselves, can a lung remain alive without its natural supply of blood and oxygen? Or, in other words, how much time did we have between the removal of a lung and its reimplantation in a body? In the case of the kidney, we had meanwhile learned the answers to this question. But the viability of the lung was still a mystery. We experimented with some one hundred dogs to determine how lungs behaved during the first forty-eight hours after their removal from an animal body. If they were cooled to 4 degrees centigrade, they remained viable for two hours and would resume their function after implantation. But two hours was the longest period outside the body we could achieve. It was better if we did not attempt any 'storage' at all, but transplanted the lung directly, as fast as possible, from one animal to the other.

"As soon as the lung was separated from the donor's pulmonary artery, it had to be perfused with cold Ringer's solution and heparin, in order to cool the tissues and prevent clotting. During the entire period in which the lung was disconnected from the body, it also had to be kept in motion with oxygen. As soon as the separation from the bronchial stem was completed, we connected the lung to a tube and pumped oxygen into it with a rhythmic movement. Then it was carried over to the recipient, and the pumping of oxygen ceased only after the lung had been sutured to the recipient's bronchial stem. In this way the lungs regularly functioned for approximately seven days in the body of the new animal. Then they were rejected.

"By this time we had reached the year 1961–62, and we heard about the recent experiences with Imuran. We gave Imuran to thirty-four dogs with new lungs; twenty of these lived for thirty days. That was toward the end of 1962—and that was a magnificent moment for us. . . . For we remembered the patient who had died because his lung was temporarily paralyzed by stomach acids. If we could have kept him alive not thirty, but only four or five days, on one lobe of his lung, the other would have begun to function again and he would have been saved. . . . So I said to my assistants: 'Gentlemen, we have put in several years now on several hundred lung transplants. The time has come. If we come to a similar case, we're going to do it.' "

John Richard Russell was a medical case, not a surgical case, and he was treated by the hospital internists. He still had no notion of what might be wrong with him. Perhaps he thought of cancer once or twice, because he had been a heavy smoker all his life and there had been so much on television about cancer from smoking. But he had repressed the thought; besides, he did not really care. The only thing that mattered to him was to be able to breathe again, at least for a while.

Actually, he felt considerably better during his first few days at the hospital. He was given medicines that got rid of some of the fluid accumulated in his legs. His heart was treated, and that, too, made his breathing easier. But his left lung made scarcely any respiratory noises; the left side of his chest was rigid. There were foci of infection in his lung. Emphysema had developed, causing a loss of elasticity in the lung tissue and destruction of the pulmonary vesicles. His respiratory capacity was only one-third of normal. This could be explained by the emphysema, but the X rays also indicated that something else was behind it: a malignant tumor of the lung. After he had been in the hospital for ten days, a bronchoscope examination was undertaken; that is, an instrument was pushed into his bronchi, enabling the doctors to inspect the bronchial tubes and take samples of tissue.

This procedure is particularly harrowing. It took Russell days to recover from it. He would have felt even worse if they had let him know the result of the examination. In the left side stem of his bronchial system was a cancerous tumor which was spreading into the left lobe of the lung. It could not be determined to what extent the carcinoma had spread to other organs.

Since Russell's kidneys also showed symptoms of severe disturbances, it seemed likely that metastases had formed there as well. Kidney biopsies showed that this was not the case. Instead, Russell was suffering from advanced glomerulonephritis. The total clinical picture was hopeless. If Russell did not die of his lung cancer, he would fall victim to the kidney disease. But it appeared that the glomerulonephritis would give him some time, whereas the cancer of the lung would surely kill him within a few weeks. Since radiation had no prospect of success, the doctors considered removing the cancerous parts of the left bronchi and the left lobe of the lung. Thus Russell became a case for the surgical division of the hospital.

During the last days of April, Russell was told the truth. He accepted it, at least outwardly, with his characteristic apathy, showing no signs of fright or horror. All he did was to ask more emphatically what could be done about his difficulty in breathing. Would the cancer suffocate him? he kept asking anxiously. When he was told that the tumor would be removed, he did not ask whether the operation would save his life. All he asked was: "Will I be able to breathe a little easier after it?"

James D. Hardy in retrospect:

"Anybody in the transplant field has taken a certain amount of static, let's face it. When we first wanted to do kidneys here, even on patients dying, absolutely dying, many people took the position that it was just outrageous, it was malpractice, it was amoral. . . . We could say, well, so what, just ignore them. Well, you can't just ignore them; it affects the department and many things involved, grants, resident applications, all sorts of things. . . . By the time we got to lungs, things weren't so bad by far. In 1963, after more animal experiments, we set up certain criteria for the first attempt at a lung transplant on human beings. These criteria were: (1) the patient must have a probably fatal disease, so that in the event untoward results were encountered his life would not have been materially shortened; (2) there must be a reasonable possibility that the patient would be benefited by the lung transplant; (3) the removal of the patient's own lung must not result in the sacrifice of any of his own functioning lung tissue; (4) transplantation of the left lung had been found to be somewhat simpler technically than transplantation of the right, and thus it was elected to initiate the clinical phase of the work by transplanting a left lung. . . .

"When Russell showed up, he had all the things that we had written down ahead of time, and I made the decision. . . . There just has to be someone who will make a decision. All surgery is based on someone making a decision."

When James D. Hardy first saw John Russell in the prisoners' ward, he did not know why the man had been sentenced to life imprisonment, and he did not ask. Patients from Parchman were not convicts to him; they were just patients, whatever their crimes. Later Hardy said: "He was not a combative type of person. He had been ill for a long time; he may have been a dashing rogue at one time, but I found him to be very placid. He was very short of breath."

In the course of the month of May, Hardy became convinced that Russell was the patient he and his associates had been waiting for. Even if the man's left lung were removed, he would die within a short time, either of the further spread of cancer or of his kidney disease. But if the surgeons limited themselves to extirpation of the lobe of the lung, it was doubtful whether the emphysematous right lung could take over the burden of breathing. The chances were that Russell would be able to live only on artificial respiration. On the other hand, there was the prospect that a new lung would considerably relieve Russell's tormented breathing and make the last phase of his life at least somewhat more human. Did not that alone provide a justification, a humanitarian basis, for this first experiment in lung transplantation on a human being?

Hardy by no means overlooked the fact that there were no such reassuring answers to some other questions. What, for example, would happen if Russell's kidney disease made treatment with Imuran impossible? What would happen if the lung were rejected, so that shortly after the first operation they had to operate again to remove the rejected lung? That would be too much for any organism—especially for this mortally sick man.

Hardy consulted the hospital's kidney specialists. They, too, had their doubts. But in the end they concluded that Russell's kidneys would survive both the operation and the postoperative treatment, though it might be necessary to support them at some point with peritoneal dialysis. On the basis of this verdict Hardy decided to take the step into the unknown—if he had further doubts, he repressed them. Early in June he went to have a talk with the quiet patient in the prisoners' ward and explain to him the nature of this last, extreme, unusual chance he had to offer.

James D. Hardy in the Journal of the American Medical Association, *December 21, 1963:*

"The entire situation was outlined carefully to the patient by means of discussion and sketches. . . . He was willing to accept the transplant."

James D. Hardy in retrospect:

"When I told him about the operation, he said he wanted to think about it and then he said: 'Well, do you think it will help my shortness of breath?' "

John Richard Russell listened attentively, although even listening was an effort for him. He heard that there was a chance for postponement of death by a simple operation. And he heard about a second chance for postponement *and* relief by means of an entirely new kind of operation. Hardy said he could show him animals that had survived a transplant. Russell also heard that he would be the first human being to undergo such an operation, and Hardy said he could not promise success. It is not clear how much Russell understood of the ideas behind a lung transplant. But he gathered that, in any case, it meant a chance he would not otherwise have to be freed for a while from his struggle for breath. He asked for a little time to think it over and said he would like to see his wife and all his children.

To Hardy's relief, Russell did not say a word about the frequent reports in newspapers of convicts who were pardoned in return for having made themselves available for medical experiments. Hardy did not want Russell's consent at the price of commutation of his sentence. He did not want to undertake his novel operation as the result of a swap. Neither did he want to bring on the spiteful commentary that his experiment was typical of southern medicine and that there was only one missing element: Hardy's "guinea pig" was not a black.

But as he looked down at his patient, Hardy decided of his own accord to approach the governor of Mississippi and ask for a commutation of Russell's sentence if the operation was carried out and the patient survived. Hardy also saw to it that Russell's son, James, received a furlough and was flown back from Germany. James came to visit his father, and Louise Russell, Mary Ellis, and Fay came from Kosciusko and Carthage.

As Louise sat by his bed and he slowly told her about the impending operation, she understood only that it was something dangerous. Later she said: "He said he didn't know whether it would turn out all right. But he didn't say once he was afraid. . . . I didn't want him to go ahead. But he said he wanted to do it—and so he did it."

James D. Hardy in retrospect:

"Once a decision for lung transplantation had been made . . . a protocol for the management of the donor and of the recipient was drawn up and distributed to everyone involved. Our two teams, the first consisting of Dr. Martin L. Dalton, Dr. Gordon Robinson, and Dr. Benton M. Hilbun for the removal of the lung, the second of Dr. Watts R. Webb, Dr. George R. Walker, and myself for the implantation, were kept on constant alert. . . . Almost a week was to elapse before a suitable donor lung became available. At approximately 7:30 P.M. on the evening of June 11, 1963, a patient entered the emergency room of the University Hospital in shock and with pulmonary edema secondary to a massive myocardial infarction. When it proved impossible to effect resuscitation with endotracheal tube ventilation, closed-chest cardiac massage, and other measures, we were informed. The internists weren't certain whether the lung would be ideal for our purposes because of the accumulation of fluid in it. But the family had come to the hospital with the dying man, and we were told they would consent to an autopsy and donation of an organ. So one of us hurried down as fast as possible to obtain permission for using the lung, and we brought the dead man into an operating room.

"Throughout this period the closed cardiac massage was continued, and rhythmical ventilation of the lung with pure oxygen by means of the endotracheal tube. Heparin was injected into the heart. . . . A blood specimen was drawn for future cross-matching with that of the recipient, and it was subsequently found that the donor . . . shared eight of thirteen groups tested with the recipient. . . . By this time the recipient team had been alerted, and after anesthesia . . . the left hemithorax was entered at approximately 8:30 P.M."

The operation was difficult, not only because it was the first of its kind, but also because Hardy and Webb encountered unexpected conditions. While they were exposing the left lung, they found such heavy adhesions between the lung and the pleura that they feared they might have to abandon the operation. Standing beside the operating table, in a state of high psychological tension, they discussed all the remaining options. Finally they succeeded in making an opening through which they could reach the lung.

They found accumulations of pus and numerous infected sites. The lung tissue was scarcely movable, even when the anesthetist pumped oxygen under pressure. Between the aorta and the esophagus were cancerous metastases that had moved from the lung into the surrounding tissue. It was apparent that removal of the left lung could not possibly save Russell's life. The left bronchial stem was so overgrown with cancer that the surgeons found it difficult to locate an unaffected area to which they could suture the new lung. Because of the heavy suppuration, Hardy did not dare to remove a part of the atrium of the heart along with the ends of the veins, as he had done in his animals. He was afraid that if he did so, he would open the way for infection to strike the heart. He severed the pulmonary artery and bronchial connection, and lifted out the destroyed lobe.

It was by now 9:30 P.M. Hardy beckoned, and Dr. Dalton brought the donor lung from the adjacent operating room. Within a few minutes Hardy and Webb found themselves facing a new complication, again one they had not foreseen. Russell and the donor were about the same stature, but as a consequence of the destruction of Russell's left lung, the thoracic cavity on his left side had shrunk. The donor lung was too big.

This was a moment of despair. If there were not enough room for the lung, all hopes would have to be abandoned. Once more the surgeons consulted at the operating table. But Hardy decided to continue by forcing the right lung back to make room for the new left lung. Nevertheless, the size of the new lung made it extraordinarily difficult to complete the suturing of the blood vessels—all the more difficult because the lung had to be kept connected to the oxygen apparatus through the bronchial opening. It took forty-five minutes before the last stitch was in place. The oxygen tube was removed and the lung sutured to the left bronchial stem. Fifteen minutes later the anesthetist took over the respiration of the new lung. It expanded completely, dissipating the fears that it might have been damaged by the donor's cardiac infarct.

Hardy needed another hour to close the thoracic cavity and perform a tracheotomy so that Russell could be supplied with air during the first postoperative days. At 11:30 the operation was finished. Russell was taken to a small room on the fifth floor that had been equipped with the usual facilities for limiting the danger of infection. He awoke within an hour and took some time to grasp what he was being told: that he had a new lung. Then he smiled and fell asleep again, while Hardy, Webb, and the rest of the team suddenly were overcome by the total exhaustion that often follows great achievements.

They had little time to yield to fatigue. At the moment, to be sure, they felt exaltation springing from the knowledge that for the first time they had demonstrated the technical practicability of lung transplantation in man. But the lung was not yet breathing independently; it was attached to a respirator. They still did not know whether it would respond to the nerve reflexes that controlled the right lung and so would go on breathing when the respirator was shut off.

On the day after the operation, Hardy had an angiocardiogram done in order to check on the blood supply to the new lung. The perfusion with blood was so surprisingly good that he decided to see whether the lung could breathe without support. He was delighted to find that it functioned without difficulty.

Russell endured the effort and pain of the tests with the silent, uncom-

plaining patience that was characteristic of him. Then suddenly he became aware that he was breathing by himself again. His impassive face
came to life. His eyes opened wide. He tried to move his arms, which were
attached to infusion tubes, as if he wanted to touch his chest and feel it
rising and falling.

James D. Hardy in retrospect:

"He was very pleased with himself; in the first place, he was less short
of breath. He had a tracheotomy; we would put him on it to make sure his
lung stayed well inflated, and then we would take him off. He did very
well without it."

For John Richard Russell, it was one of his greatest experiences. He
could feel the air entering his lungs again. His breathing was by no means
that of a healthy person. But he had long ago forgotten what really
healthy breathing was. For him the slightest improvement was a wonderful gift. He began to believe a miracle was taking place, and even Hardy
could not entirely close his mind to the hope of a miracle.

James D. Hardy in retrospect:

"He looked great; I thought we were in for a long run. And he got
better as time went on."

The tests showed that Russell's blood was being enriched with oxygen,
that the new lung was actually doing its work better from day to day. The
fever subsided, because along with the old lung the source of infection
had been removed. For the time being no signs of rejection could be discovered.

The one factor that worried Hardy was that Russell's kidneys were
functioning more poorly than the nephrologists had judged. The urea level
began to rise. It seemed truly the irony of fate. Russell was the first human
being to be breathing with a new lung. But his life was threatened by a
kidney failure—a problem medical science had already conquered, at least
on the theoretical level. Hardy hoped he would be able to balance out the
kidney failure by peritoneal dialysis.

James D. Hardy in retrospect:

"We put him on peritoneal dialysis. And that's one thing—in blood
dialysis you can practically guarantee the thing will work, but on some
patients you just cannot get the peritoneal dialysis to work, and we didn't

have a blood dialysis [artificial kidney], and so we started peritoneal dialysis. But it never really did work."

The new lung breathed, the incisions healed—and the uremia continued inexorably to increase. Once more fluid began accumulating in Russell's legs. The new lung breathed—but intestinal obstructions made it impossible to nourish the patient. Russell lay helpless, only a little skim milk dripping through a tube into his body, which grew weaker and less resistant. The joy of being able to breathe sheltered him from the awareness that his life was ebbing away. At the beginning of the seventeenth day his lung was still functioning. But a few hours later uremia and exhaustion produced a loss of consciousness. On June 29 he took his last breath. The autopsy showed that the new lung displayed no indications of rejection.

James D. Hardy in retrospect:

"This experience affords justification for several conclusions. First, clinical homotransplantation of a lung is readily accomplished technically. Second, a homotransplanted lung can participate in respiratory support of the patient. Third, immunological response in our patient was suppressed with available drugs during the eighteen days that the patient survived, though advanced renal disease may have supplemented the effectiveness of these agents. Fourth, experience with this case opens the way to further careful exploration of lung transplantation in man."

John Richard Russell was not around to learn of the contribution he had made to a world that had treated him badly most of his life, raising him in poverty and ignorance and finally rejecting him. But the world, too, was only dimly aware of what had happened in Jackson. For on the day the University of Mississippi Medical Center released the news of the first lung transplant in history, the newspaper headlines were dominated by events that seemed to the citizens of Mississippi and the rest of the country far more important than any medical experiment, no matter how unusual.

On June 12, the day on which Russell awoke in his hospital bed and realized that he was able to breathe again, an unknown white man murdered the black leader Medgar Evers outside his home in Jackson, shooting him from ambush and leaving the murder weapon, a rifle, behind. One of the greatest manhunts in the history of the city of Jackson began. Not only the FBI participated; the citizens of Mississippi and Jackson were also determined to find the killer, for they wanted to prove that the unrest in their state had been caused by "outside agitators" and that Evers's murder was the work of a stranger.

There was little newspaper space for Hardy's unique operation—it was submerged by the tumult of race troubles. By the time that tumult briefly subsided and it was proved that not a Mississippian but a Californian had killed Evers, John Richard Russell was already buried and Hardy's operation was no longer news.

A few months later, however, an event occurred that might have served to recall the life and death of John Richard Russell. Ross Barnett, the Governor of Mississippi, signed a document commuting Russell's sentence. The text read: "Subject, desiring to be of help to humanity and with full knowledge of the various ramifications of his condition, believing in the professional skills of the surgeons and staff of the hospital and knowing that said surgeons and staff desired to do everything possible to prolong his life, agreed in writing that a lung from another person be substituted for subject's impaired left lung. By reason of the subject's great contribution, coupled with the skill of surgeons and staff of the University Hospital, this historic operation has brought much acclaim and no doubt will redound to alleviate human misery and suffering in the years to come."

But posthumous commutations are not uncommon. Their news value was considered small, and so for many years the story of John Richard Russell went largely unnoticed, along with Hardy's bold plunge into the unknown.

From a Rivista Scientifica *interview, June 1968*
(questions by Robert Hall, answers by Dr. Seibert):

QUESTION: Hardy's first lung transplant took place on June 11, 1963, his first heart transplant on January 23, 1964. Was it after the lung transplant that he decided to venture the transplantation of a heart, or did he, at the time of the earlier operation, already have in mind his next step?

ANSWER: Hardy began his heart transplant preparations at the same time that he was engaged in laboratory experiments leading to lung transplantation. By the time he actually attempted the lung transplant in Jackson, the heart work had advanced very far. The operation on Russell no doubt accelerated the transition from animal experimentation to an attempt to transplant a heart in man.

QUESTION: Then the laboratory experiments went on for some eight years?

ANSWER: Approximately. As in the case of the lung, the background history is much longer. In 1905, Guthrie transplanted hearts from dog to dog. Now, the heart has a double connection with the circulatory system, of course. In the first place, there is the connection of the heart's coronary arteries with the general circulation. These arteries serve only to nourish the heart muscle and preserve its vigor. On the other hand, the heart is the pump that keeps the entire circulation going. Guthrie first connected the coronary circulation of his dogs with the carotid artery and vein of other animals, in order to determine whether the heart could be nourished in this way. Once he had proved that this was possible, he carried his experiments further, artificially connecting the ventricles and atria of the heart with the carotid arteries and veins of other dogs. In his experiments he removed the hearts; they were outside the animals' bodies. But he succeeded in getting them to beat. Several beat eighty-eight times per minute for two hours. Then the blood coagulated in the ventricles—since at that time there was no heparin. The next significant experiments were performed by Vladimir Demikhov in the Soviet Union. They began in 1940.

QUESTION: Is that the same Demikhov who also undertook experiments with artificial hearts?

ANSWER: Yes, but that is another story. Demikhov transplanted hearts directly into the bodies of other animals, implanting them as additional hearts alongside the natural heart. He removed parts of the lung in order to make room for this second heart. From 1946 to 1958 he undertook 250 experiments. Most of the animals died on the operating table, or afterward from blood clots and lung infections. But enough survived to prove that hearts that were at rest during the transplanting operation could be made to beat again by attachment to the new circulation and by electric shocks. In one of his dogs a second heart beat for thirty-two days before it failed by fibrillation. Demikhov was without the apparatus needed to carry out a real heart transplant—above all, he did not have the heart-lung machine. Only with that could the recipient be kept alive during the period in which he was without a heart. Consequently, the really decisive experiments were made in England and in the United States, by, among others, Russell Brock in London, Adrian Kantrowitz in New York, Richard Lower and Norman Shumway at Stanford University in Palo Alto, and by the man we have been talking about, James D. Hardy, and Watts R. Webb in Mississippi.

QUESTION: Were they all working in the same direction?

ANSWER: Fundamentally, yes. Once the heart-lung machine made it possible to excise a human being's entire heart and nevertheless keep him alive for hours, three questions remained to be solved: (1) How could a heart removed from a dead donor be kept viable during the time it took to connect it to the recipient's blood vessels? (2) How and how quickly could surgeons attend to the multiple anastomoses between the new heart and these vessels? After all, no less than five blood vessels are involved: the vena cava, the two pulmonary veins, the aorta, and the pulmonary artery. (3) How would the new hearts receive the nerve impulses from the brain which regulate the human heart as well as the lung, adjusting it to changing needs of the body? Brock, Lower, and Shumway had considered this problem as early as 1959. They did not remove the recipient's entire heart, but left the part of the atrium with the mouths of the great veins. The corresponding atrial portion was excised from the donor heart and the surfaces connected at implantation. Then all that was needed was to establish the connections with the pulmonary artery and the aorta. This method also preserved an important nerve center in the posterior wall of the atrium.

QUESTION: What was Hardy's approach?

ANSWER: After many losses of animals in the early years after 1956, Hardy's and Webb's experiments proceeded in the same direction. In order to keep the donor hearts viable, Hardy and Webb initially employed hypothermia, cooling the heart to 4 degrees centigrade. Hearts cooled in this way began to beat, after an electric shock, in ten dogs; they continued to beat for from thirty minutes to seven and a half hours. But in experiments with calves, whose hearts are larger, Hardy found a more effective technique. As soon as the donor heart had been removed, he thrust a catheter into the coronary arteries and rinsed them with cooled, oxygen-enriched blood.

QUESTION: In other words, similar to the technique used for transplanting lungs?

ANSWER: Yes. Altogether Hardy and his closest associate, Webb, carried out some 300 experiments on animals. Later they practiced the transplantation technique on human cadavers until they had learned to perform the blood vessel anastomoses in less than an hour. By 1963 they were ready to go further. As in the case of lung transplantation, the problem of rejection now seemed soluble. Strictly speaking, by this time all the other experimenters, at least in America, had reached about the same stage of technical preparation. Who would be the first to venture a heart transplant was no longer a question of technique. It was simply a question of who would have the courage to break through the high moral barriers that surrounded the human heart, not only in public opinion, but also for the majority of the medical profession.

Ever since Aristotle the heart has been considered as virtually equivalent to life itself and therefore possessing a spiritual and divine aspect; it has rarely been envisaged as just a pump that can be transferred from one human being to another. It was different with the kidneys—vital though the kidney was to the organism, it had never acquired that kind of spiritual association. Besides, the kidney is a paired organ, which makes it somewhat more expendable. Since the human being has only one heart, the idea of heart transplantation sounded monstrous even to nonreligious persons. The sinister image was of surgeons cutting still-living hearts out of the dying. There is no doubt that Hardy, in the relative isolation of Jackson, was the first to trace his way through all the psychological and moral scruples that have continued to be associated with heart transplants. He faced these issues between July of 1963 and January of 1964, when he found his first feasible heart patient: Boyd Rush.

Early in the afternoon the green 1956 Chevrolet was still standing, locked and untouched, beside the mobile home on the southern edge of the trailer camp near Hattiesburg. Jane Colanski, who lived with her husband and children in an adjacent trailer, had been watching this car since the preceding day. It was Monday, January 20, 1964, and it was highly unusual for the car to be standing there, for its owner was ordinarily a man of strict habits. Every working day, at the same time in the morning, he left the trailer, in which he lived alone, carefully cleaned the windows of the Chevrolet, sat down at the wheel rather stiffly, in an old man's way, and drove off cautiously toward Hattiesburg. He seemed hale and hearty, though getting on to seventy; his bespectacled, rather flushed face was usually good-natured and friendly. Whenever he saw any of the other residents of the camp, he would greet them with a certain solemnity, tipping his hat and smiling. But he never said a word, for he was a deaf-mute, though he could understand others by reading their lips.

Toward five o'clock in winter and six o'clock in summer he returned, went into his trailer, took off the suit he wore even in the sweltering temperatures of Mississippi and changed into older clothing, and came out again to wash his car until there was no longer a speck of dust on it. This work was evidently hard on him, for he would breathe heavily as he plied the hose and brush. But he would go on until he was done, and then return to his trailer, prepare his supper, wash his dishes, and sit for a while reading before going to bed. Only Sundays brought a change in this schedule. He would leave his trailer somewhat later in the morning, always carefully dressed, and drive to a church in Hattiesburg where services were held for deaf-mutes—the minister there knew sign language.

Jane Colanski had been at the camp for five months. But she had never seen the old man deviate from his habits or omit his drives to Hattiesburg, where he worked as a door-to-door pedlar. His stock in trade consisted of pots and pans, kitchen knives, brushes, and sewing needles; the earnings added a bit to the small pension he received. When she drove to Hattiesburg to shop, Jane would occasionally see him ringing doorbells, tipping his hat, and holding out the card that said he was deaf and dumb. His expression was so friendly that hardly anyone turned him away; most people looked at his merchandise and bought some trifle. Each item of his wares had a price tag, and whenever anyone asked him a question, he read the lip movements fluently and wrote down the answer on a pad he carried.

When Jane Colanski looked out the window of her trailer again at 4:00 P.M. and saw the Chevrolet still standing there, it occurred to her for the first time that something might have happened to the old man. She knew little about him, scarcely more than his name: Boyd Rush. She had also heard that he had a relative, a sister or stepsister, somewhere in the northwestern part of Mississippi, who had helped him buy his trailer. He had visited this sister once during the summer, and as far as Jane recalled, that was the only time he had been gone for several days.

When Jane knocked at his door, there was no answer. She knocked louder and then tried to open the door. It was locked. The curtains were drawn over the windows, so that she could not see in. Finally she ran to the manager of the camp and brought him over to help. He was able to open the door with a skeleton key—and they found Boyd Rush lying on the floor. He was dressed for church. Evidently he had climbed on a chair to fix a damaged spot on the ceiling of the trailer and had fallen. Probably he had been lying helpless on the floor since Sunday morning. He was still breathing, but very weakly, and showed no other sign of life.

"He has a sister," Jane Colanski said. But the manager searched the trailer in vain for the sister's address. Finally he did the only thing he could do in such a case; he called the community hospital in Laurel, twenty-five miles away. Toward six o'clock the ambulance arrived with howling siren, and the driver and his assistant carried Boyd Rush into it. They asked whether any relatives or friends wanted to come along. When no one spoke up, they drove off. Only after the red light of the ambulance had vanished into the night did Jane Colanski realize that in all the excitement she had forgotten something. She should have told the ambulance men that Boyd Rush was a deaf-mute. Now it was too late.

On the night of January 20, 1964, while the ambulance was speeding down Highway 11, its crew convinced that they would be delivering a dead man to the hospital, James D. Hardy was ready. For at least seven months, since the lung transplant, he had been determined to take the next step: transplantaton of a heart in a human being. He knew quite well that it was a much more risky undertaking than the lung transplant had been. But he believed firmly in the necessity for this next step. That step lay in the future, he was convinced, and must be taken.

James D. Hardy to Jerry LeBlanc, 1970:

"I was talking at a meeting in Atlanta on heart transplants. Dog transplants are expensive, and this fellow at the meeting wanted to know just why we were wasting all this time and the government's money on something that was a fantastic pursuit. . . . I knew that no answer was going to satisfy that fellow anyway, but I said: 'Have you heard the fable about the king who was going to have a man beheaded if he couldn't teach his horse to fly? His friend came with the man to see the king and he begged for three months more. And the king says: "Well, I'm going to give you three months more, but if you don't teach him to fly, well, then you've had it." Then the friend said to the threatened victim: "I can't take this any longer. I've been here with you time and time again, and I just can't go through the strain any more. If I were you, I wouldn't be able to stand these three months more of hopeless waiting for death." Then the other man said: "Well, there are three reasons why I don't just let him behead me. In the first place, the king might die and I have reason to believe his son is more lenient. In the second place, I might die and might not have to face it anyway. And in the third place, we just might teach this horse to fly." Well, the fact is, my horse—the heart transplant—is flying, just slightly, and he'll fly better as time goes by.' "

James D. Hardy in the Journal of the American Medical Association, *June 29, 1964:*

"As the laboratory work continued and animal heart transplants came to exceed 200 in number, considerable reflection was devoted to a definition of the clinical circumstances under which heart transplantation might be ethically carried out. It was fully appreciated that, while the clinical transplantation of a nonpaired organ such as the liver had been widely accepted, transplantation of the heart would involve basic emotional factors. . . . The question . . . was therefore discussed with many thoughtful persons, both physicians and laymen."

James D. Hardy to Jerry LeBlanc, 1970:

"I said there's going to be a lot of shellfire for transplanting a heart at all. I said the American public doesn't realize it can be done in dogs, and the psychological impact is going to be big because people look upon the heart as something a little different, the seat of the spirit."

James D. Hardy in the Journal of the American Medical
Association, *June 29, 1964:*

"All agreed that a rigid set of circumstances must exist. The donor
hearts presumably would be derived from a relatively young patient dying
of brain damage, and the recipient must be a patient dying of terminal
myocardial failure. . . . But how soon after 'death' of the donor could
the heart be removed? If it were not done promptly, irreversible damage
might have occurred. To minimize such damage it was planned to insert
catheters into the femoral vessels and begin total body perfusion the instant death was announced by a physician not associated with the transplant team. It was believed that if the relatives were willing to permit use
of the heart for transplantation, they probably would not object to
heparinization and insertion of the peripheral catheters using local anesthesia at some point just prior to cardiorespiratory arrest. In this way oxy-
genation of the body tissues could be affected while thoracotomy was performed to excise the donor heart and begin coronary sinus perfusion."

James D. Hardy to Jerry LeBlanc, 1970:

"People said to me, if your heart transplant doesn't make it, you're
dead. . . . I talked to the lawyer of the state medical association, and he
said he didn't think state medical would be outraged. He said that he
would sort of plant the seed around a little bit so that it wouldn't be a
complete surprise. . . . This was in the summer of 1963, somewhere
around June or July."

James D. Hardy in the Journal of the American Medical
Association, *June 29, 1964:*

"At the outset it was expected that months, or perhaps even years,
might elapse before an acceptable donor and recipient died simultaneously in the relatively small University Hospital. . . . Yet . . . in fairly
rapid succession three young men were admitted in either the University
Hospital or the adjacent veterans' hospital with fatal head lesions. . . .
Oblique inquiry disclosed that the responsible relatives of two of these
three neurosurgical patients were willing for either the heart or the kidneys to be used for transplantation. Each of these patients died after vari-
able periods of mechanical pulmonary ventilation, a fact that raised a disturbing moral problem: when, if ever, would a physician be justified in
switching off the ventilator in a patient whose voluntary respiratory effort

had long since ceased, to permit the hypoxia that would be followed by cardiac arrest? We were not able to conclude that we would be willing to do this, despite the fact that at some point fruitless resuscitation efforts must cease if a viable kidney, heart, or other organ is to be obtained for transplantation to a recipient."

The ambulance driver made the twenty-five miles to Laurel in record time. The sick man's breathing had that irregular sound so familiar to him as the respiration of the dying shortly before the end. But the patient was still alive when they carried him into the emergency room, where an over-worked young doctor examined the unconscious old man. Neither the driver nor the assistant could answer any of the doctor's questions about the circumstances or the identity of the patient. In his pocket they found a driver's license giving his name as Boyd Rush and the year of his birth as 1896. They also discovered a bottle of digitalis tablets; but the label was so smudged that neither the druggist nor the name of the doctor who had prescribed the heart stimulant could be deciphered. The young doctor found that Boyd Rush's heart was beating with extreme irregularity and that his blood pressure was too low to be measured. He had the old man placed in a ward, ordered an intravenous infusion of norepinephrine to raise the blood pressure, and turned to other patients.

To his surprise, by morning the old man had recovered considerably. Since the doctor was going off duty, he turned his patient over to his successor, an older resident, who now undertook a more thorough examination, X-rayed the chest, and had an electrocardiogram prepared. He also telephoned the manager of the trailer camp and learned something about Boyd Rush's circumstances. The heart was in so desperate a condition that it seemed a mystery how Rush could have lived for so long alone in his trailer. The coronary vessels displayed extreme changes. The heart muscle had evidently suffered a series of infarcts some time before. Until someone could find out what doctors had treated Boyd Rush previously, or if he had had any treatment, it could not be ascertained whether these attacks had been noticed or whether they were so-called "silent infarcts."

When the resident tested the patient's reflexes, he found that Rush, though unconscious, could move all his limbs if the stimulus was sufficiently painful. His left thigh, however, was cold and discolored. Un-doubtedly an interruption of circulation had produced a gangrenous de-struction of tissue, which would force amputation unless the circulation could soon be restored. The doctor was convinced that a blood clot had formed in the patient's heart; it must have reached his crural artery, and possibly a cerebral artery also, blocking circulation. Since he saw no way to help the man by internal medicine, he informed the surgeon, Dr. Sam L. Robinson.

Robinson was a young man who had learned surgery under James D. Hardy in Jackson and had imbibed some of Hardy's belief in the progress of medicine. Before moving to Laurel he had participated in Hardy's laboratory experiments in lung and heart transplants. As he worked on Boyd Rush, he soon realized that the man had only a few days to live at best. Nevertheless, he made an attempt to save the leg. The old man was so deeply unconscious that only a light local anesthetic was needed for him to expose the femoral artery, insert a probe, and remove a blood clot that might have been responsible for the gangrene. It was now noon on January 21. Robinson decided to give Rush additional circulatory drugs and wait to see how the leg responded.

At this time James D. Hardy, a hundred miles away in Jackson, was going through a period of suspense such as he had not experienced since the days of the lung transplant. The reason for this state of mind can be found in the recollections of one of his associates:

"It was around October or November 1963 when all of us realized, with a certain degree of frustration, that we were asking too much of fate to expect that a cardiac patient would be dying at the very same time as a convenient donor. Our pessimism was deepened by various things that happened with cardiac patients we had in mind as recipients. For example, doctors in the emergency room reported the delivery of a dying man after a cardiac infarct and proposed him as a recipient. But the man, supposedly as good as dead, recovered. . . . This incident taught us that a heart recipient would have to be a patient with a severe chronic heart disease going back many years, a disease that had entered its last, fatal stage in which there would be no surprising recovery. . . .

"Such was the situation when Hardy heard from New Orleans that Dr. Reemtsma had succeeded in transplanting chimpanzee kidneys to human beings and that one of his patients, Jefferson Davis, had survived the operation and was doing amazingly well. Reemtsma had been a pupil of Hardy's when the latter was teaching surgery in Pennsylvania. On November 18, 1963, Hardy flew to New Orleans to visit Reemtsma. On this occasion he saw Jefferson Davis, who seemed to be recovering, and returned to Jackson profoundly impressed.

"Next day he proposed a new idea which filled us with excitement. If the transplantation of chimpanzee kidneys to a human being is possible, he said, chimpanzee hearts should also be transplantable. Of course, chimpanzee hearts are smaller than human hearts and at best could pump no more than about 4 liters per minute; but the cardiac performance of severely ill patients is so small that transplantation of a chimpanzee heart would in any case lead to some improvement in circulation. On the flight back from New Orleans, Hardy had considered buying several chimpanzees for our hospital. He thought that in a future case of potential heart transplant he might be able to resort to a chimpanzee heart if no donor turned up in time, and so could carry out the operation. Since we already feared violent reactions to the transplantation of a human heart, we could only expect that using an ape heart would intensify these reactions. But Hardy decided to take the risk.

"Since we had only small dog cages, he had several chimp cages with strong bars set up in the basement of the old medical school building. In December, with aid from the Jackson Zoo, he bought four large chimpanzees. They came from Texas, cost between $500 and $800 apiece, and were so strong and unruly that one of them broke out of its cage and had to be subdued by using a rifle that fired narcotic bullets. Unfortunately the narcotic dose was too high, and so we lost the valuable animal. But in any case, the idea of using a chimpanzee organ gave new impetus to the whole transplant idea.

"During all of December and the beginning of January we practiced a kind of transplantation alert. Two teams were set up, one for the donor and one for the recipient. There were certain difficulties, because Dr. Webb, who had been Hardy's closest associate since 1956, moved to Southwestern Medical School and Dr. Carlos Chavez took his place. That imposed fresh burdens on Hardy. . . . In January 1964 he deliberately started to air his plan for a heart transplant around the Medical Center. Hardy wanted the idea to be discussed as thoroughly as possible. He wanted to prepare both other doctors and the public, for, as he told us: 'I've discovered that people who are informed about a surprising event in advance react much less violently.'

"On January 18 we went through a kind of dress rehearsal of a very special sort. A week earlier, on January 11, a former pupil of Dr. Hardy's, Dr. Robinson of the South Mississippi Charity Hospital in Laurel, had sent us an unusually tragic cardiac case, a thirty-six-year-old black named William H. Paige, from Lumberton. Paige had been in Houston in the spring of 1963. He got into some kind of fight—I don't know how and where—and was stabbed in the heart. He was operated on at the old Jefferson Davis Hospital in Houston, the heart wound was sewed up, and he was sent home. But the injured left ventricle began forming blood clots. It was like a gruesome game of Russian roulette: the clots were pumped into his circulation. One clot blocked a cerebral artery, so that Paige was paralyzed on his left side and remained mentally confused. Then his left leg died and had to be amputated. The horrible process continued; the same thing happened later to his right leg. After that clots blocked an intestinal artery, producing grave damage. . . . In despair, Paige's mother took her son to Laurel. There he recovered somewhat—if you can speak of recovery for a man in such a condition. But any moment some other disaster might take place, unless that source of clots inside the heart could be eliminated.

"Dr. Robinson telephoned Hardy on January 10. Since he knew about our heart transplant plans, he asked whether Hardy was prepared to make the try. Transplantation, he said, was the only way to deliver Paige from the heart that was killing him. And on January 11, Paige, now no more than the helpless torso of a man, was brought to Jackson.

"Hardy was eager. But as soon as he saw Paige he decided that this was not a case for the first attempt at a heart transplant. I recall his saying: 'It's possible that an aneurysm has formed on the scar in the heart and that we can prevent further embolisms by repairing the suture.' As chance would have it, on January 18, just as we were about to operate, a patient was delivered to the hospital who was dying of a severe brain injury. His heart continued beating only under artificial respiration. But the brain was dead and he was doomed; it was only a matter of time before his heart would stop.

"Thus Hardy had the opportunity for a dress rehearsal. Everything was ready in the improbable event that Paige's heart failed during the operation. In that case, either he would receive the heart of the man with the injured brain or else (if the man hung on) the heart of our heaviest chimpanzee, which weighed 96 pounds, more than Paige's legless body.

"The operation on Paige succeeded. Hardy removed the source of the embolism. Paige came out of the anesthesia and there was no reason for transplantation. It was an irony of fate that in this case the possible donor's heart stood still at the exact moment that Paige's heart was exposed and the exchange of hearts could have taken place. Paige recovered and later returned home to his mother. But in the Medical Center the rumor went around that Hardy had carried out a heart transplant.

"Hardy was convinced that as a result of the operation on Paige we were better than ever prepared for an actual heart transplant. Still, nobody wanted sensational newspaper accounts. We tried to suppress the rumor, but in vain; it reached the outside. Reporters started telephoning, accusing us of withholding important news. We even received telephone calls from Czechoslovakia and Japan. But there was nothing we could do about it. At least we were glad to have reached the stage of being fully prepared, psychologically and technically. At the same time, the waiting became a kind of torture. It was like getting a horse ready to jump a hurdle and then holding it down before the leap."

By late afternoon on January 21, Dr. Robinson realized that removal of the clot from Boyd Rush's femoral artery had not sufficed to restore circulation in the leg. The gangrene was advancing; amputation could scarcely be postponed for more than twenty-four hours. Meanwhile, however, Robinson had made a closer study of the patient's general condition, and of his heart in particular. The more he learned, the more he became convinced that Boyd Rush was an ideal patient for his former teacher in Jackson. He knew Hardy's criteria: that a candidate for transplantation must be in the last stage of a long-lasting chronic heart disease. Unquestionably the unconscious old man from the trailer camp in Hattiesburg had reached that stage.

Recollections of a former employee of the South Mississippi Charity Hospital in Laurel:

"Dr. Robinson later left Laurel and moved to another state. But I remember that he telephoned Dr. Hardy, and they decided to have the patient from Hattiesburg taken to Jackson for the amputation, but what was mainly involved was the possibility of a heart transplant. The thing was, we knew hardly anything about Boyd Rush besides his name, and it was impossible to go ahead with an operation on an unconscious man without the consent of his relatives. That would have led to all sorts of wild rumors about misuse of a helpless dying man. So that afternoon or evening we began trying to find relatives. We couldn't learn anything at the trailer camp. But then in a corner of Rush's wallet somebody found a scrap of paper or a letter with the telephone number of a Mrs. J. H. Thompson, in Cleveland, Mississippi. And then everything was simple. She answered and turned out to be his stepsister, maybe his only living relative. Of course, Dr. Robinson didn't say anything about a possible transplant, but only talked about moving her brother or stepbrother to Jackson for amputation and that they needed her consent. She answered that she would come herself, she'd drive to Jackson immediately to see her brother. And then came the surprise: she told us that Boyd Rush was a deaf-mute. On January 22 he was transferred to Jackson."

Cleveland, in the northwestern part of Mississippi, is about 130 miles from Jackson and 230 miles from Laurel. Mrs. J. H. Thompson had been living in these parts twenty-five years, somewhat on the outskirts of the small town, in a brick and frame house a short distance off Highway 8. She was now fifty-seven years old and had been born when her stepbrother, Boyd, was eleven and attending a school for deaf-mutes in Jackson. The two had different fathers and the same mother, and during her childhood she had seen Boyd only when he came home on vacations. Even as a child she had felt solicitude for him, perhaps because he was born with a handicap, had lost his father at the age of four, and ever since had had to live in an institution full of other deaf-mute children. But she had also never met a sweeter-tempered, kindlier person, and she had learned his sign language so that she could communicate with him.

Later he had moved to Baton Rouge, Louisiana, where he worked as an upholsterer at a shop in the town's bus depot. There he met and married his wife, Nora. The pair lived quietly in a small house and had no children: a peaceable couple who regularly attended a Baptist church for deaf-mutes. Indeed, strange as it seems, both of them sang in church. Their singing consisted of mutely following the movements of lips and fingers. Boyd had a natural feeling for notes and read the sounds of the instruments from the movements of the players.

In 1961, when Boyd reached the age of sixty-five, he retired from his job in Baton Rouge. He and his wife moved to Grenada, a small town of about a thousand inhabitants sixty miles to the east of Cleveland. Nora had relatives in Grenada. But after two years there Nora had died. Boyd was left alone and despondent. He longed for a church community, and since there were no services for deaf-mutes in Grenada, he again moved south, finally settling in Hattiesburg. Because he could not afford to rent a house or apartment, he bought a trailer. His stepsister helped him find a used car and locate the camp. In a phase of desperate loneliness he had married again, but his stepsister had never met this second wife. She had lived with Boyd only a few weeks and then cleared out.

Boyd Rush had never been one to complain. If he had been ill for a long time, as Dr. Robinson said, he had never reported this to his stepsister. All she knew was that he suffered from high blood pressure. At Christmas he had mentioned that he did not feel very well. But that was all she knew. After all, she and Boyd were separated by 250 miles, and she herself hadn't grown any younger or more mobile. Yet as soon as she heard that he was in the hospital and realized how helpless and alone he must feel, she packed a few things and on the morning of January 22 set out for Jackson.

James D. Hardy in the American Journal of Cardiology, *December 1968:*

"Still stuporous when hospitalized in Jackson, he was promptly evaluated by the cardiologist, who found atrial fibrillation with rapid ventricular rate and inadequate respiration. He had marked cardiomegaly [enlargement of the heart] . . . and relative low blood pressure. . . . A tracheotomy was performed and mechanical ventilatory assistance initiated."

. . .

When Mrs. Thompson arrived at the Medical Center Hospital she was shown to a small white room on the fifth floor where Boyd Rush had been placed after his arrival from Laurel. She could not restrain her tears when she saw the breathing tube inserted into the incision in his throat, and his sunken features, distorted but still showing that sweet-tempered look that had always been his. Sorrowfully, she realized that Boyd was very far away from her, though still alive. It no longer mattered that he was deaf and dumb, or that anyone watching beside his bed could understand his sign language. His inability to hear or speak had erected a wall between him and the outside world all his life. But as long as his mind had been alert and his dark, warmhearted eyes able to look around, that wall had not been insuperable. Now his eyes no longer saw anything.

She sat with him for a long time, hoping that he would come to, recognize her, and tell her what had happened to him in his trailer in Hattiesburg. In vain. Half attentively, she listened to the explanations of several doctors. She did not doubt that these doctors would do everything humanly possible to keep Boyd alive. And since she did not want to be in their way, she finally asked them to telephone her at her motel as soon as Boyd's condition changed and there was even the slightest chance that she could talk with him in sign language. Then she left the hospital to wait. She did not know that Boyd's removal to a private room was a sign that the doctors attached a special importance to him. And certainly the word or the idea of a heart transplantation was utterly remote from her thoughts.

James D. Hardy in the American Journal of Cardiology, *December 1968:*

"The blood pressure remained unstable. . . . Brief episodes of apparent semiconsciousness were spaced between long periods when he could be aroused only by painful stimuli. Respiration was irregular and inadequate without mechanical assistance. Both lower extremities were edematous. . . . The cardiologist again recorded the presence of Cheyne-Stokes respiration and found the heart sounds muffled. . . . A lumbar puncture was performed to exclude subarachnoid hemorrhage as the cause of the semicoma which persisted. The cerebrospinal fluid pressure was normal, the fluid was clear. . . . It was decided that mental deficit was due to previous shock, to a persistent systolic blood pressure level ranging from 90 to 100 mm. Hg in a previously hypertensive subject, to cerebral thrombosis, or to emboli arising from the left side of the heart, as presumably had the one which had produced gangrene of the left lower leg and foot.

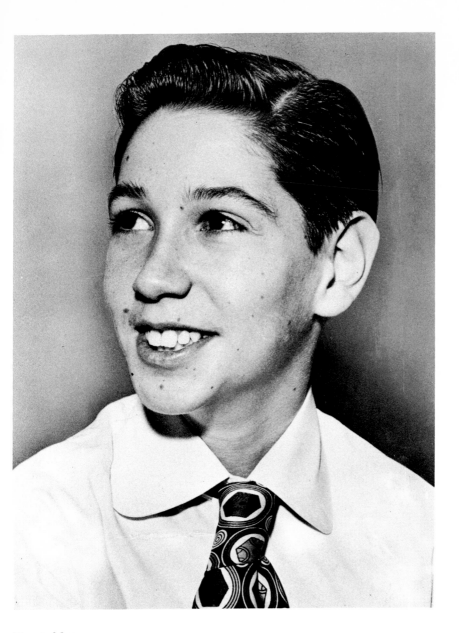

Marvin Mason

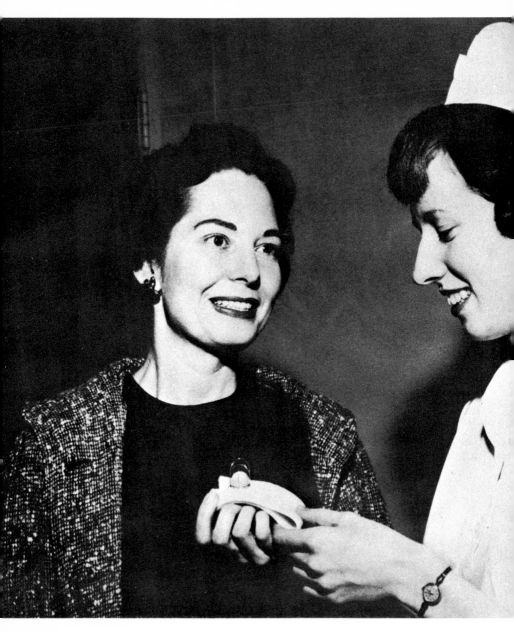

Mary Richardson, 1963, after the last of her four operations.
The nurse shows her an artificial aortic valve.

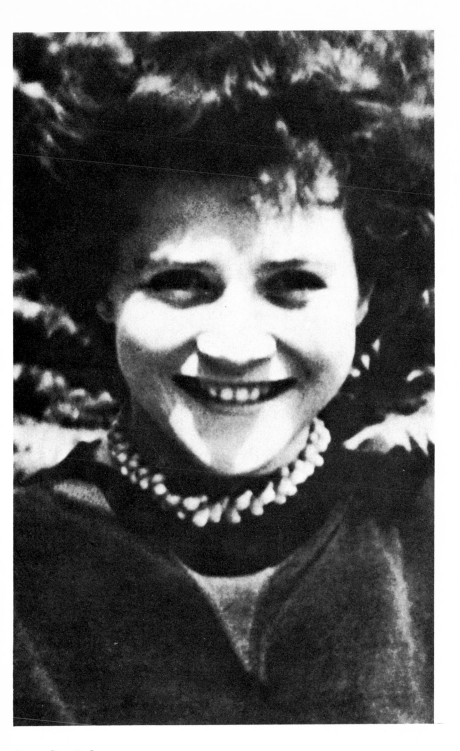

Jacqueline Cado, 1950

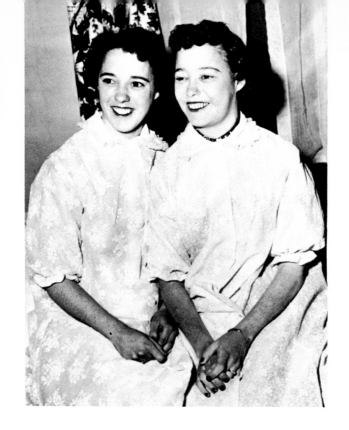

The twins Edith Helm
and Wanda Foster, 1961

Left, Lee and Edith Helm; next to Edith, Wanda with her four sons; third from right, Edith's son, John, twelve; far right, her daughter, Vicki, ten, 1971

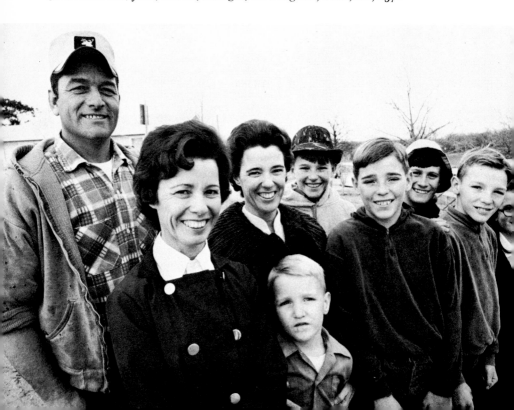

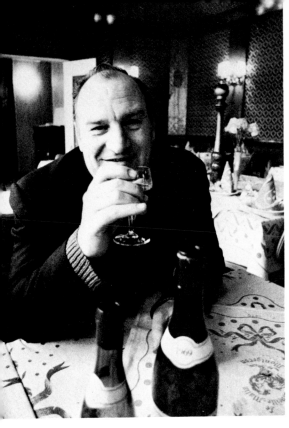

Georges Siméon, 1970

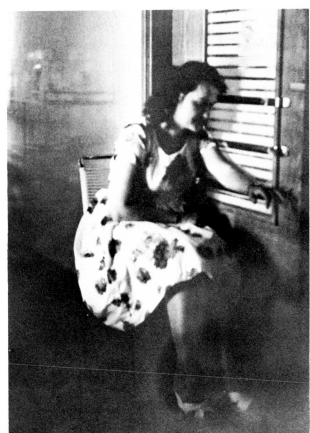

His wife, Armande,
in July 1959, outside
the isolation room
at Necker Hospital

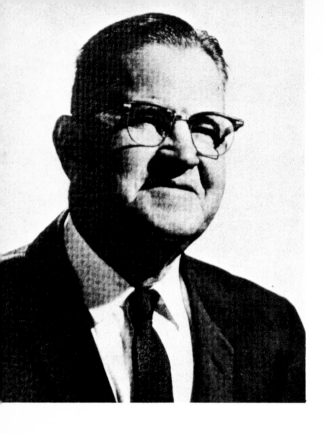

Boyd Rush, 1963, and the permit signed by his step-sister, Mrs. Thompson

OPERATIVE PERMIT

I hereby give full permission for left leg amputation and heart surgery on

Boyd Rush. I understand that any clots present will be removed from the heart to

stop them from going to still more arteries of his body. I further understand that

heart is in extremely poor condition. If for any unanticipated reason the heart

fail completely during either operation and it should be impossible to start it, I

to the insertion of a suitable heart transplant if such should be available at the

I further understand that hundreds of heart transplants have been performed in

laboratories throughout the world but that any heart transplant would represent

initial transplant in man.

Signed (for family) _Mrs. J. M. Thompson_ (sister

Witnessed _Maurice C. Turner_

Witnessed _Ophelia Ann Ward R. N_

January 23,

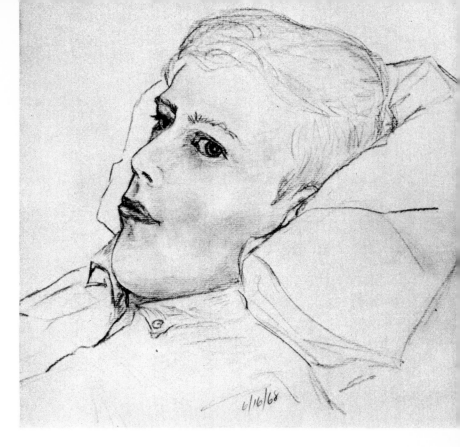

Tommy Gorence, 1968, after the liver transplant operation,
in a drawing by his mother, Joan Gorence Knapp

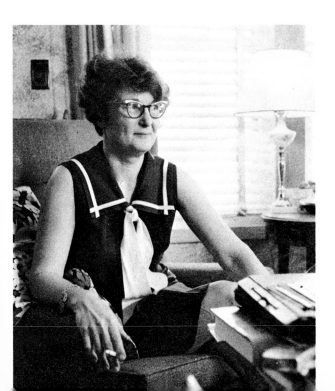

Mrs. Knapp, 1970

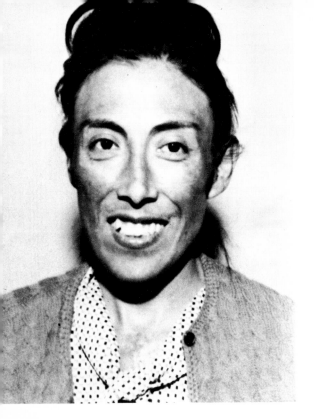

Esperanza del Valle Vásquez, 1966

With her son, Pepe, 1970

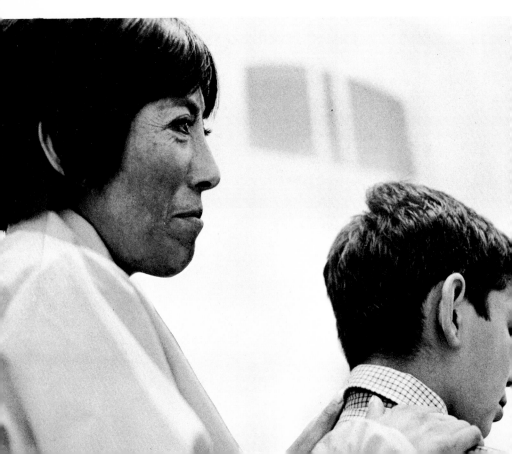

The cardiac output was determined by the dye method and was found to be 3.6 liters per minute.

"The conclusions of the cardiologist were: '. . . By all rules, life expectancy can be measured in this case in hours only.' "

After the first examinations of Boyd Rush, it was clear to Hardy that the patient could no longer be helped by either medicine or surgery. He knew that Boyd Rush presented all the criteria he had set up for his first heart transplant subject. Nevertheless, for a brief moment he felt something like a sense of relief when, on January 22 and then on January 23, there were no patients in the hospital who might serve as donors of a heart. At the same time he could not help wishing that fate would push him over the threshold into the heart transplantation he had been working toward for so long. He decided to keep Boyd Rush alive as long as possible. If in the interval fate provided a donor, he would act—using either the heart of the human donor or, if no donor was available, the heart of a chimpanzee.

Shortly after coming to this decision, he learned that a young man with fatal brain injuries had been taken to the intensive-care unit. An attempt had been made to keep him alive with artificial respiration. But the brain function had ceased, and only the mechanical respiration was keeping his heart going. As always, it was impossible to know how long it would continue to beat. This news from the intensive-care unit swung the decision.

James D. Hardy in retrospect:

"I called my crew together and said: 'Now, look, we might have to face the issue tonight.' "

Hardy sent for Mrs. Thompson to obtain her consent for a heart transplant. He knew that he might encounter incredulity, stunned incomprehension, or indignation; it was also possible that the woman would react with calm thoughtfulness, or simply with submission to the opinion of a noted surgeon. He was well aware that the proposal he was going to make had never before been put to the relatives of any patient. For the present, he decided, he would ask permission for amputation and for a surgical attempt to remove the blood clots from Boyd Rush's heart. Then he could explain that this effort might well be hopeless and propose, as an extreme chance to save Boyd, or at least to bring him back briefly to consciousness, the possibility of—a new heart.

James D. Hardy in Transplantation Proceedings, *June 1969:*

"The problem was discussed in detail with the relatives, including the fact that heart transplantation was being considered only if all else failed. . . . The possibility of using a lower primate heart was acknowledged in discussion with the recipient's relatives, should the anticipated death of the patient with massive brain injury not occur. Furthermore it was candidly stated that while we and others had performed many heart transplants in animals, this would represent the first heart transplant in man."

The relatives in the plural was a slight exaggeration—the only relative was Mrs. J. H. Thompson. But since she believed that men who stood so high in the ranks of Mississippi surgery and medicine as Dr. Hardy must be judging and acting rightly, she signed the following document:

OPERATIVE PERMIT

I hereby give full permission for left leg amputation and heart surgery on Boyd Rush. I understand that any clots present will be removed from the heart to stop them from going to still more arteries of his body. I further understand that his heart is in extremely poor condition. If for any unanticipated reason the heart should fail completely during either operation and it should be impossible to start it, I agree to the insertion of a suitable heart transplant if such should be available at the time. I further understand that hundreds of heart transplants have been performed in laboratories throughout the world but that any heart transplant would represent the initial transplant in man.

Signed (for family) *Mrs. J. H. Thompson* (sister)

The document was witnessed by Maurine Twiss of the public relations department of the Medical Center and by Phoebe Ward, a nurse. The words "suitable heart transplant" opened the way for implantation of either a human or a chimpanzee heart.

The amputation of Boyd Rush's leg formed only a minor prelude to the great event. Light narcosis administered through the tracheotomy tube sufficed, and the doctors were able to carry out the amputation with remarkable speed.

Hardy hoped to be able to keep Rush alive until the donor's heart stopped beating; then he would begin at once with the transplantation. While both his teams waited, he sent one of his anesthetists to the intensive-care unit at regular intervals to check the condition of the donor's heart. Hour after hour, the man returned with word that the heart was still beating vigorously. Meanwhile, Boyd Rush's condition steadily deteriorated. His breathing weakened, portending the imminent collapse of the heart-lung system. Even large quantities of drugs no longer sufficed to maintain a blood pressure of at least 90. Then—toward six o'clock in the evening—came a sudden alarm. Rush had fallen into shock. His blood pressure dropped to 40. As soon as the mechanical respiration was interrupted, his breathing stopped.

James D. Hardy in retrospect:

"Obviously Boyd Rush's heart was going to arrest momentarily, so my total energies were concentrated on getting him to Operating Room 6 . . . and . . . on the pump in very short order, or we wouldn't have any possibility of transplanting anything."

Hardy, Dr. Carlos M. Chavez, Dr. William A. Neely, Dr. Fred D. Kurrus, Dr. Allen U. Hollis, Dr. Robert D. Williams, Dr. Thaddeus D. Labecki (the anesthetist), Dr. Leonard W. Fabian, Dr. Don Turner (the physiologist), Helen W. Carr (the heart-lung pump technician), and Hardy's operating room nurses, Joyce F. Caracci and Ruby Nell Winters, were assembled in Operating Room 6 within the shortest possible time. Twenty minutes later Boyd Rush's feebly twitching heart had been exposed. The operation truly took place at the last minute, for at the very moment the heart-lung machine took over his circulation, his heart stopped.

Hurriedly, Hardy had the donor's condition checked. But the anesthetist who ran to the intensive-care unit reported that no failure of the heartbeat could be expected—unless the mechanical respiration were switched off. Since this was considered inconceivable, two possibilities remained. Either the heart-lung machine would be disconnected and Boyd Rush would die in the operating room, or a chimpanzee heart would have to be implanted.

Hardy gave orders to have the largest of his chimpanzees stunned sufficiently so that he could be brought to Operating Room 5 and placed under anesthesia. Simultaneously, the key members of his two teams, Dr. Neely, Dr. Fabian, Dr. Chavez, and Dr. Labecki, gathered beside the operating table where Boyd Rush lay with his already arrested heart.

It was 7:50 P.M. when Hardy began clamping off the blood vessels that connected Boyd Rush's circulation with his heart and removing the heart in the same way that he had practiced so many times. At the same time the chimpanzee lay in Operating Room 5. There Chavez headed the team. Within twenty-five minutes he had severed the chimpanzee's pulmonary artery and aorta and removed a part of the atrium, along with the vena cava and the pulmonary veins. The operation followed the procedures worked out for years. A catheter was introduced into the coronary vessels. After a rinsing with Ringer's solution, oxygen-enriched blood was pumped through, and Chavez carried the slightly fibrillating heart into Room 6, where Hardy was working.

At 8:15 P.M. Hardy began the implantation of the chimpanzee heart into the empty, blood-flecked space where Boyd Rush's heart had been feebly beating a short time before. He connected the matching surfaces of the atria, then the pulmonary artery and aorta. The whole operation went much more smoothly than he had imagined, because Boyd Rush's blood vessels were larger than the vessels of the experimental animals. At nine o'clock he removed the catheter from the coronary artery and opened the clamps around Rush's cardiac blood vessels. Next moment, the blood pumped by the heart-lung machine streamed into the new heart.

James D. Hardy in retrospect:

"All the while I was under terrible tension. Because, you see, Dr. Webb and I had done all the hearts together, but just in December he had taken the chair at Southwestern Medical School in Dallas. . . . With him not here, it was pretty much on me. . . . I was afraid the heart wouldn't start."

But Hardy's fears were unfounded. A few seconds after Boyd Rush's warm blood poured into the chimpanzee heart, the ventricles began violently fibrillating. A single shock with the electric defibrillator sufficed to produce a regular heartbeat. Boyd Rush's heart began pumping at 80 beats per minute.

It was an indescribable moment: the first foreign heart beating in a human chest.

The heart continued to beat regularly, and bit by bit Hardy reduced the support of the heart-lung machine. At 8:45 P.M. the last connecting catheter was removed. The first act of the fantastic adventure, of the push into new dimensions, seemed successfully completed.

Then, only minutes later, the heart began to swell, and its beat faltered. Hardy injected digitalis to increase performance. Anxiously, he asked himself: was the chimpanzee heart, in spite of its capacity of 4.2 liters of blood per minute, too weak to receive the venous stream from Boyd Rush's body and return it to the circulatory system?

In order to increase the beat, Hardy sewed the electrodes of a Chardack pacemaker into the wall of the heart. The beat was set at 100 per minute—and the chimpanzee heart obediently followed the impulses. Yet even at a hundred beats it was capable of maintaining the blood pressure only between 60 and 90. Between 10:00 and 10:30 P.M. Hardy began desperate cardiac massage. But half an hour later it became irrevocably clear that the chimpanzee heart did not have the strength to maintain human circulation. At eleven o'clock Hardy, exhausted, abandoned the massage. The heart beat on for a while, regularly, but more and more feebly, until it stopped. The Imuran, which was to have prevented Boyd Rush's body from rejecting the new heart, remained unused on an instrument table.

When Hardy left the operating room, he found himself facing some twenty hospital doctors who had gathered, at the rumor of a heart transplant, outside Operating Rooms 5 and 6. Their attitude gave him a foretaste of what he assumed he would have to face: curiosity, surprise, horror, agreement, doubt, or pensiveness. At the moment he had no idea that as far as public reverberations were concerned, his operation would meet the same fate as his lung transplant: it would be ignored or quickly forgotten. When the public relations department of the Medical Center issued a press release on the heart transplant on the morning of January 24, it forgot to state explicitly that a chimpanzee rather than a human heart had been transplanted. While the first newspaper reports were coming out, it sent in its correction. But the enthusiasm of press and radio had quickly died with the death of the patient, and few of the corrections were printed. Hardy encountered none of the violent emotional uproar he had feared from the general public.

He did, however, have to face storms within the medical profession. When he flew to New Orleans on January 24 to attend a meeting of the Southern Society of Clinical Investigation, he was encouraged by Keith Reemtsma. Reemtsma had lost Jefferson Davis, but his optimism was now based on his next patient, Edith Parker. When Hardy discussed the transplant at a dinner with Reemtsma and several other surgeons from Tulane Medical Center, Reemtsma said:

"If it beat for two hours, someday it will go on beating."

Two weeks later, on February 8, Hardy went to New York to face the Sixth International Transplantation Congress. From the majority of those present he encountered outright hostility and condemnation. But he had expected to be attacked, and replied: "Yes, my patient did not live long. He did not come out of the anesthesia. But I have proved for the first time that a heart can be transplanted into a human being and will begin to beat again. If an animal heart beats in man, a human heart certainly will. It is only a question of time before I or you transplant a human heart, and it will beat not for a short time, but for much longer. If what I have done prompts all of us to concern ourselves more intensely with the new horizon of heart transplantation, then I have brought medicine closer to this horizon."

By the time he left New York and flew back to Jackson, he was convinced that the storm of indignation would only promote further work and accelerate the march into the future. But even as he was boarding the plane, the New York medical world was overtaken by a scandal that had broken around the time Boyd Rush was taken to Jackson. The scandal involved the Jewish Chronic Disease Hospital in Brooklyn. There, in July 1963, doctors under the direction of Dr. Chester M. Southam had injected cancer cells into patients who did not have cancer, allegedly without their knowledge. While Hardy was flying back to Mississippi, the waves of this scandal surged as far as Washington. The result was a strong reaction against any medical experiments using human beings as subjects. Any further development of heart transplantation was suspended. And so America, where most of the basic research had been carried out, for a time bowed out of the endeavor.

When Hardy arrived back in Mississippi, he found a note informing him that Boyd Rush had been given a quiet burial.

2 / Louis Washkansky
Philip Blaiberg

Journal of the American Medical Association, *November 20, 1967:*

" 'We think the way is clear for trial of human heart transplantation,' says surgeon Norman E. Shumway (Stanford University).

" 'We have achieved a degree of experience with heart transplantation in the laboratory with which we feel confident we can take appropriate care of the patient with a cardiac transplant. . . . Although animal work should and will continue, we are more or less at the threshold of clinical application.' "

Newsweek, *December 18, 1967:*

THE HEART: MIRACLE IN CAPE TOWN

"Early Sunday morning, December 3, in Cape Town, South Africa, Dr. Christian Neethling Barnard and a 30-man surgical team at Groote Schuur Hospital . . . removed [Louis] Washkansky's own incurably diseased heart and replaced it with a healthy heart from Denise Ann Darvall, an automobile-accident victim."

Louis Washkansky was a baby when the soldiers of the Czar came, declared that all the inhabitants of Slabodka were spies for the Germans, loaded them into cattle cars, and transported them across Russia in a journey that lasted seven days. Slabodka was the Jewish quarter of Kovno, in the Lithuanian province of the Czarist Empire; and the animosity of the Czar made life so difficult for Jews that, at the beginning of 1914, Louis's father had emigrated to South Africa where, he had heard, Jews were able to live in freedom. Washkansky, a dealer in groceries, had never paid close attention to politics; even if he had, it surely would not have occurred to him that a world war and a revolution were about to break out and separate him from his family.

As the cattle cars rolled over the endless plains, Louis's mother and elder sisters, Tevja, Leah, and Anna, feared that the journey would end in Siberia. They were immensely relieved when the doors were at last unlocked and they found themselves in Melitopol, in the Crimea. They located a cottage and opened up a small shop in which they sold stockings. Sometimes hungry, sometimes freezing, sometimes healthy, sometimes sick, they endured four years of war and two years of revolution. They survived looting and mistreatment from the White Guard and from Bolsheviks. After six years they set out on the endless homeward journey to Slabodka, where they found nothing but their vacant house. There were two more years to get through until at last they were able to take ship to the Cape of Good Hope.

Louis was now nine years old. In those nine years he had lost the ability to cry when he was beaten or whimper when he was hungry and cold. He had seen more of the cruelty and unpredictability of life than millions of older persons, and he had learned such stoicism that hardly anything could get him down. At the same time he had grasped the idea that every chance must be seized and every good moment enjoyed as if there were no tomorrow.

From the moment he entered his new home in the Gardens District of Cape Town, Louis discovered that poverty and hunger were not, after all, unalterable facts of life. But by then the foundations of his character had been formed. He did not become a bookish person. In the Physical Culture Palace of Cape Town he trained himself to be an athlete who could "take it" physically as well as psychologically and who was quite ready to fight with his fists if necessary.

He grew up into a tall, broad-shouldered young man with a vigorous nose, wide mouth, and strong hands—no beauty, but a man like a rock. Like his father, he went into the grocery trade, and worked for a wholesaler. His exuberance and his gift of gab made him popular wherever he went. Among his many friends there was a saying that nobody could ever get "Washy" down. He was the kind of man, they said, who could be dropped in a desert without water and would come riding home on a camel with a case of beer.

Louis Washkansky proved the truth of that saying in 1940, when he joined a unit of South African engineers that fought in Kenya, Egypt, and Italy. Although he was in many hard battles, he returned home without a scratch. Back in Cape Town he met the sister of a friend, a pretty girl with a motherly disposition named Ann Sklar. They married. Louis opened a business of his own and lost it when it was bought out by a large firm. Without complaint he started out afresh as a salesman, driving about the countryside in his red car. He worked like a demon, had a good house for Ann and his son, Michael, in Sea Point, and evidently enjoyed every second of his life. In his world of salesmen and sportsmen, a party was a party only when "Washy" was there.

In 1955, at the age of forty-one, he suddenly began suffering from acute thirst. When Ann at last made him go to a doctor, it turned out that he had diabetes. Thereafter he took his pills dutifully, but gave no thought to letting up on his work. In 1959, at the age of forty-five, while driving to see a customer, he suddenly had a bout of sickness behind the wheel. The pain in his chest was terrible. But he kept on driving and saw his man, and not until a year later did it come out that he had suffered a heart attack. In December 1960 he had another—this time after a Saturday-night barbecue party. At seven o'clock in the morning Ann found him in the dining room, pacing around and around the table and waving his arms. He said he had a pain between his shoulder blades. When she asked whether she should call a doctor and he nodded, she guessed that something really unusual had happened. For ordinarily Louis wanted nothing to do with doctors.

The doctor said he was suffering from angina pectoris and must be rushed to a hospital. Louis refused; all he needed was to rest in his own bed, he insisted. After a few weeks in bed, he got up again, took some new pills, and resumed driving about as usual.

He refused to recognize that he now tired quickly, had frequent chest pains, and sometimes had to stop by the side of the road. For five years he continued in this way. Then, in 1965, while he was driving in Rondebosch, he was stricken by such terrible pains in his left arm that even his capacity for "taking it" reached its limit. He stumbled into a store and asked the owner to take him to the nearest doctor. But the doctor was out on call. Another doctor was likewise not at home. It was an hour before they reached the Rondebosch Cottage Hospital. There Louis got out of the car and staggered, ferociously determined to stay on his feet, up a flight of stairs. At the top he keeled over like a felled tree. He had suffered his third heart attack and finally done grave damage to his heart muscle.

Nevertheless, it was impossible to keep him in bed for more than a few weeks. He mutinied, and would get up whenever he was not being watched. At the end of the third or fourth week he was discharged, supposedly because the hospital was no longer willing to take responsibility for him. By now he had changed outwardly; he was short of breath and often had swollen feet. Yet he still refused to admit that there was anything wrong with his heart. He swallowed new medicines and continued to crawl into the driver's seat of his car to visit his customers. When they asked him about his health, he replied: "I won't let a little thing like that bother me. How about another drink—and what can I provide you with this week?"

In 1966 the nights became an ordeal for him. His gasping for breath would awaken Ann; she would be sure he was dying. After a few weeks he told her: "There's nothing wrong with me. But since it worries you so much, let's go see a doctor." And so they went to Dr. Kaplan. Kaplan found damaged coronary vessels and signs of several past heart attacks, incipient kidney failure, lung congestion, and the beginnings of dropsy. He said he was afraid Louis Washkansky would not survive more than a few months unless he went to a hospital. But Washkansky replied that he had better things to do than lie around in a hospital. He knew nothing whatsoever about heart disease and was not of a mind to learn. All he would take from the doctor were prescriptions for new pills; then he went back to work. It took him longer to make his rounds, and the number of customers he could visit in a day steadily diminished.

By the end of 1966, Washkansky was no longer able to get into his car. He spat blood. Fluid accumulated in his legs. But as soon as he succeeded in purging the fluid by taking a murderous quantity of Lasix, he would be on his way again, or he would take Ann to a soccer game or a party where he would announce: "Washkansky is feeling fine."

In February 1967 he collapsed, losing consciousness several times. Now he could no longer conceal his condition from Ann. Kaplan made him promise to go to Groote Schuur Hospital for an examination. Ann drove him to the huge, red-roofed "building of a thousand beds" which towers over the districts of Observatory, Salt River, and Woodstock. Louis settled into a bed in Dr. Velva ("Val") Schrire's cardiac clinic with the intransigent announcement that he would be back home in a few days.

Kaplan knew that the hospital had an outstanding heart-surgery team under a young doctor named Barnard. Barnard had gone all the way to America to learn open-heart surgery in Minneapolis and had brought the first heart-lung machine to Cape Town. In the past several years he had carried out a large number of heart operations, mostly repairs of valve defects, and had several times removed aneurysms from hearts. Since Kaplan assumed that Washkansky had probably developed an aneurysm, he hoped that this capable cardiac man might be able to do something for his patient.

Schrire's assistants refused to let Washkansky go home after a few days, however much he blustered. The findings of the angiocardiogram were fearful. The greater part of the muscle in the left ventricle had been destroyed. The heart was immensely enlarged. It was also swollen by an aneurysm. Instead of the normal quantity of about 15 liters, it was pumping only 2.5 liters of blood per minute. Two coronary arteries were completely blocked, and the third was so stenotic that the heart muscle was barely receiving enough blood and oxygen to keep going. Dr. Barnard, the heart surgeon, did not even see Washkansky. On being shown the results of the examination, he refused to operate because he was sure the patient would die on the table. Since Schrire saw no way to do anything for Washkansky, he sent him home as incurable.

But no sooner was Washkansky back home than he again began telephoning his customers. He assured everybody that he was perfectly all right. He did, however, take one measure because of his illness: he wrote to the South African police reserve asking to have his name removed from the list of reservists because he was not entirely up to the work.

By September 14 so much fluid had accumulated in his body that he was afraid he would soon be unable to breathe at all. This time he was docile about going to the hospital. Schrire's staff tried everything to reduce the quantity of fluid. Finally they resorted to an old and brutal method of treatment: they sat Washkansky in a chair, placed his feet in basins, and inserted needles under the skin. For almost a week Washkansky sat while incredible quantities of water dripped from his legs. But he assured his wife: "Don't worry. I'll make it." He tried to conceal from her the fact that one of his hands was shaking—the consequence of a slight stroke.

After he had been put back to bed, he became delirious. The needle wounds on his left leg became inflamed; the doctors expected his death at any moment. But he did not die. Early in November he lay drowsing in a ward. Professor Schrire informed Ann that he would have to be transferred to a home for terminal cases; he certainly could not be allowed to go back home. Weeping, Ann signed permission for Louis's transfer to the Conradie Nursing Home. At her next visit Ann finally got up the courage to tell Louis where he was being sent. He knew the Conradie Nursing Home and knew, also, that it was opposite the Jewish Cemetery. When he saw Ann crying, he tried to laugh—although the effort produced only a grimace—and said: "Why, that's fine. When the time comes I won't have far to go, just across the street."

That was November 10, 1967. The following night he sat half upright in bed, because it was easier for him to breathe that way, and smoked a cigarette. He was not supposed to smoke, of course, but the doctors and nurses had given up trying to stop him. His inflamed leg lay outside the blanket, resting on a chair. He was not expecting any more visits; Ann and his niece Chava had already gone. Suddenly the door opened. Dr. Kaplan came in, and with a curious earnestness sat down beside the bed and said he had something to discuss with him.

He had talked with Professor Schrire, Kaplan said, and Schrire said there was a chance to replace Washkansky's heart with a healthy heart from another person.

Washkansky looked at Kaplan under his heavy eyebrows; there was a greater keenness in his eyes, but no sign of emotion. Then he said: "If that's the only chance, I'll take it."

He did not ask what was involved. Perhaps he was no more interested in this than in all the other medical matters, which he regarded chiefly as things done to him rather than for him. He had simply accepted these painful measures as he did all the inevitable buffets of life. Perhaps he also did not ask because he intuitively realized that another person would have to die for him to have a new heart, and he was repressing all thoughts about the origins of this heart.

Kaplan asked him to think the matter over and told him that no such heart transplant had ever been done. This would be the first time, he said. But Washkansky stuck to his guns; if this was the only chance, he wanted to take it.

After Kaplan, still astonished at his lack of curiosity, had left, Washkansky turned to the other patients in the room. "Did you hear that?" he said. "They're going to give me a new heart."

The others thought he was delirious again and did not take him seriously.

Next day Professor Schrire, thin, bespectacled, and grave, appeared at Washkansky's bed. He had to assure himself that Kaplan had reported the conversation correctly, for he could hardly believe that a patient would have said yes to such a proposal, without alarm at the monstrous notion, without any anxious questions. But Washkansky asked Schrire only if it was true that they wanted to give him a new heart, and added that he wanted one.

A few hours later he was sitting in bed trying to read. Ever since he had been forced to accept the fact that he was a doomed man, Ann had been bringing him mystery stories. And he read whenever he was not feeling too weak.

A young man in a white smock entered the room. Washkansky had never seen him before.

He was a very skinny fellow and had thin, rather irregular features. His right ear was higher than his left, and his jaw, too, seemed slightly askew. A strand of dark hair hung over his forehead. He brushed it back after he had closed the door behind him, and came up to Washkansky's bed. He said that he was Professor Barnard, the heart surgeon, and that he intended to do the heart transplant that Professor Schrire and Dr. Kaplan had told him about. If Washkansky was still willing, he would transfer him to his own ward.

Washkansky laid the detective story on his blanket and looked at his visitor over the rim of his glasses. The fellow seemed very young to be a professor. But, after all, new things generally came from young people.

With an effort he said: "That's fine with me—I'm ready and waiting for it."

He saw that the skinny young man with the light blue eyes was looking at him with the same surprise that Schrire had shown. The young professor offered to explain whatever he would like to know about transplanting a new heart. Professor Schrire had done everything he could to help Washkansky, he said, but in vain. If he wanted to lead a normal life, there was only one chance: to remove his ruined heart and replace it with a new one.

Washkansky replied that he had heard all that before. What was the need of explanations? It was all logical and clear. If part of a machine was ruined, no amount of repairs would help. The ruined part had to be replaced. Anybody could understand that. And he repeated: "So, I'm ready to go ahead."

These words sounded so final that Barnard could only take his leave. "Well then, good-bye," he said.

When Ann came to visit shortly afterward, Washkansky said to her: "The big bugs came to see me. They're going to give me a brand-new heart."

For a moment Ann Washkansky thought he was delirious again. The way people doubted him was so irritating; he struggled for air to tell them so. To calm him, they pretended to believe every word. And next day he told other visitors the same story. All thought he no longer knew what he was saying; but they pretended to believe him in order to keep him calm.

Twenty-four hours later Ann came to the hospital and found him absent from the room he had occupied for two months. Terrified that he had died, she ran about looking for someone to ask. She was told that he had been shifted upstairs to Ward C-2. She found him in a private room. Only then did she realize that he had not been having fantasies, but had told her the truth—or, at any rate, she realized that something unusual was afoot. Before she could pull herself together, a young doctor whom she had not seen before entered the room. He came up to her and introduced himself as Dr. Barnard. He added that he was the man who wanted to give Louis a new heart. As he spoke, she felt horrified, not only by what he was saying, but also because he looked so boyish. How could this boy think of doing something so inconceivable?

The doctor saw her recoil and tried to explain what a heart transplant involved. But she broke in with a terrified question: had he ever done such an operation before?

"No," he replied, and spoke about animal experiments. It was Louis's only chance, he said. Shakily she asked him: "Suppose it fails?"

"Even a tonsillectomy can fail," he replied.

"Professor Barnard, what chance do you give him?" Ann asked.

"An 80-per-cent chance," Barnard replied.

After Barnard had left Ann bent over Louis. "Louis, for heaven's sake, do you know what you're doing?" she asked.

"I want the new heart," Louis said with an effort.

From an unpublished review of the book One Life, *by Christiaan Barnard and Curtis Bill Pepper (New York: The Macmillan Company, 1969):*

"Here, then, we have the story of the man who in November 1967 undertook the first human heart transplant on Louis Washkansky.

"As far as the facts of his life are concerned, this book at first seems to offer little that is new to us. Once more we have the story, told over and over again in thousands of articles since 1967, of the poor boy Christiaan Barnard who was born in 1922 in a settlement of the South African semi-desert, the Karoo. We meet father Adam Barnard, the impecunious Afrikaans minister who preaches to a colored congregation. There is Elizabeth Barnard, the mother of four barefoot sons, all of whom she sends to the university. And there is Christiaan himself; the medical student in Cape Town who never goes to a movie and daily walks four miles to school to save fare. In 1946 he becomes a doctor, in 1948 he marries the nurse Louwtjie, practices in the provincial town of Ceres, by 1950 realizes his vocation as a surgeon and researcher, and returns, wretchedly poor, to Cape Town. In City Hospital he develops a new treatment for meningitis; in 1954, in Groote Schuur Hospital, working in a third-rate animal laboratory, he discovers a surgical method for curing a congenital intestinal defect; in 1955 he receives an American fellowship. We see the young man scrubbing floors in Minneapolis and earning his doctorate in half the normal time. With C. Walton Lillehei he learns open-heart surgery, is given a heart-lung machine when he returns to South Africa, and in July 1958 performs the first heart-valve operation in Cape Town, on the colored South African woman Joan Pick.

"In 1962, at the age of forty, he is appointed professor, later chief of the department of thoracic surgery. By now our poor boy has become world-famous. He builds his group of heart surgeons into a transplant team because he is thinking of doing kidney transplants. Once again, in 1966, he receives a fellowship from America to study kidney transplantation under Dr. Hume in Richmond. There he meets Dr. Richard Lower, who worked for ten years with Norman E. Shumway in Palo Alto developing the methods for heart transplantation. Christiaan learns how a heart might be transplanted were it not for so many biological and ethical problems. The rest of the story involves the hero's perception that here is a vast realm that can be explored for the benefit of mankind. He returns to Cape Town and begins his courageous endeavors toward the first human heart transplant.

"Viewed in this light, we do not seem to be learning anything from *One Life* that has not been wearisomely told and retold. And yet, for the attentive reader, there is a good deal that is new here. For the book contains the first real answer to the question of why the first human heart transplant was not done in America, where all the preliminary research was undertaken. Men like Shumway or Lower or even Kantrowitz in New York were like swimmers standing around a pool. The question was, which would be the first to overcome the last moral scruples and dive in.

"The answer is implicit in *One Life*, for the book is the story of a consuming passion for success. Here is a boy whose mother impressed upon him that he must always be first, never second; a boy who never bowed to the fact that he could not catch up to the best runner in his school. When he passes an examination in physics, he asks his teacher to let him repeat it, because his mark was not high enough. He loses his first girl friend not because he is poor, but because she charges him: 'You've disciplined yourself like a machine.' As a young practitioner in Ceres he cannot stand his rejection by the townspeople and plunges into the world of medical research in order to compensate. As a young surgeon, he diagnoses arthritis in his own hands—and is compelled to even greater efforts to win success before it is too late. Temporarily frustrated on his way 'to the top,' he pours his ambition into the career of his daughter Deirdre who has a talent for water-skiing. He tries to make her a world champion and is able to analyse his own motives unsparingly:

She had, I felt, the making of a champion. At that point, I was hooked on her career. I did not know how far I would eventually go in heart surgery. . . . Maybe we would make it, maybe not. There was no doubt, however, about this little girl. . . . Deirdre's picture was in all the papers. I was wreathed in her glory. . . . At the same time I became concerned about Deirdre ever reaching the top. She was, I feared, too nice a girl. She did not have the killer instinct needed to become a world champion. . . . Deirdre had the natural ability to become a champion. Yet it also required drive and discipline, and I had thought I could make up for any she lacked. But it was becoming clear you could not transfer that to someone else. . . . I had failed to transplant into her my own hunger for victory. . . . The time had come to cease using my daughter to satisfy my own ambitions. . . . No longer compelled to transfer myself into my daughter's career, I could concentrate on a far larger transplant.

"The audacity of this young man is amazing. With what he had learned in America, after only a few animal experiments of his own and a single kidney transplant, with what today seems a naïve understanding of rejection problems, he went to Professor Val Schrire in October 1967 and asked him for a patient for a heart transplant. He describes his discussion with the professor as follows:

"Everything is ready," I said. "We have the team and we know how to do it."

"How do you know? . . . Your dogs don't live very long. You should get longer survivors before you try this." . . .

"I'm not trying to get longer survivors in dogs. I can't nurse a dog like a human being. I can't handle a dog on immunosuppressive drugs as I can a human being."

"I don't know."

"Well, I know. I studied it in Richmond, and we have applied it here successfully with the kidney transplant. I know how to handle such a patient. All we need now is for you to give us one."

"We have first to consider all the risks."

"What risks are you talking about?" I asked, trying to control myself. "We're preparing to do this on a patient with irreversible disease who is beyond hope of recovery, and who has only a few days or hours of life—you call that a risk?"

"Some people will."

"Not the man who's about to die—and you know it, Val. He will beg you for it. He'll beg you for the chance. Because that's what it means to him—a chance, not a risk." . . .

All through the last two weeks of October I kept after Professor Schrire—plaguing him day and night.

"Finally we come to the point in the story when a hesitant Professor Schrire turns over the needed patient: the stoically dying Louis Washkansky. Barnard writes of the patient in his coolly analytical manner:

Since then, many people have said it was very brave of Louis Washkansky to accept a heart transplant. They really mean it would be brave for them to accept one—not Washkansky. For a dying man, it is not a difficult decision because he knows he is at an end. If a lion chases you to the bank of a river filled with crocodiles, you will leap into the water convinced you have a chance to swim to the other side. But you would never accept such odds if there were no lion.

"After the self-portrait emerging from these quotations, we know why Barnard was the first to jump into the pool while the Americans, well prepared though they were, stood hesitantly around it. He knew less about what awaited him in the way of medical and biological surprises, but he surpassed all rivals in his consuming drive for success, in the determination to be the first, to shatter the taboos that had hampered whole generations of doctors."

.   .   .

On November 14, 1967, Louis Washkansky began his wait for a new heart. He knew quite well that death was lurking around the next corner, though he denied his knowledge, and that the new heart was his last and almost incredible chance for life. He was afraid he might die before this young doctor could give it to him. But he kept up his spirits with an outward brashness. When Barnard and another doctor came to see him, on the second day after his transfer to Barnard's ward, he joked—in a voice so changed by his shortness of breath that it was barely recognizable: "Where's the new heart? When you came in, I thought you had it with you."

Medical notes, November 14–22, 1967:

After patient's consent had been obtained, preparations for the heart transplant were begun.

1. Preparatory measures for tissue-compatibility determination.
   a. Washkansky's blood group is A Rhesus-positive.
   b. Dr. Marthinius Botha, the immunologist, has employed the method recently developed by van Rood and Teraski for tissue matching.
2. International experience with kidney transplants shows that weakening of the immunological defenses by antirejection drugs can lead to fatal infections caused not only by outside agents, but also by bacteria normally present and harmless in or on the recipient's body. Dr. Forder, the bacteriologist, is carrying out continuous checks of Washkansky's own germs. Swabs of skin, nose, ear, throat, mouth, ureter, and rectum have been taken and cultured. The whole body is being repeatedly washed with antiseptic solutions. One source of danger is the infection of the left leg. Klebsiella germs have been detected here. Treatment with antibiotics has not eliminated this focus of infection. It remains a danger.
3. Room 270 is being prepared as an aseptic room for Washkansky after the operation.
4. All personnel who will be caring for the patient are being checked for virulent organisms.
5. Dr. LeRoux is building a temporary mobile cobalt radiation apparatus. If necessary, every available antirejection method will be employed, including cobalt radiation.
6. Review of all reports from America and England on the signs of incipient rejection. The conclusions are more confusing than informative. Shumway believes that certain changes in the EKG indicate the onset of rejection.

7. Because of this uncertainty, constant studies of Washkansky's blood status, electrolyte balance, enzymes, liver, kidneys, lung function, and EKG are being carried out. Changes in these after transplantation may be indications of beginning rejection. It remains difficult to distinguish between incipient rejection and infection.

8. Preparations are being made for a daily conference of the hospital's specialists after transplantation, to discuss the patient's condition and the possibility of rejection and infection. In addition to Dr. Christiaan Barnard, Dr. Botha, Dr. Arderne Forder, and Professor Schrire, participants will be Professor Palmer (X ray), Professor James Kench (biochemistry), Dr. Reuben Mibashan (hematology), Dr. Geoffrey Thatcher (nephrology), Dr. William Jackson (diabetes), and Dr. Simcha Banks (gastroenterology).

9. The emergency room and the department of neurosurgery (Dr. Peter Rose-Innes) have been requested to report the next patient suitable as a heart donor and after contacting the relatives to transfer him to Ward C-2.

10. It has been decided to transfer the donor, after determination of brain death, to Operating Room B and Washkansky to Operating Room A. As soon as Washkansky is prepared for implantation of the heart, artificial respiration of the donor will be interrupted. The heart will then be removed and transplanted to the recipient. Recipient operating team: Professor Christiaan Barnard, Dr. Rodnew Hewitson, Dr. François Hitchcock, Dr. Siebert Bosman, Dr. Joseph Ozinsky (anesthesia).
Donor operating team: Dr. Marius Barnard, Dr. Terry O'Donovan, Dr. Coert Venter, Dr. Cecil Moss (anesthesia).

For a few days Washkansky let up on his everlasting demands for a new heart. It was clear enough that something was being done. Doctors, technicians, and nurses swarmed around his bed. But soon his temperamental impatience reasserted itself. "Why are you stuffing me with so many pills for my old heart if you're going to give me a spare?" he would demand. Or he would declare: "As soon as the new pump is working Washkansky's going to give a party and teach you how to dance." While red streaks from his leg moved ominously up toward his abdomen, he continued to insist—but always in his characteristically proud, oblique fashion. "Washkansky's getting the hell out of here," he would announce. "This comedy has gone on long enough."

Washkansky did not know that Barnard himself, because he could see the patient's rapid decline, was waiting in near despair for a donor. Barnard's state of tension kept discharging against everyone around him, so that the whole team rejoiced when, on November 23, a seventeen-year-old boy named Hendrick Tobias, who had been run over by a car, was brought dying into the Groote Schuur Hospital. Dr. Rose-Innes declared that Tobias's brain was dead. Barnard called together his team, and one of the assistants rushed into Washkansky's room to tell him: "We have the heart."

Washkansky was washed with antiseptic solution. His chest and belly were shaved. Then hour after hour passed, and still he was not taken to the operating room. It had proved impossible to get in touch with the boy's parents, and without their consent the heart could not be used. By the time they were reached, hours had passed, and in spite of artificial respiration the condition of Tobias's heart had so deteriorated that it could no longer be used. By six o'clock in the evening the transplant had to be canceled. No one wanted to tell Washkansky, and so Barnard, painfully concealing his own disappointment and exhaustion, had to do it. When Ann entered the room a short time later, she found Louis livid with helpless anger. He said: "I'm getting out of here!" although, in fact, he was incapable of moving.

It was a long time before he calmed down. His temper became worse on the following weekend. For he knew that most of the doctors were going to the country, and he was therefore convinced that for at least another two days nobody would give a thought to his new heart. He refused to calm down even when he was told that every doctor could be reached immediately and rushed back to the hospital as soon as a heart was available.

During the entire week that began on Monday, November 27, Washkansky continued to rebel. At times he was unconscious, but as soon as he came to again he took up his complaint: "Where's my heart?" Or he would pant: "What do you think my customers would say if I kept my promises the way you do yours?"

As the weekend of December 2–3 approached, a new wave of the despair he usually managed to conceal came over him. "Now they're all going to play golf," he whispered. "And Washkansky just lies here and waits." When Barnard said good-bye on Saturday, Washkansky was barely strong enough to put a handkerchief to his mouth. Nevertheless he grumbled: "Everybody's left. Even Frumilla from the lab is going to a party tonight. I suppose you're going sailing or fishing, too."

When Ann and Washkansky's sister, Anne Taibel, came to visit, they could scarcely get a word out of him. "I tell you, they're going to make me wait the same way next week," he whispered. "But not Washkansky. They can't do this to Washkansky." Ann prolonged her visit until he had calmed down somewhat; then she set out for home with her sister-in-law. On Main Road, in the vicinity of Coppenberg's Wrench Town Bakery, they saw a crowd and realized that there had been a traffic accident. They saw two women lying in the street. The police waved them on, and they drove past without for a moment thinking that there might be any connection between this accident and the heart that Louis was waiting for so desperately.

Washkansky himself lay dozing after an injection. He woke up occasionally and then fell asleep again, until sometime late in the evening he saw the figure of a doctor standing by his bed and dimly heard the words: "Louis, we have the heart." He woke up and, struggling for breath, replied: "I don't believe you any more. You told me that before. I want to see the professor. Don't think I'll let you do anything to me until I see the professor."

But when a nurse came and began shaving and preparing him, he did not fend her off. And when Barnard, pale with tension, stepped to his bedside for a moment, he began to believe that this time it was the real thing. Later, toward one o'clock in the morning, Dr. Ozinsky came to his room. The anesthetist, a young man with a broad, friendly face, accompanied him to the operating room. Because of his shortness of breath, he had to be kept sitting upright in his bed, which was wheeled directly into the elevator.

In Operating Room A he waited on the table, still sitting, until Barnard came to see him once more. He still felt or pretended to feel a touch of mistrust, for he asked in a whisper whether he was really going to be given the new heart now. Only after Barnard said yes did he lie back to receive the anesthesia. He went under at 1:30 A.M.

Cape Town, Saturday, December 2, 1967, 3:20 P.M., to Sunday, December 3, 1967, 6:50 A.M.; from a factual summary:

DECEMBER 2, 1967

3:20 P.M.   Denise Darvall, 25, a bank employee in Cape Town, goes for a drive with her father, Edward George Darvall, 66, her mother, Myrtle Ann Darvall, 53, and her brother, Keith.

3:30 P.M.   Denise Darvall parks on Main Road and with her mother crosses the street to the baker to buy doughnuts.

3:40 P.M.   On the way back both women are struck by a car driven by Frederick Prins, 36, and mortally injured.

3:52 P.M.   Ambulance brings the two women and Edward Darvall to the emergency room at Groote Schuur. Dr. Rose-Innes, the neurosurgeon, examines the victims. Myrtle Ann Darvall is found to be dead. Denise Darvall: broken bones, severe skull fracture with brain exuding. Artificial respiration administered.

5:30 P.M. Denise Darvall's reflexes cease. Rigid pupils, flat electroencephalogram. Cessation of brain activity. With continuing artificial respiration, heartbeat remains virtually normal. Dr. Rose-Innes informs the cardiac surgery ward of potential heart donor.

6:00 P.M. Dr. Bosman and Dr. Venter transfer Denise Darvall to Room 283 in the cardiac ward. Artificial respiration continued. Stimulation of the heart by infusion of aludrine and supervision with an electrocardiographic monitor.

7:00 P.M. Dr. Botha informed and samples of Denise Darvall's blood turned over to him for blood group determination and tissue matching. Dr. Botha establishes relative compatibility within the limits of the tests he can make so quickly.

8:00 P.M. Dr. Bosman informs Barnard of the presence of a potential donor.

10:00 P.M. Dr. Bosman and Dr. Venter go to see Edward George Darvall, who has collapsed and is lying in a doctor's office. They tell him his daughter cannot be saved and point out that there is a man whose life can be saved if he permits the transplantation of Denise's heart.

10:04 P.M. Edward George Darvall signs the permission.

11:10 P.M. Barnard arrives at Groote Schuur. He examines the potential donor's electrocardiograms. A potassium infusion is given to maintain the strength of the heart.

11:40 P.M. Dr. Rose-Innes confirms brain death.

11:45 P.M. Telephone alert for the heart transplant team.
Louis Washkansky is informed and prepared for the operation.

DECEMBER 3, 1967

1:00 A.M. Denise Darvall, accompanied by portable respirator, transferred to Operating Room B.
Louis Washkansky transferred to Operating Room A.

1:30 A.M. Anesthesia of Louis Washkansky initiated.

1:40 A.M. Barnard, Dr. Moss, Dr. O'Donovan, Dr. Hitchcock, Dr. Marius Barnard in Room B. Final decision made to switch off Denise Darvall's artificial respiration and induce heart stoppage as soon as Washkansky's heart is exposed and the transplant can begin.

2:00 A.M.   Barnard in Room A. Dr. Hewitson opens up Washkansky's thoracic cavity and pericardial sac. Confirmation of the diagnosis: irreparable destruction of the coronary vessels and both ventricles. Washkansky attached to heart-lung machine No. 1.

2:10 A.M.   Barnard in Room B. Artificial respiration switched off. Cessation of support of the donor heart by aludrine, potassium, and isoprenaline. Continuing heartbeat. Discussion of possibility of immediately opening the thoracic cavity and exposing the heart, or waiting for final cessation of heartbeat. Decision to wait. Cessation of heartbeat after fifteen minutes. Injection of heparin. Opening of thoracic cavity. Attachment of Denise Darvall to heart-lung machine No. 2 to maintain blood supply of heart muscle. Hypothermia to 28 degrees centigrade.

2:36 A.M.   Barnard in Room A. Heart-lung machine No. 1 switched on. Incident: sclerotic changes in Washkansky's femoral artery interrupt the blood supply to the machine. In changing to a direct attachment of the machine to the aorta, a connection blows, spilling blood on the floor. Reconnection is managed seconds before Washkansky suffers fatal brain damage. Barnard in Room B. Removal of Denise Darvall's heart. It is placed in a basin of cold Ringer's solution.

3:01 A.M.   Heart is carried to Room A. Attached to a special pump that pumps Washkansky's chilled blood from the heart-lung machine through the coronary vessels. Removal of Washkansky's heart by the Shumway method, slightly varied. Insertion of the donor heart by same method.

5:15 A.M.   To permit the last sutures at the aorta, donor heart is cut off from coronary supply of blood, interrupting oxygen supply to the heart. Time of suture: 19 minutes.

5:34 A.M.   Unclamping of the aorta. Warmed blood pours into the new heart. Fibrillation. Infusion of Scoline, aludrine, potassium.

5:36–6:13 A.M.   Shock with defibrillator. Washkansky arches up from the shock. Beginning of heart activity. Pulse 100, blood pressure 85.

Heart-lung machine switched off. Heartbeat stops, blood pressure falls. Machine switched on again. Slow recovery of blood pressure. Fears that new heart will not act independently.

6:13–6:24 A.M.   Third attempt to switch off machine. Heart finally begins to beat more regularly. Barnard exclaims: *"Dit gaan werk!"* ("It's going to work!")

Infusion of protamine and hydrocortisone.

6:36 A.M.   Barnard informs the medical superintendent of the hospital, Dr. Jacobus Burger, that a heart transplant has been done.

CONCLUSION

1. In terms of surgical technique, the heart transplant performed on Louis Washkansky involved no important innovation. It represented primarily the application of principles already worked out in the United States.

2. The innovation lay in the realm of ethics and philosophy. Barnard crossed the frontier at which James D. Hardy had halted in 1964 and which all Americans hesitated to cross until the time of Barnard's operation. At 2:15 A.M. on the morning of December 3, Barnard, by switching off Denise Darvall's artificial respiration, brought about the cessation of her heartbeat. Even then he and his assistant O'Donovan shrank from the logical consequences of this act, which would have been to open the donor's thoracic cavity without waiting for the complete cessation of heartbeat, thus securing a more viable heart. In waiting they paid a last small tribute to the old notions of the connection between the heart and death. But fundamentally Barnard shattered these emotionally governed ethical taboos.

On the morning of December 3, 1967, Louis Washkansky, lying on the operating table, opened his eyes briefly. But he was still unconscious. As he was lifted to a sterile bed, Dr. Bosman stretched a tent over the bed to protect him from germs during the short ride back to his new, sterile room. Arrived there, Washkansky lay on his back, white and immobile. Through a tube running into his nose, a respirator drove oxygen into his lungs. A second tube through his nose extended into his stomach. Three plastic tubes came out of his veins. Drainage tubes connected his thoracic cavity with suction machines. Lines and pipes led to manometers, urine collectors, thermometers, and other measuring instruments. Electrodes and wires transmitted the impulses of his heart to the viewing screen of the electrocardiograph.

Through the tubes into his veins, blood and glucose flowed, along with hydrocortisone, prednisone, and Imuran, the defensive weapons against kidney rejection, which were now, for the first time in history, being used to combat rejection of a heart. In addition, aludrine, isoprenaline, lignocardine, and potassium to regulate the new heart were being dripped into Washkansky's blood vessels, increasing the stream of drugs that for years had been flooding his body.

Meanwhile, the new heart beat 120 times per minute. Now and then there were spells of atrial flutter and the ventricles changed their rhythm. But the heart was beating.

Washington Daily News, *December 4, 1967:*

"It's going to work. Dying African gets girl's heart and lives."

Times *of London:*

"Dead girl's heart transplanted—sick man given new hope after unique operation."

Medical Proceedings:

"Are we in sight of the day when surgeons can sew a kind of Joseph's coat out of many different parts, when failing hearts and heads can be renewed, and a kind of immortality on earth can ultimately be achieved?"

Pravda, *Moscow:*

"In spite of South Africa's reactionary position in the community of nations, it seems, as Dr. Christiaan Barnard's tremendous endeavor proves, to contain creative forces."

Hardy had braced himself for it in 1964: public excitement, moral outrage and charges. But he had never imagined such a storm as burst on Monday and Tuesday, December 4 and 5, and roared over the greater part of the inhabited globe. When South African radio issued the first reports (without details and names) at noon on Sunday, December 3, a United Press International correspondent transmitted the item, and by afternoon it lay on the desks of all the news media throughout the world. If the news had come from Boston, Palo Alto, New York, or Houston, the editors would have reacted immediately. But because this incredible item came from South Africa, they were dubious.

It was Monday before they could check the report. Then the storm broke. It began with the landing in Cape Town of a special plane carrying a television crew from CBS. Reporters from all over the world besieged the Groote Schuur Hospital. They scurried through the corridors, and the staff had all they could do protecting the room in which Washkansky still slept. In no time the reporters had dug up the name and address of Denise Darvall. They crowded in on her shattered father, who was filled with doubts about whether he had done right to assent to the doctors' request at a moment of confusion and despair. With equal speed, the reporters found out the name of the first human being to carry another's heart within his body. They besieged Ann Washkansky's home and ferreted out Louis's life story.

They had a comparatively easy time of it with Dr. Botha, Dr. Bosman, and Dr. Marius Barnard. As far as they were concerned, these men were "provincials" who, never having dealt with hard-boiled reporters before, could be coaxed into giving out whatever was wanted: one piece of information or another, a statement, or an inside story. Christiaan Barnard, too, played right into their hands. He was a man who through long years of obscurity and ambition had been made ripe for the temptations of publicity.

Within forty-eight hours the tempest of multimedia journalism had made Barnard the "greatest physician of the age" and Louis Washkansky a world celebrity. France had once prayed for Marius Renard and his mother; Oklahoma had taken a keen interest in the fate of Edith Helm. But never before had the name of a patient been bruited from one end of the world to the other. The moral indignation and the philosophical dismay at the transplantation of a human heart, which Hardy had feared, also became a reality. But the ordinary man did not listen to these arguments. He knew that millions like him were dying every year of ruined hearts, that he himself might suffer the same fate any day. His interest was riveted upon the news of Louis Washkansky's new heart and new life, for these stood for the possibility of a longer life, perhaps of immortality.

A cross section of "man-in-the-street" interviews on radio and television concerning the heart transplant in South Africa:

A salesgirl in London: "Good Lord, in a few years there won't be any more heart patients."

A secretary in New York: "Fabulous—soon they'll be able to give everybody with heart disease a new heart."

A workman in Milan: "I've been having trouble with my heart for a long time. But now I'm not worried about the future."

A teacher in Chicago: "All the churches should get together and ensure that such games with God's noblest creation are not repeated."

A schoolgirl in Berlin: "I'm young, but I think about death sometimes. It helps to know that my generation won't have to die of heart diseases."

A professor in Athens: "Barnard is a filthy ghoul. Death is one of the laws of life. This kind of artificial prolongation of life is a crime against nature."

A hippie girl in San Francisco: "Fantastic, man, that's cool. This is the kind of thing that means something to us, because it's not for war, it's for life, life, life."

A bus driver in Mexico City: "I telegraphed Louis Washkansky to tell him he's got to live a long time. If he lives, we'll all live longer."

An engineer in Frankfurt: "Trip to the moon and a new heart—it's worth living in these times."

A pop singer in Los Angeles: "I'm writing a song about new hearts and people living forever."

About six o'clock in the morning on Monday, December 4, Louis Washkansky opened his eyes for several minutes. He observed two figures in smocks, hoods, and masks standing like ghosts by his bed. Then he dropped off to sleep again. He awoke for the second time when another ghost asked him: "Louis, how are you?" He wanted to answer, but could not because of the tubes in his nose and throat. Later he awoke for the third time because someone was pulling wires or tubes through his nose and arranging a transparent tent around him. From somewhere he could hear the faint hissing of air that was good to breathe, and a few seconds later he made his first sound. He now recognized one of the ghosts as Barnard, who again asked how he felt.

Washkansky whispered: "Fine." As he painfully formed the word, his memory returned, and in a short while he asked, word by word: "You promised me a new heart. . . . I suppose you gave it to me?"

Barnard bent over him and replied: "Yes, we did."

There was a moment's pause. Then Washkansky's face twisted into a smile—and he dozed off once more. Thereafter he was aware only now and then that the gowned figures were taking his blood pressure and temperature every fifteen minutes, were drawing samples of blood from his arm, fingers, or ear lobes every hour, were dosing the infusion bottle with drugs or injecting them directly into his veins, and were rolling him over on his right or left side every two hours to clear his lungs. Dimly, he noticed that a man with a camera was pleading with one of the shrouded figures; he went on pleading until at last he was permitted to approach Louis's bed and take the first photograph of the man with a new heart. He certainly did not realize that the flash had provided light for a picture that the stranger with the camera (his name was Jim McLagan) would have printed in many newspapers all over the world. He also did not hear the clamorings of other reporters and photographers, nor was he aware of their efforts to climb trees and direct telescopic lenses at the window of his room.

Medical notes:

Heart activity has been somewhat unsteady since the end of the operation. The EKG shows simultaneously the rhythm of the remaining part of the atrium from Washkansky's old heart and the natural rhythm of the new heart. Pulse at times reaches the alarmingly high figure of 140. Continuing atrial flutter and several extrasystoles of the new ventricles. At the same time rise in the enzyme levels. Divergent opinions among the members of the medical staff: was this rise a sign of rejection or not?

On the morning of December 5, Louis Washkansky awoke after a restless night of being rolled from side to side, having ghostly figures fuss with his arms and stick needles into him. But after waking he remembered that he had a new heart, that it must be beating under the white bandage and the wires that covered his chest. At the same time he experienced an ease in breathing that seemed like a resurrection, although he was infinitely weak and tired. Finally, he felt hungry. One of the nurses brought him buttered toast and milk; and the taste of the toast on his dry tongue made him aware again that he was alive. Then he dozed off once more. But the constant measuring and rolling woke him so often that something of the old Washkansky spirit was aroused. "What a hotel, where they don't let you sleep for five minutes," he whispered. He asked to see Ann. Told that her first visit would have to wait a while, he sent her a message that he was as good as new. Then he noticed a machine being pushed over him. He was forced to lie perfectly still for a long time. He did not yet know that an X ray of his heart was being taken.

Later, a press photographer made his way to the door. He had begged hour after hour for a shot in Washkansky's room and had for a time contented himself with filming the old heart, which was being preserved in alcohol. Now he took a color picture of Louis "with his new heart." The picture displaced Audrey Hepburn, the movie star, from the cover of *Life* magazine. While the picture was being taken, Washkansky briefly opened his eyes. But he was still too far removed from the world outside to know that everyone was clamoring for his picture and that the *Life* shot made his blunt features world-famous.

Medical notes:

At a press conference the staff informs a crowd of reporters that Washkansky's heart is behaving "beautifully."

Actually, there are still problems. Considerable atrial flutter in the evening. Irregular ventricular activity. Sudden drop in pulse frequency. The medical conferences cannot decide whether these symptoms indicate rejection. For safety's sake a first irradiation of the heart with 100 roentgens is carried out. Great difficulties because the cobalt source in the mobile radiation apparatus is too feeble. The two-hour duration of the radiation imposes considerable strain on the patient.

On the morning of December 6, Washkansky's face for the first time since the operation took on some color. He was still lying under the oxygen tent. Another two-hour irradiation session wore him out. But he revived later, beckoned to the nurse on duty, and whispered: "Washkansky, the new Frankenstein."

Medical notes:

Rise in pulse to above 130. Atrial flutter and further rise in the enzymes. Persisting uncertainty over whether rejection has set in. Possibility that enzyme increase is due to the radiation treatment. Nevertheless, a second radiation with 85 roentgens. This is so hard on Washkansky that the doctors decide to carry out further radiation in the radiotherapy department, where it can be done quickly, in spite of the risk of infection.

Louis Washkansky was unaware of the sometimes alarming galloping of his heart. He felt the incision pains of all patients who have undergone major operations, suffered from the continual disturbances—measurements, blood samplings, infusions, being rolled over. But he remained unaware that his new heart occasionally pounded too fast, or fluttered. He was likewise unaware that he had become a world sensation. When Dr. Bosman told him so, Washkansky scoffed. He began to grasp it only after a new sterile tent was draped around him, the oxygen tank was attached to his bed, and he was rolled a quarter of a mile to the radiotherapy department. This time the radiation treatment, with 200 roentgens, lasted only forty minutes. But as he was moved to and fro he caught glimpses of the photographers who were lying in wait for him like highwaymen for a man with a treasure.

When he was returned to his room, a newspaperman had made his way in. He was the medical consultant for *France-Soir,* and had flown from Paris to Cape Town; as a physician, he had been able to persuade the staff to let him come to Washkansky's bed. What he mostly inquired about was whether Louis felt the foreign heart to be his own. Louis still knew nothing about the origin of the heart, or about the fate of Denise Darvall. But in answering the question he used the phrase "my new heart." From which the *France-Soir* man concluded that no vestige of another soul or other emotions had accompanied the heart. That would have been even more patent had he known the real Washkansky. For on being told that everyone in Paris was awaiting each new report with the greatest suspense, Washkansky replied with a wink: "Then tell them to take up a collection for the trip and they can see Washkansky in person." That was Washkansky speaking, not Denise Darvall.

A while later Dr. Bosman came in with a sterile microphone. He could no longer hold out against the South African Broadcasting Corporation, which was insisting on a direct interview with Washkansky. While the radio men outside taped the conversation, Bosman asked: "How are you now, Mr. Washkansky?" And then, for the first time since the operation, Washkansky's voice, weak but clearly audible, reached the outside world, proving to all and sundry that he was really alive: "I feel fine."

"What would you like to eat tonight?"

"Something light. Nothing heavy yet."

"How does it feel to be a famous man?"

"I'm not famous," Washkansky retorted, still somewhat dubious. "The doctor is famous." Then he added, borrowing a trite phrase from "doctor novels" he may once have read: "The man with the golden hands."

The conversation lasted half a minute. To the world, every word seemed like revelation.

Shortly afterward Ann—her plump, maternal figure unmistakable even under the sterile gown and mask—visited her husband for a few minutes. In some corner of her mind she had been afraid that the new heart might have changed Louis. She felt enormous relief when he addressed her through the tent as he always did: "Hello, kid." And she knew he was the old Louis when, in response to her telling him how famous he was and how reporters from all over the world were asking for stories about his life, he said: "What have I done? Nothing."

Medical notes:

The behavior of the heart becomes alarming by late afternoon. Pulse 160 and more. Decision to administer digitalis to slow the heart. Kidney excretion diminishing in spite of diuretics. High increase in enzymes. Fear of rejection grows, although no agreement can be reached on the significance of the symptoms.

On December 8, the sixth day of his new life, Louis Washkansky awoke feeling exhausted. Had he been a little stronger he probably would have resorted to the phrase he had used so many times while he was waiting for his new heart: "Washkansky is getting out of here." But he was too tired even for that. He merely said: "I've had enough. Leave me alone," and turned on his side to watch the monitor that constantly drew graphs of the rhythm of his heart. He did not see in it what Barnard or Bosman saw— the leveling off of the peaks, which indicated a drop in voltage. He turned his back on all the doctors and nurses in helpless anger, because their constant checks gave him no rest.

Barnard was called and promised the patient they would let him alone as much as possible. He was given an injection and slept from ten o'clock in the morning until two in the afternoon. He awoke somewhat refreshed. When Ann visited, she thought he looked better than he had in the past four years. She said so to the waiting reporters—with no idea that the reality was very different.

Medical notes:

EKG changes and Washkansky's irritability are attributed to his exhaustion from the incessant tests. But later there is sudden deterioration. Pulse over 160. Further drop in cardiac voltage. On the basis of American experiments, this may be interpreted as a sign of rejection. Differences of opinion among the members of the team. Barnard decides it is rejection and orders a massive increase of antirejection drugs, including actinomycin. Bacteriologists are concerned because of probable total destruction of the body's immunological resistance to infection. Mention is made of klebsiella bacteria which have been found in the orifices of Washkansky's body. These might spread. Decision, as a precaution, to apply the antibiotic gentamycin also.

Suspenseful night, December 8–9. Early in the morning surprising change in the patient. Beginning of the normalization of EKG. Pulse drops to normal. The team is convinced that there actually was an attempted rejection which has now been overcome. Continued dosing with Imuran, actinomycin, etc. In addition a fourth radiation treatment of the heart, 200 roentgens.

December 9 was a day of miracles. Even before Barnard visited his patient, Louis practiced typical Washkansky kidding on nurses Hall and Papendieck. He invited them to his first dance after returning home. His voice was now clearer and stronger. He insisted they take away the "candy wrapping"—meaning the oxygen tent. He could breathe all the air he wanted, he said.

Barnard hesitated at first, but then consented to removal of the tent and the last infusion tubes.

On December 10, Washkansky asked for newspapers and a radio; they were given to him after being carefully sterilized. A few hours later he learned, from the newspapers, the story of Denise Darvall. For a while he became very quiet. But after his own fashion he indicated that he was thinking about the girl's heart implanted in him, for he jokingly asked whether his skin might get to be as soft as a woman's. Over the radio he also learned something about the rejection process that threatened his heart. His face turned a little gray, so that the nurse on duty was prompted to remark: "You don't have to take that seriously. They've been saying that every day." But Louis had already overcome his initial qualm and characteristically blustered: "If they think I'm giving up this heart, they're nuts."

Later, he asked whether he could go home soon. Barnard assured him that if he went on the way he was going, he could be home for Christmas. And on Monday, December 11, he felt so well that Barnard and Bosman again yielded to the rabid demands of the reporters. However, they now transferred Washkansky to another sterile room, No. 284, which had a long balcony running along it so that entry could be more easily controlled.

Medical notes:

Improvement continues. Normalization of the heart now beyond doubt. Improvement in kidney function likewise remarkable. It has proved possible to keep the diabetes in check despite the side effects of the cortisone. Even if W. should die, his case has already provided valuable experience. Barnard makes this point in speaking to reporters, but insists that the remark be kept off the record because W. is now reading the newspapers. Barnard also declares that if there is no rejection in the next three months, there probably will be none ever.

On December 13, Louis Washkansky laid aside the latest batch of newspapers, remarking: "We've had enough of that now." He found all this fame gratifying, but his stoicism shielded him from overestimating himself. He sensed that the fame was not accorded to him personally, but to his new heart; that was clear from a question he asked: "I wonder how many people want a heart like mine?"

On Thursday, December 14, he was up for the first time, was helped to walk to the balcony door, and sat for a short time in the sun. To a radio reporter he said: "I feel a hundred per cent." But when asked his plans about the future, he replied that it was premature to talk about it. Shortly afterward, while relatives were visiting him, he suddenly complained about pains in his stomach and said that he was fearfully tired.

From an unpublished review of Christiaan Barnard's One Life:

"Although this book has been heavily criticized, I do not doubt that its concluding chapters will someday be considered among the classics of medical literature.

"They start with the evening of December 14. It is somewhat harrowing to read of the conferences of the specialists. They confer over the results of the innumerable tests taken in the course of the day, over a breakdown of red blood cells, a rise in leucocytes and lymphocytes, creatinine clearance. They compare the acid and alkaline balance, sugar in the blood and sugar in the urine. They try to interpret mineral status, kidney status, enzyme levels, bacterial cultures, X rays, and electrocardiograms. But they do not know why Louis Washkansky has suddenly begun to talk about stomach pains and immediately afterward is overcome by extreme fatigue.

"The stomach pains might be attributable to the cortisone, which frequently produces stomach ulcers. The leucocytes indicate strange signs of disintegration. What is the hematologist's opinion? These symptoms might be those of rejection, but they might also mean the beginning of an infection. The levels of lactate dehydrogenase have doubled. What does the biochemist think? He, too, believes the cortisone may be responsible. But the symptom could also be a belated consequence of damage to the blood from the heart-lung machine. On the other hand, the pain and fatigue might indicate that the heart is being rejected after all. There has also been a morbid rise in the coproporphyrin level in Washkansky's urine. No one can say whether this means rejection or infection or a toxic condition produced by the drugs. All of them can only hope that the patient's fatigue will pass.

"Next day, December 15, does not bring the hoped-for recurrence of Washkansky's 'resurrection.' Louis speaks of pain in one shoulder. Some imperceptible change is taking place in his attitude. He who has never complained, but denied his sufferings, is now complaining in an almost inaudible voice about pain and weakness.

"X rays of his shoulder show nothing. The new day's flood of tests do not present a clear picture. Barnard, grasping at a straw, concludes that his patient is merely overstrained by all the visitors. But he does not forbid the visits scheduled for this day, including those from a South African cabinet minister and a German reporter. The latter sees Washkansky only through the window from the balcony and scarcely recognizes him. He asks: 'How are you, Mr. Washkansky?' The sight of the reporter in the sunlight of the balcony briefly stirs in Washkansky his naïve awareness of the importance of his recovery to Barnard and to millions of people throughout the world. He replies that he is fine. But he does not sound convincing.

"He is no better during the afternoon, although Ann visits—she has had a cold and been unable to come for the past five days. When she sees him, she starts in fright. She had been listening to the radio and hearing of nothing but his triumphant restoration to new life. His appearance seems to belie such reports. She decides that he has had a cold, although he says he hasn't. With his wife, too, he tries to cling to the euphoria of the previous week. 'Ah,' he says, 'she's at me already. I've got a cold. I don't happen to have one, but if it makes her happy I've got one.'

"Once more the reader is troubled—the persistent perplexity of the doctors is upsetting. Again they sit in their conference room trying to make sense of all the analyses of Washkansky's body fluids. Shortly afterward Dr. Bosman finds shadows on a photograph of the lungs. The other doctors have also seen these shadows, but—concentrating as they are on the possible rejection of the heart—have paid them little attention. Washkansky is now complaining about pains in his chest. He runs a slight fever. The possibility of pulmonary complications, which afflict so many kidney transplant cases, seems too obvious to be missed. But Barnard takes refuge in the idea that the pains are aftereffects of the operation. Perhaps he does not want to believe that the period of triumph is nearly over.

"On Saturday, December 16, there is no longer any dodging the issue. Washkansky is running a high fever and coughing. X rays of the chest show that the shadows of the previous day have spread to both lungs. Once again the doctors measure, filter, peer into their microscopes. But throughout the day they confront one uncertainty after the other. Is the problem of pulmonary infection the penalty for Barnard's concentrating on the fight against rejection of the heart and battering Washkansky's defenses with massive radiation and saturating him with drugs? Was the 'resurrection' nothing more than a temporary effect of the cortisone, one of those deceptive euphorias often produced by this drug? In the seesaw struggle between rejection and infection, has the team forgotten some of the painfully garnered experiences of kidney transplants? Or is a heart transplant a different case entirely?

"The doctors cannot even agree whether the trouble is a pulmonary infection. Washkansky coughs, but he does not cough up any mucus that Dr. Forder, the bacteriologist, could study for infectious agents. From smears taken from nasal mucus, he cultures klebsiella bacteria, which have occurred before. But he does not know whether they have penetrated the defenseless lungs, or whether the difficulty is an ordinary pneumococcus infection. In fact, until he has secretions from the lungs he cannot say definitely whether there is a lung infection. There are perils as well as blessings in treatment with antibiotics. If penicillin is given—which works against pneumococci but not against klebsiella—and it turns out that there are no pneumococci, more harm than good may be done. Penicillin can open the way for the klebsiella germs to invade the lungs. In case of a lung infection, it is essential to reduce the amounts of Imuran and cortisone, thus giving the body's immunological defenses a chance to recover. If, however, it is not an infection, reducing the anti-immunological drugs will again increase the danger of heart rejection. And if there is no lung infection, the shadows in the lungs, the pain, fever, and coughing, might be caused by blood clots. To combat these, the chief weapon is heparin.

"The majority of the doctors are finally inclined to diagnose infection, but cannot absolutely exclude an infarct. Barnard decides to treat for infarct—perhaps because his main fear is the rejection of the heart he has transplanted, and so he does not want to lower the dosage of antirejection drugs. He administers heparin, and as a compromise more gentamycin to combat the klebsiella germs that have been found in Washkansky's nostrils.

"Toward noon Louis coughs up sputum for the first time. The color indicates that he has a lung infection. Late in the afternoon the bacteriologist discovers pneumococci. Immediately, 20 million units of penicillin are dripped into Washkansky's body. The patient's breathing accelerates. The cortisone is reduced, the Imuran likewise. Barnard reports his feeling 'that we finally had this crisis under control.'

"December 17 marks the fourteenth day of Louis Washkansky's 'new life.' While the world still imagines that all is going well with him, he loses control of his bladder function—thus experiencing, though only half consciously, one of the most humiliating signs of physical decline. His respiration has reached a rate of more than 30 breaths per minute. His temperature is 103.5, his pulse 106. Barnard comforts himself with the thought that Louis's old heart would have collapsed during the first few hours of such a lung infection, whereas the new heart is holding firm. He tries to communicate this comfort to Washkansky. But the man he speaks to is no longer the old indomitable Louis. This patient listens absently; he seems to have given up hope.

"There seems little doubt that the penicillin is not doing its job. For although the bacteriologist finds the number of pneumococci diminishing, the fever remains high and the lungs appear not to have cleared. Once again each of the specialists offers another opinion. The bacteriologist points out that he has discovered klebsiella and pseudomonas organisms in the sputum. It is possible that these bacteria have invaded the lungs from the nose and mouth. But their numbers are still small. Hence, they could have entered the sputum only as it passed through the mouth. On the other hand, the lung infection might be caused by a virus or fungus; these frequently spread when antibiotics have destroyed their rivals, the bacteria. But viruses are invisible; and although the bacteriologist can find fungi on Louis's skin, there are none detectable in the sputum.

"Barnard decides to add the powerful antibiotic cephaloridine, which is effective against pseudomonas, to the penicillin and gentamycin already being administered. This flood of antibiotics brings Washkansky's already overdrugged digestive tract to the brink of collapse. For the rest, Barnard decides to wait one more night. If the antibiotics show no effect by morning, he is prepared to accept a diagnosis of 'transplant lung.' This is a condition that has been noted in England and America as a complication of kidney transplants. In this case, renewed treatment with Imuran, cortisone, and actinomycin is indicated.

"In fact, the antibiotics prove ineffective. On December 18 the fever continues. X rays of the lungs show spreading lesions. Circulation in the limbs slows, and the skin becomes cyanotic. Barnard therefore decides on another bombardment with 100 milligrams of cortisone, 200 milligrams of prednisone, 250 milligrams of Imuran, and 200 milligrams of actinomycin.

"To the reader, this must seem like an act of desperation. At one point in his book Barnard mentions that before the operation he promised Washkansky to do everything possible to save his life; he felt that he must leave nothing untried. And he reports that at the beginning of this renewed antirejection bombardment he went to Washkansky's bed and could read in his eyes the question: do I still have a chance? He assured the patient: yes, we are beginning a new treatment. But it is also evident that by this time some of his closest associates are wondering if Barnard is still acting rationally. He is obsessively pushing on with treatment out of his own determination not to lose his patient, although it is plain to them that the limits of what is humanly possible have already been reached.

"Louis Washkansky's lungs become more and more incapable of transmitting oxygen to his blood. Once more he is isolated from his surroundings by an oxygen tent. On the morning of December 19 the white blood cell count drops precipitously from 22,200 to 5,640. Dr. Forder finds that the lungs are swamped with klebsiella and pseudomonas organisms; the question of infection is now definitely settled. The cortisone, Imuran, and actinomycin bombardment have destroyed Washkansky's last defensive resources. Again the specialists confer and come to no decision. The oxygen tent no longer suffices. Once again Washkansky is connected to the respirator; oxygen is forcibly pumped into his lungs, so that he is no longer able to speak. Barnard sends for Ann and begs her to encourage Washkansky not to give up the fight, to go on fighting with him, Barnard. But Washkansky barely has the strength to press his wife's hand.

"Barnard pumps blood and concentrated leucocytes into the dying man's failing circulation, in order to force an increase in the number of white blood cells that are fighting the lung infection. All antibiotics known to be effective against klebsiella and pseudomonas bacteria are simultaneously dripped into the patient's veins: gentamycin, cephaloridine, carbenicilline.

"Washkansky's body is now purple. It is late at night on December 20. Barnard still clings to the belief that all that counts is to keep Washkansky alive until the antibiotics can deal with the lung infection. He goes on believing this even though the number of white blood corpuscles steadily diminishes and all defensive ability is vanishing. Toward three o'clock in the morning the discoloration of Washkansky's tormented body intensifies, although he is now receiving pure oxygen. Barnard, to cite Ann Washkansky, is behaving 'like a madman.' Evidently the fact that the transplanted heart continues beating makes it impossible for him to give up. He cannot admit that incomprehensible biological processes are making a mockery of his technically successful work. His closest associates are appalled when he proposes connecting Washkansky to the heart-lung machine again. He wants to open the thorax once more, either in the operating room or, if necessary, in Room 284, and hook the patient's circulation to the machine in order to gain some time for the antibiotics to work. Barnard goes to Professor Schrire, the cardiologist, with this plan and cannot understand Schrire's horror. To his credit, he reproduces his conversation with Schrire:

"*Schrire:* 'Chris, you have no more time. It was up yesterday or maybe even the day before. It's all over.'

"*Barnard:* 'My God, how can you say that?'

"*Schrire:* 'Listen, Chris, Washkansky is clinically lost. Everybody knows it except you. . . .'

"*Barnard:* 'Everybody doesn't know it. We had a chance until tonight, and we still have a chance. . . .'

"*Schrire:* '. . . To put him back on the pump is madness. You'll increase his agony, and torment everybody else.'

"Barnard reports that he did not know how to reply. He admits that he no longer knew what his aim was. Was he prolonging Washkansky's agony only because he himself could not bear to give up? At any rate, it is Schrire who restrains Barnard from an act of medical madness. Even now, Barnard does not give up all hope, for at five o'clock in the morning he is still injecting potassium. But toward 6:30 A.M. on December 21, Louis Washkansky's new heart fails, after having kept beating for eighteen days."

Notes of an Italian correspondent in Cape Town, 1967–1968:

"I arrived at Cape Town on December 21. My assignment was to replace a colleague who had until then been reporting on Washkansky. I had relatives in Cape Town and had studied medicine for a few semesters, so my editors thought I was the right person for this assignment. Besides, I was young and like most of our readers believed in the idea of a transplanted heart, whereas my male colleague was a skeptic. And you can't sell skepticism to a world that wants to believe.

"I arrived too late, for Washkansky had died early in the morning. That was a bitter disappointment, but I was firmly convinced that this would not be the end of heart transplantation. If Washkansky had lived for eighteen days, the next patient would live longer, and I hoped that Barnard would not give up, that he would try again.

"When I called on my colleague in his hotel, he gave me a briefing. 'And how he'll try again,' he said. 'You don't know this man Barnard. He's staked his career on heart transplantation, and he believes that sooner or later transplanting hearts will be like changing the fuel pump on an old car.' He started packing his typewriter and camera, meanwhile adding: 'The fellow will learn someday that human beings are not cars and hearts aren't fuel pumps. It's clear that Washkansky's death hasn't made much of an impression on him, to judge by his announcement this afternoon. He says the autopsy results provided no evidence against continuing heart transplants, and that he means to perform the next one as soon as he is back from a speaking engagement in America and has another heart patient available. As a matter of fact, we know that the next guinea pig has already been lined up. His name is Philip Blaiberg and they have him in Groote Schuur Hospital. You won't have long to wait for the next transplant show.'

"Naturally the first thing I did was to arrange a meeting with Philip Blaiberg, Barnard's second heart patient. He was a rather portly, round-faced, good-natured, very ordinary looking person, a dentist by profession. I found him in Ward D-1 at Groote Schuur, with eighteen other patients.

"It was pure chance, of course, that like Washkansky he was the son of Jewish emigrants from Russia. His mother came from Lithuania; at the beginning of the century his father had emigrated from Krajewo in Russian Poland to England, and later to South Africa, where he became a small shopkeeper. Blaiberg had spent his youth near the rather wretched railroad stop of Uniondale Road, and later in provincial Oudtshoorn, between Cape Town and Port Elizabeth. He'd been a druggist's apprentice and later studied dentistry in Johannesburg and London. In 1936 he married Eileen Abel of Oudtshoorn, and was just establishing his dental practice in Cape Town when the Second World War broke out. His war service as a military dentist in South Africa and later in Italy, usually in camps behind the front, was just as uneventful as the rest of his life. His most distinctive trait was that he had always been a good fellow. He returned to Cape Town after the war, opened a new office, later bought a house in Rondebosch, and lived a thoroughly average life centering on work, good food, beer, a few friends, and a mild passion for sports, which consisted mainly of memories of playing rugby in England. In later life he liked to go swimming or would occasionally climb up Lion's Head and Devil's Peak, on Table Mountain.

"Shortly after one such climb in 1955—he was then forty-six and thought himself pretty fit, though a bit overweight—he had his first heart attack. In 1956 he was treated by Professor Schrire at Groote Schuur Hospital for angina pectoris pains and atrial flutter. Schrire observed changes in the coronary vessels, enlargement of the heart, extensive infarct damage of the heart muscle, and high blood pressure. He treated Blaiberg with anticoagulants and digitalis. But efforts to take him off the digitalis failed; each time his heart weakened dangerously. Between 1960 and the beginning of 1967 he slowly became a cardiac cripple. Probably the death of his son, Harris, contributed to his deterioration; in 1960 Harris, aged twenty-two, was found in a friend's house dead of a bullet wound. The circumstances were never clarified. This tragedy shattered the harmony of the family's life. Blaiberg submerged himself more and more in work; his wife, Eileen, sought distraction by taking a job as a secretary.

"On April 5, 1967, Blaiberg suffered another severe attack, with atrial flutter, pulmonary edema, and shortness of breath. He was taken to Groote Schuur Hospital again. An aneurysm had formed; several of his coronary arteries were completely blocked. Schrire considered an aneurysm operation and sent the results of his tests to the Cleveland Clinic in the United States for a prognosis. But the reply was that the case was hopeless. Schrire therefore sent Blaiberg home with prescriptions for still larger quantities of digoxin, aminophylline, and erosemide. At the same time he informed Eileen that the case was hopeless.

"Blaiberg gave up his practice, sold the house, and moved into an apartment in Wynberg. By early December 1967 he was no longer able to utter a brief sentence without acute shortness of breath. It took him an hour to recover from the small exertion of going to the toilet. Half dozing, on December 3, 1967, he heard radio bulletins about the operation on Washkansky, and like a drowning man seized upon the idea of having a heart transplant himself. Thereafter he talked—almost every word punctuated by gasping for breath—of nothing but the operation. The talking affected his condition so badly that Eileen had to appeal to Schrire for help once more. Schrire himself called at their apartment and told Eileen he had already discussed the matter with Dr. Kohn, their family doctor. After the success Barnard had just had with Washkansky, there was now a possibility to save her husband—by transplantation. Everything depended on Blaiberg's decision, however. The moment Blaiberg heard about this, he gave his consent without considering for a moment. He demanded the operation—'the sooner, the better.' Eileen was still hesitant; her husband made her promise that she, too, would consent.

"Somebody at Groote Schuur Hospital—I don't know who it was, since I was not there at the time—incautiously hinted to one of the many reporters who besieged the place that Barnard's next heart transplant patient would be a retired dentist from Wynberg. Within a few days the correspondents had tracked down Blaiberg's name and address and begun watching his home. Schrire had intended to move Blaiberg to the hospital on December 16, but the dentist's condition deteriorated so rapidly that he had to be brought in to Ward D-1 on December 14. By next day he was no longer able to move in bed or even to wipe his nose.

"That same day—the day that marked the fateful turning point for Washkansky, although Barnard did not yet realize it—Barnard visited Blaiberg for the first time in order to obtain his consent in person. Blaiberg repeated almost inaudibly: 'The sooner, the better.' Those words bespoke not only his own desperation; they were also characteristic of the naïve, boundlessly hopeful mood of that period, after Washkansky's good days. Barnard came again on December 21 and informed Blaiberg that Washkansky had died, although the cause was pneumonia, not failure of the new heart. Did Blaiberg want to withdraw his consent? Struggling so hard for air that he could scarcely speak, Blaiberg repeated what had become his single theme: he wanted the operation. His sole concern was that Barnard might not return soon enough from his trip to America. My predecessor had told me about that trip, adding a few spiteful remarks.

"In the first flush of Washkansky's apparent recovery, Barnard had been invited to the United States by CBS to appear on 'Face the Nation,' together with Professor DeBakey from Houston and Kantrowitz from New York. He had at once accepted. But shortly before Washkansky's death he had begun to hesitate, not relishing the idea of facing 20 million Americans as a surgeon with a dead patient. On the day Washkansky breathed his last, however, Barnard realized that the tide of hope was still running high, that he was still regarded as a medical pioneer. He had therefore decided to keep his engagement.

"He was fully aware that he would not encounter undivided agreement and sympathy from his American colleagues. Kantrowitz, it is true, had cabled congratulations. But on December 6, three days after Barnard, Kantrowitz himself had attempted the first human heart transplant in America, at Maimonides Hospital. His patient was a seventeen-day-old boy, the donor a child who had died of brain damage. The heart had functioned only for a few hours. It was only natural, moreover, that American medicine, which could fairly claim having initiated most of the heart transplant research, would receive the outsider from Cape Town with a degree of reserve. But Barnard sensed that the enthusiastic masses would be behind him. And his own faith in heart transplantation, together with the publicity fever that had seized him, apparently induced him not to miss this first great public appearance of his life.

"On Friday, December 22, while Louis Washkansky was being buried in the Pinelands Jewish Cemetery, crowds of reporters and the curious gathered at Malan Airport to see Barnard depart for America. Another crowd was waiting at Johannesburg, where the plane made a stopover, and still another in London. Barnard's next six days in America were a triumphal tour. With his flair for public relations, he was quick to declare, from the moment he landed in New York, that he had acquired 90 per cent of his knowledge in America. Thus he took the wind out of his denigrators' sails. With skillful sophism he disposed of the unsolved question of rejection cautiously raised by DeBakey and Kantrowitz. In New York he was greeted by Mayor Lindsay; he visited jazz master Wilbur de Paris in Greenwich Village; and in Washington he announced that he would perform his next heart transplant in January. President Johnson invited him to his Texas ranch; and wherever Barnard went he had praise for America ('I stand on the shoulders of many American doctors').

"Meanwhile, back in Cape Town, we learned that Blaiberg's condition was daily deteriorating. He was transferred to the intensive coronary unit, received steadily increasing quantities of mercury drugs and oxygen, sank into states of collapse in which his blood pressure became no longer measurable, and began to cough blood. Everyone feared that he would die if Barnard did not hurry. Barnard, in New York, was informed, and on December 30 he flew back. London's newspapers ran headlines such as BARNARD FLYING TO NEXT HEART OPERATION. On January 1 we waited for him again at Malan Airport. After two hours of sleep he drove to Groote Schuur Hospital, where more crowds were waiting.

"It was as though a decree from on high had arranged everything in his favor. On New Year's Day, a very special holiday for the coloreds of South Africa, many colored families drove out to the beaches for picnics. Among them were a twenty-four-year-old textile worker named Clive Haupt and his wife, Dorothy. Shortly after nine o'clock Clive suddenly collapsed unconscious and was taken to Victoria Hospital, where Dr. Basil

Sacks diagnosed a massive cerebral hemorrhage. Sacks began artificial respiration, but saw clearly that there was little hope and informed Dr. Venter in Groote Schuur Hospital that he probably had a heart donor for Blaiberg. Venter implored him to keep the young man alive as long as possible, and had Haupt transferred to Groote Schuur, where he arrived at five o'clock in the afternoon, accompanied by Dorothy and his mother, Muriel, a cleaning woman. At seven o'clock Venter talked with Dorothy and Muriel Haupt. He told them there was no longer any hope for Clive and asked for permission to take his heart. Dorothy Haupt was far too distraught to make any decision. Clive's mother decided for her. What she supposedly said sounds rather grandiloquent; probably some reporter added a flourish, turning a sobbed consent into: 'If you can save the life of another person, then take my son's heart.'

"By this time Blaiberg's condition was moribund. When informed about the impending operation, he was supposedly asked whether he had an objection to a colored heart and supposedly he answered: 'At last you rotters are doing something. I was beginning to think you never would.' Today I don't believe these words were ever spoken; they sound too much like imitation Washkansky. But at the time we greedily printed everything we could pick up, no matter how trite and implausible.

"In any case, it was not until the morning of January 2 that Haupt's brain death was determined, the respirator switched off, and the heart stopped. Throughout the night Groote Schuur Hospital had been besieged by curiosity seekers and reporters. Around eleven o'clock in the morning word finally came that the operation was in progress. It was finished by three in the afternoon. As we now know, it differed in no way from the operation on Washkansky—with the exception that Blaiberg's new heart at once began beating strongly and regularly after a single electric shock.

"This seemed a favorable omen, and so we stood around waiting for Barnard to leave the hospital. When he emerged from a side exit at six o'clock he shook hands, kissed two little girls, and told us that the operation was a great success and Blaiberg was already feeling well in an isolation room. His brother Marius remarked that the team had learned a good deal from the experience with Washkansky. They would not again be lured into applying the wrong therapy by supposed signs of rejection. Other correspondents, who were meanwhile keeping track of Eileen Blaiberg, reported that she was celebrating at home with friends and relatives, and that champagne corks were popping. I, too, believed that this time Barnard had succeeded and that before long thousands of hearts would be transplanted throughout the world.

"In order to protect Blaiberg against infections more effectively than had been the case with Washkansky, during Barnard's absence an isolation ward had been hastily set up in one of the ear-nose-throat sections. Except for medical personnel, no one at all was permitted to see Blaiberg. Naturally, this cut off our sources of information and made the battle for news more unscrupulous than it had been in Washkansky's case. But even with sterile walls completely surrounding Blaiberg, there were plenty of opportunities to question nurses, doctors, and hospital employees, and above all to woo Eileen Blaiberg, invite her to restaurants and night clubs all over Cape Town, and pump her for news. This hitherto uncelebrated woman so suddenly raised to prominence succumbed to many of these temptations.

"The great question, of course, was whether Blaiberg would survive longer than Washkansky. Every additional day was hailed as a victory. Blaiberg was in an oxygen tent; then the tent was removed. He began to eat, to do breathing exercises, to move around. On the tenth day the first alarm came. Blaiberg developed a sore throat. At once the specter of a spreading infection arose. After two days of suspense we heard that he was well again. His mucus membranes had merely been irritated by some tart beverage, it was said. In reality it had been a fungus infection, but it had been knocked out by drugs.

"The next dramatic day was January 20, because this was the eighteenth day of survival, the day on which Washkansky had died. The fact that Blaiberg survived the day and actually drank a glass of beer diluted with lemonade made the big story for January 21. The waiting reporters were overwhelmed to learn that Blaiberg, talking to his wife through the speaker system, told her not to sell his car as they had intended because he was sure he would be driving again.

"We reported in detail on Blaiberg's first efforts to stand. Eileen, coached by the journalists, put some questions to him. When would he be climbing Lion's Head again? He replied that he wouldn't be climbing Lion's Head but Devil's Peak (the higher peak); at this point he could not yet walk a few steps unaided. By then, in all probability, his feeling that he had a mission to fulfill was already beginning to develop. I mean, his sense of obligation that he must become a symbol of successful heart transplantation, and that by every word and gesture he must represent a new, healthy life with a second heart.

"Thereafter every day became the 'twenty-first day,' the 'twenty-second day,' as if Blaiberg had been born on January 2. On January 27 there was another crisis, with rising temperature, rapid pulse, and weakness. But after the fateful consequences of massive antirejection treatment in Washkansky's case, Barnard's team was much more cautious. X rays showed an enlargement of the heart. That could simply mean that the pericardial sac had filled with secretions from the incision. The sac was punctured and 400 grams of fluid drawn out. Blaiberg's 'twenty-sixth day' could begin.

"In the meantime the Americans had made two new attempts at heart transplant, and failed in both cases. In Palo Alto, Shumway, for so many years the pioneer of heart transplantation, had operated on Mike Kasperak, a fifty-four-year-old steelworker incapacitated by heart trouble. On January 6, Shumway had implanted in Kasperak the heart of Virginia White, a Santa Clara housewife who had died of a sudden cerebral hemorrhage. Her husband stated to the press that only a few days before he and Virginia had been talking about the heart transplants and she had exclaimed: 'How wonderful to be able to give someone else a chance to live.' But immediately after the operation severe complications had set in. Kasperak's lungs had been damaged by his heart disease. Oxygen balance could not be maintained. Then internal hemorrhages began. Kasperak's liver was diseased; his gall duct was blocked by clotting and had to be replaced by a plastic tube in the course of a second operation. There followed hemorrhages from stomach and intestinal ulcers. A third operation was necessary to remove parts of the stomach and spleen. Then Kasperak's kidneys also failed, and he died on January 21, after fifteen days with his new heart.

"On January 10, Kantrowitz in New York undertook a second transplant; his patient this time was a fireman named Louis Block. Kantrowitz and his patient were even less fortunate than Shumway and Kasperak. Block was dead eight hours after the operation, and Kantrowitz blurted out: 'I don't think any heart operation can be regarded as successful until the patient goes home.'

"The failures in America increased South Africa's pride in Blaiberg's 'second life,' and even gave rise to a certain amount of gloating. Confidence increased in Cape Town when, on February 14, a photographer was permitted to take a first picture of Blaiberg shaving himself. The picture, captioned 'Twenty-four Days Old,' proved a sensation. That same day teams from America and Germany were allowed to set up sterilized floodlights in Blaiberg's room, to film Blaiberg through the window, and to interview him through a sterile microphone. His voice was feeble. But he answered all questions optimistically, announced that he would soon be home, and sang in a brittle but quite audible voice the first lines of a song to prove that his new heart allowed him to breathe vigorously again.

"Barnard, meanwhile, was traveling about the world like a missionary for heart transplantation. He threw himself into the publicity scene with such enthusiasm that for the first time remonstrances began to be heard in international medical circles. These protests struck me as sparked by envy of a young revolutionary who had changed the whole nature of cardiac medicine and was also breaking personally with the traditional proprieties of his profession. In Paris, Barnard appeared in the Crazy Horse, a strip-tease joint. In Monaco, 900 millionaires paid sizable entry fees just to see him. Princess Grace danced the first dance with him at a ball. In Rome the Pope received him in private audience; so did Gina Lollobrigida and Sophia Loren. A private bank in Vienna put out gold coins with his portrait. In London the participants in the Miss Universe contest voted him the most important man in the world. On February 15, before flying off on another tour, he visited Blaiberg to say good-bye to the living symbol of his success.

"While Washkansky was still living, Barnard, I now learned, had told a journalist that the best press photograph would show Washkansky looking at his own heart. Now, on this February 15, he made a reality of this conceit. He called on Blaiberg holding a jar in which Blaiberg's old heart was preserved in alcohol. Blaiberg looked at his heart (smiling as if to signalize his victory over death) while Barnard asked: 'Are you aware that you are the first man in the history of the human race who has been able to look at his own dead heart?'

"A day later Dr. P. K. Sen in Bombay attempted a heart transplant on a young farmer, Bodham Chithan. Within a few hours the patient was dead. This failure only emphasized once more the remarkable fact of Blaiberg's continuing survival. On February 29, Blaiberg came to a window in his ward for the first time, holding up two fingers in the V-for-victory sign.

"That was the fifty-eighth day. Around March 10 word got out that he would shortly be discharged to go home. The team was only waiting for Barnard's return, so that he would not miss the triumph of bidding Blaiberg good-bye at the hospital door. The great day came on March 16. Blaiberg was still too weak to walk any considerable distance. He was helped to dress and placed in a wheel chair. But at the exit, before he emerged into the sunlight and faced the crowd, he stood up—filled, no doubt, with the sense that he was more than Philip Blaiberg, dentist—he was a historic symbol who must appear erect and victorious to the world. He went through the scene of parting with Barnard and walked to the resplendent car that was to drive him home to Wynberg. There the reporters had meanwhile photographed everything, down to the easy chair in which he was going to sit.

"Once inside the door of his apartment house, Blaiberg had to be helped up the steps to the elevator. Then—because he could be seen from outside again—he walked the longest distance of that day, down an outside gallery to his apartment. Next day millions upon millions read detailed descriptions of his homecoming, and torrents of telegrams and letters arrived in Wynberg. Kantrowitz's comment that success could be claimed only if a patient went home had become a reality—and faith in heart transplants was, accordingly, greater than ever.

"Blaiberg mostly stayed at home thereafter. But the stream of news reports flowed as thickly as ever. Agents now entered the picture, demanding fees from each representative of the mass media before granting an interview with Philip or Eileen Blaiberg. On the other hand, there were no longer any sterile walls. Visitors were required only to remain at some distance from Blaiberg and to wear surgical masks. We learned practically everything of inconsequence: the story of his first haircut, what he had for breakfast, lunch, and dinner, the drama of his first bath, his portentous opinions on the issues of the day, the names of the innumerable medicines he washed down with his milk, the results of the examinations for which Eileen took him to Groote Schuur Hospital, the visits of celebrities such as the American pianist Liberace.

"Early in April, Philip Blaiberg was seen for the first time at the beach, and a few days later he made his first attempt to drive his car. His sense of mission grew; he flared up angrily whenever, anywhere in the world, someone expressed doubts about his recovery or vitality. Whoever the doubter was, Blaiberg invited him to come to Cape Town where he, Blaiberg, would personally meet him at the airport and drive him to his apartment. And he would add: 'We'll sit in my living room, have a drink, and you'll be able to see for yourself how well I feel and how fantastic it is to be living again.'

"That was how things stood by the end of April 1968. I recalled my colleague's skepticism. To me it seemed that he had been badly mistaken and that Blaiberg was the living embodiment of the greatest triumph in the history of medicine."

3 / Everett C. Thomas

From a letter by Dr. P.M.:

"Birmingham, April 8, 1968
"Dear J.T.:
". . . All this is hysteria, understandable only when you remember that in the United States alone 500,000 persons die of heart diseases every year, and none of them want to die. They are clinging to the illusion that they may have a chance to be Blaibergs if their own hearts stop functioning someday. Yet even the greatest transplant optimists know that—if only because of the different types of heart disease—only a few thousand of that half million could ever be considered for a heart transplant. But hardly anyone is saying that, and if anyone says it, nobody listens.

"The newspapers are going crazy. The readers are going crazy. Patients all over the world are beginning to go crazy. Before long the doctors will go crazy, too, and start an international heart transplant olympics. Public opinion in their countries will force them into the contest, because not only America, Russia, France, England, or Germany, but Cameroun or Afghanistan as well will insist on having their Barnards and Blaibergs."

From a letter by Dr. P.M.:

"Toronto, June 6, 1968
"Dear J.T.:
". . . Remember what I wrote in April about the 'olympics' in heart transplants? If you have been following the world-wide reports for the past month, you'll agree, I think, that the olympics have begun. They evidently started in Stanford on May 2. On that day Professor Shumway undertook his second heart transplant, on a carpenter, Joseph Rizor, from Salinas, California, who had suffered three heart attacks since 1961. After hearing about Barnard's operation on Washkansky, he declared, according to his wife: 'I wish it had been me.' The donor was a telephone worker, Rudolph Anderson, who was struck by a fatal cerebral hemorrhage. His wife, Maggie, told newspapermen: 'I know he would be proud to have a

290

part in a transplant operation.' This time, too, Shumway was unfortunate; Rizor died on May 6.

"Since May 2, however, one heart transplant has followed another. Within a month I've counted thirteen, and I may have overlooked a few more. On May 3, Dr. Donald Ross of the National Heart Hospital in London made the first attempt in England. This was rather surprising because before Barnard's operations Ross had remarked that the technical problems of transplantation had been solved, but the problems of rejection not at all, and that it would probably take a decade before they were. His patient was a truck driver, Frederic West, forty-five years old. West is still alive, but obviously going through one severe crisis after another. On May 8, Professor Negre in Montpellier, France, implanted a heart into a woman named Elie Reynes; she died two days later. On May 12, Professor Dubost attempted a heart transplant in Paris. His patient was a Dominican monk, Jean-Marie Boulogne, the donor a man of forty named Jean-Claude Gaugiraud. On May 25 it was the turn of Dr. Richard Lower, who had participated in Shumway's heart studies at Palo Alto and who had also been Barnard's teacher. His patient, Joseph Klett, survived only six days.

"On May 26 the Brazilians entered the race, with Professor Zerbini of São Paulo as surgeon and a cattle drover, João Ferreira da Cunha, as recipient. I've heard that this operation was regarded as a 'milestone for medicine in South America.' I've also heard that Cunha did not know what was being done to him; he learned afterward that he had received a new heart. On May 31 two olympic teams entered the ring simultaneously: Dr. Belizzi in Buenos Aires and Pierre Grondin in Montreal. Belizzi implanted a new heart in a noodle salesman, Antonio Serrano, who died on the fifth postoperative day. Grondin operated on a fifty-eight-year-old butcher, Albert Murphy, whose new heart stopped after one day.

"On May 31, C. W. Lillehei, the pioneer of open-heart surgery, operated on Ronald Smith, a black policeman, in New York. Smith died the same day.

"All in all, what we have here is an impressively macabre series. But it hardly compares with the events that took place in Houston between May 3 and 21. In this period of less than three weeks Professor Denton A. Cooley performed heart transplants four times. On May 3 he implanted the heart of a sixteen-year-old girl into Everett Thomas, an Arizona public accountant. On May 5 he operated on James Cobb, on May 7 on John Stuckwish, and on May 21 on Louis Fierro. Cobb and Stuckwish survived for only a few days. Louis Fierro and Everett Thomas are at the moment the only surviving American heart transplant patients.

"Whether the reasons are personal, nationalistic, or scientific ambition, a wave of operations has started such as the world has never seen before."

When Everett Claire Thomas, on an April morning in 1968, left his small, green-painted house in the northeastern part of Phoenix, Arizona, he did not know whether he would see it again.

He was a tall, lean man of forty-seven with a sensitive, bespectacled face under thinning hair, in no way distinguishable from the average office worker, salesman, or accountant, except perhaps in his friendly, devout peacefulness, which might not have escaped a keen observer. As he crossed his lawn toward the car that would take him to the Phoenix airport, he showed no signs of agitation.

His wife, Helen, and Mark, his twenty-year-old son, were going with him to the airport; he said good-bye to his other two boys, Paul and Charles, aged sixteen and twelve. Both were old enough to know about their father's condition and his destination.

As the car started Everett Thomas looked back at the two boys standing in front of the house. In the past twenty-five years his life had not been easy. In 1943, at the age of twenty-two, he had contracted scarlet fever while in the service, and ever since had had heart trouble. For at least fifteen years he had known that three of his heart valves were calcified. But his parents had impressed him with the "power of positive thinking," and in whatever befell him, he looked for the bright side of things. So it was with his scarlet fever. He had been a bombardier in the air force, and he told himself that if it had not been for the disease he might have been shot down over Europe or in the Pacific. God's will had preserved his life by making him sick. Helen took much the same view. She came from Falls City, a small town in Nebraska, and had married him in Oakland, California, shortly after he was released from service for reasons of health. She had been a pretty, fragile girl, slim as a reed. Her face was rather haggard now, and it was clear that the twenty-two years of marriage had been marked by work and anxiety. But she, too, had not complained; she, too, believed in bearing "her portion."

Shortly after their marriage they had moved to Phoenix, hoping that the mild climate of Arizona would help Everett. They had also been lured to Phoenix as a rapidly expanding metropolis with plenty of employment opportunities—for Everett, like tens of thousands of other Americans after the war, had to establish himself in civilian life. It was not until 1947, at the age of twenty-seven, that Everett began learning a profession. He passed his examination in accountancy, and henceforth ran his affairs with an accountant's precision. They bought a house, raised the children, and by the time Everett found out from his doctor, Joe Ehrlich, how sick he really was, he had established his family life so solidly that, he felt, God could call him any day. He had paid his bills, his insurance premiums, his mortgage installments punctually and saved whatever he could, so that his sons' educations would be provided for and they would be in a position to care for themselves and their mother.

As the car drove past Dr. Ehrlich's office at the Osborn Medical Center, Everett thought of the moment, two years ago, when Ehrlich had told him that his heart with its crippled valves was about done for after a twenty-three-year struggle, and that the only possible salvation for him, if there was one, would be a valve operation. Dr. Ehrlich had frankly told him that it would be a gamble if three heart valves had to be operated on simultaneously, and that very few patients could withstand such an operation. Everett Thomas had returned home and decided to postpone the operation, not because he was afraid but because he felt he still had to secure the future of his family. He wanted to see Mark through his four years at Arizona State University. He persuaded Helen to take courses there also, so that she could get a job as a teacher if he did not survive.

But the previous December, shortly before Christmas, he discovered that Providence would not be giving him as much time as he had hoped for. A blood clot that had formed at one of his diseased heart valves had reached a cerebral artery, and a stroke had almost totally paralyzed him. He spent three weeks in Good Samaritan Hospital. Dr. Ehrlich feared this might be the end. But Everett knew that he had not yet attained his goal, and by the end of January he was on his feet again. His paralysis gradually receded, and he struggled against it with a rare doggedness. By March, however, he realized that he was no longer able to be useful to his family. He was a cripple, still able to move about but with a heart so weak that he could not work at all. Consequently, he decided that he must no longer be a burden to Helen and the children. He would seek the way out that this operation possibly offered. If God willed, he would recover; if not it was better to die.

He had asked Ehrlich to tell him where to go for the operation. Around April 15 the doctor told him that in his opinion the best person was Dr. Denton A. Cooley at St. Luke's Hospital in Houston. He promised to telephone Cooley and, if Cooley was willing to risk a triple valve operation, to make the necessary preparations.

These had all been made, and on this Sunday, April 28, 1968, Everett was on his way. He had insisted on flying to Houston alone; neither Helen nor Mark should be taking time off from their studies. Sick and weak as he was, he had not forgotten that Helen had several exams coming up, and he did not want her to miss them. That fact governed his decision. He made Helen and the children understand that they could not help him at all; the only person who could was Dr. Cooley. They had yielded to his decision, contenting themselves with his promise to let them know in time what day was set for the operation.

Everett Thomas's destination, St. Luke's Hospital in Houston, was a part of the Texas Medical Center, a "$150 million creation" which had brought together some of the most distinguished men in American medicine. What had won it world fame, however, was the presence of two men, DeBakey and Cooley.

Michael Ellis DeBakey had come to Texas from Louisiana. His father had emigrated to the United States from Lebanon. He had opened a drugstore in Lake Charles and had raised six children in the belief that work was the true meaning of life and any waste of time sinful. DeBakey trained and practiced at Tulane University and at the Charity Hospital in New Orleans—where in 1902 the surgeon Rudolph Matas had first ventured to attack a vascular aneurysm with a scalpel. In 1948, after eight years as a professor in New Orleans, DeBakey had come to Houston to head—at the age of forty—the department of surgery at Baylor University College of Medicine, the scientific headquarters for the Texas Medical Center and its hospitals. That same year he had for the first time removed an aneurysm, and thereafter he had pioneered methods of operating on morbid changes in the blood vessels that would be followed by surgeons the world over. He excised and diverted arteries, replaced them by chilled arteries from cadavers and by plastic tubes. He became a master in the use of plastic materials for repair of the heart and the blood vessels.

His small, sprightly figure, his peaked face dominated by a powerful hooked nose, thick horn-rimmed glasses, and receding hair, was pictured in media throughout the world, and popularized. Nicknames such as "Texas Tornado" and "Black Mike" attempted to capture his passion for work, his contempt for private life and leisure, his perfectionism, his formidable demands upon his associates, and his outbursts of fury.

But he was more than a prima-donna surgeon and a domineering egoist; he was a thoroughgoing scientist whose ambitions went far beyond the operating tables now given over for the most part to his assistants, where he himself took a hand only at the decisive phase of an operation. The high mortality rates for cardiac and vascular diseases impelled him to look for the causes of those diseases, and to attempt the development of artificial plastic hearts. He was able to commandeer millions of dollars in federal funds from the National Heart Institute or the National Institutes of Health for his Baylor laboratories. Among the new buildings of Methodist Hospital was a "$20 million wonder," a research center for circulatory diseases with futuristic-looking operating rooms and laboratory wings filled with electronic gear. And as a man who had once known poverty, he was bold in attacking the dollar-mindedness of American doctors and advocating every man's right to health. Whether he took the role of surgeon, scientist, or social missionary, he remained the brightest star at Baylor University, Methodist Hospital and the Texas Medical Center.

Denton A. Cooley was of a different breed. In the first place he was twelve years younger than DeBakey. He was also a native Texan, and as the son of a Houston dentist had never known what it was to fight for his daily bread. He had the kind of handsomeness that would have made any movie director glad to cast him in the role of a dashing Texas Ranger. And Cooley had never been exclusively a man of books and research. At the University of Texas in Austin he had been one of the stars on the baseball team. He had learned surgery under Alfred Blalock in Baltimore and had been present in 1944 when Blalock performed the first blue-baby operation. Aside from two years in the service as a medical captain and surgeon with the U. S. Army in Europe, he had stayed at Blalock's side until 1950. That same year, knowing little about DeBakey, he had likewise performed an aneurysm operation. The following year he had come home to Houston to teach surgery, and later to work in DeBakey's department. One summer day in 1951, Cooley completed the operation on a gigantic aneurysm before DeBakey arrived in the operating room—and it became obvious that the two were rivals.

As soon as the heart-lung machine was invented, Cooley performed the first open-heart operation in Texas. His innate daring and his phenomenal skill pushed him toward new surgical targets, and he was not held back by a somewhat more scientific temper like DeBakey's. Moreover, he had not bothered his head with the need for revolutionizing social medicine. He worked with greater and greater speed, finishing five or more operations in a day. Nor did he completely bury himself in laboratories; he was often seen golfing, swimming, or water-skiing. In addition, he was an accomplished charmer who won the hearts of his associates and his patients.

It was almost inevitable that there should be tensions between him and DeBakey. The break took place in 1960. Cooley remained a professor at Baylor Medical School. But he wanted his own operating rooms, and found them in St. Luke's Hospital, only a few steps away from Methodist Hospital. In the eight years that had passed since then, he had not risen quite to the eminence of DeBakey. But he had created a medical atmosphere of his own, where even in the operating room staff members joked, and jazz or cowboy music came over the stereo speaker system. Doctors and students from all over the world sought entry to his operating room to watch the speed of his movements, the unique dexterity that ultimately made it possible for him to open the tiny hearts of newborn babies and correct congenital heart defects. He could boast of heading the fastest heart team in the world, and the most productive; he and his colleagues performed a thousand and more operations a year. "Denton cuts them open, sews them up, and sends them away," reporters wrote. Texas millionaires provided money for a new twenty-eight-story building on the grounds of St. Luke's Hospital, and Cooley was placed in charge of this Texas Heart Institute with its magnificent operating rooms and its 300 beds for cardiac patients.

The news of Barnard's first heart transplant undoubtedly affected Cooley differently from Shumway and Kantrowitz, who had devoted infinite pains to studying not only the techniques of heart transplantation, but also the problems of rejection and the moral aspects of the operation. Cooley had wasted no time on laboratory studies of rejection, nor could he have, since he had no laboratories of his own. He had observed that DeBakey was studying rejection, regarded it as inevitable, and was therefore turning to work on artificial hearts, which would presumably be perfected sometime in the distant future. Consequently, Cooley must have taken the news from South Africa as something of a blow. For Barnard, though he had nothing like Cooley's technical skills, had exceeded him in daring and decisiveness and had acted like a surgeon, undeterred by the complex problem of rejection. Since he was a fair man, Cooley had paid due tribute to the South African. But when Barnard's second transplant on January 2 succeeded and Blaiberg survived, Cooley decided not to hesitate another moment.

After a few experiments he was confident that the operation presented no technical problem for him. He could work so much faster than Barnard that it would not even be necessary to cool or perfuse the donor heart with blood to keep it viable. He would give the heart no time to deteriorate.

Shumway's and Kantrowitz's ill-fated first attempts only made him the more determined to do the first successful heart transplant in America at the Texas Heart Institute. When he heard from Denver, Colorado, that a new serum against lymphocytes had been developed and was proving effective against rejection in kidney and liver transplants, he sent one of his associates there to study possible application of the serum to a heart transplant. Ever since, he had been ready to perform the first heart transplant in Texas. He had been forced to wait, however—not for lack of moribund patients, but for lack of a donor.

He was still waiting on April 15 when a nurse told him that Dr. Joe Ehrlich was on the telephone and wanted to talk to him about a patient.

Denton A. Cooley's recollections:

"He was referred to me by Dr. Joe Ehrlich of Phoenix, Arizona, by telephone. . . . The doctor confirmed that this man was the highest risk.

Not only did he have three bad valves in his heart, but his ventricles showed very poor function. . . . So everyone was doubtful whether he could tolerate any kind of surgery. . . . There's nothing you can do to ventricles. The Lord gives you a pair of these things and you've got to make out with what's there.

"In discussing with Dr. Ehrlich I said: 'It's not inconceivable that we could do a heart transplant on him.' I told Dr. Ehrlich: 'Bring Mr. Thomas down. We'll sit on him a while and maybe a donor will come along, or, failing that, we may just go ahead in a desperate effort and try to replace his valves, even though it seems a 75-per-cent risk of his dying on the operating table.' "

Everett Thomas was prepared for anything, but not for a heart transplantation. Not that he hadn't read the newspapers, listened to the radio, and watched television broadcasts about Barnard, Washkansky, Blaiberg, Kasperak, and Block. But Dr. Ehrlich had always told him that he needed repair of his heart valves. At their last talk Ehrlich had remarked that he knew no one but Cooley whom he would trust to do whatever might conceivably be helpful. Thomas consequently looked forward to the examination by Cooley with the sense that he would be meeting an unusual doctor and a kind of last authority before God.

He had to wait patiently for several days. A St. Luke's cardiologist, Dr. Robert D. Leachman, and several other doctors put him through a course of tests such as he had never before experienced. But then, on April 30, Cooley suddenly stood beside his bed, a tower of a man with shirt open at the neck, white smock, tennis shoes, a young, enterprising, candid face and warm blue eyes. From the moment he first set eyes on Cooley, Everett Thomas had the feeling that Providence meant well by him in sending him to Houston.

He did not yet know what the tests had shown: that a valve operation on his heart would not give him even a 25-per-cent chance of survival, but something closer to 10 or 5 per cent. Nevertheless, Cooley was prepared to try the operation rather than watch Thomas die helplessly in his bed. But he also knew that Thomas was a patient suitable for the heart transplantation he had been planning for so many weeks, and it occurred to him that transplantation might provide a last chance to save the man if the valve operation failed.

Denton A. Cooley's recollections:

"Mr. Thomas was at the end of his tether. He was bordering on pulmonary edema, and there is no real problem in convincing a patient like that

that he needs something. . . . He told me that life wasn't worth anything to him the way it was. He was a burden to his family. He'd always been a breadwinner and he didn't like people to have to nurse him, and he certainly didn't want to be dependent on his family for his support. He had the courage to say: 'I'd rather be dead than the way I am.' So we talked to him about the possibility of a heart transplant."

Cooley quickly observed Thomas's composure and religious faith. He therefore explained frankly what his condition was, and that he had only the choice between death and an attempted valve operation. Even at that, the chances for a successful operation were very, very slim, Cooley said. If it failed, the only remaining chance was a new heart. He said that he himself had great hopes for the new method, which had made such a sensation in South Africa but had actually been developed in America. Was Thomas prepared, if necessary, to stake his life on a new heart? Of course, much depended on whether he would be able to find a donor during the next few days, for the heart valve operation could not be delayed much longer without throwing away all chance of success.

Denton A. Cooley's recollections:

"And he said: 'Well, use your judgment. The only reason I'm in Houston is because my doctor respected your judgment more than anyone else's in the country, and respected your skill, and thought you'd do the best thing for me in the best way it could be done. . . . We'll see if a donor will become available.' "

Cooley was moved and full of admiration for this man from Phoenix who had been placed in his hands. Before he left Thomas, he said: "You know, you're one of the bravest persons I've ever met." He decided to perform the valve operation on the coming Friday, May 3, and planned to do it late in the afternoon, after all the easier cases had been taken care of. He did not think he could postpone the operation any longer, even though operating so soon might mean there was no chance to find a donor.

Helen Thomas was informed. She and Mark took the next plane to Houston. There Everett told her for the first time about the possibility of a heart transplant. Even Helen's composure was shaken by this news. She thought of Blaiberg, but she also thought of all the others who had died. Everett assured her that she must put everything in Dr. Cooley's hands, and God's.

Cooley, who on Thursday had flown to Shreveport, Louisiana, to lecture on heart diseases, had little hope of finding a donor so soon. When a reporter for the *Shreveport Times* asked him whether he was planning a transplant, he replied honestly that heart transplantation was a fascinating field, but that he was not planning one in the near future because of the difficulty of finding donors. Then, late that afternoon, as he arrived at the Shreveport airfield to fly back to Houston, he was called to the telephone. One of his assistants in St. Luke's informed him that around three o'clock a young woman in Houston had shot herself in the head. She had been taken first to Ben Taub Hospital, but her family had insisted on her being transferred to St. Luke's because she was formerly a patient of Cooley's. Since her condition was hopeless, there was a chance that she might be a heart donor.

From the report of a former assistant at St. Luke's Hospital:

"The girl who shot herself was named Kathleen Martin. She was only sixteen and had married five months before. As a child she had suffered from aortic stenosis. Dr. Cooley operated on her successfully in 1962, when she was ten years old. Kathleen was a girl of very unstable temperament. She was still in junior high school in 1967 when she met Charlie Lee Martin, the son of a sectarian preacher in Brunswick, and married him right off, though he himself was only seventeen. Charlie found a job with General Electric, and he and Kathleen moved into a small apartment on Charrin Drive. Kathleen left school because her girl friends teased her about being married. After that she became more unstable than ever. Every heat wave, or even a gust of wind that disarranged her hairdo, could send her into a state of wild excitement.

"She and Charlie quarreled frequently, and on the afternoon of May 2 they quarreled again. Charlie started out for work, but turned back because he felt uneasy. He found Kathleen in the bathroom holding a gun against her head. She threatened to kill herself. When he tried to grab the weapon, she pressed the trigger, and the bullet shattered part of her brain. Her heart was still beating when she was brought to Ben Taub Hospital, but brain currents were no longer measurable. Nevertheless, her father thought Dr. Cooley could save her again as he had done in 1962. He insisted that she be taken to St. Luke's. By then her blood pressure was dropping rapidly and only artificial respiration was keeping her alive. Around that time Dr. Cooley arrived from Shreveport."

This opportunity for a first heart transplant had come to Cooley as a surprise, but he leaped at the chance. First of all he went to obtain the consent of the weeping husband and of Kathleen's father.

Denton A. Cooley's recollections:

"Of course we had to limit our exposure to the donor. But I was involved with the donor, too, to some extent. . . . The fact that I was the surgeon for the girl at the time helped considerably in our getting permission to use her as a donor. . . . So it was a heart that I had known before. And here it was two of my patients ending up at what was really one patient. A very gratifying and unusual experience; I don't know if I'll ever have another one just like it."

As soon as the permission came through, Leachman and Cooley made sure that Kathleen Martin's heart was in good condition in spite of the earlier operation. An enlargement of the heart that had resulted from the aortic stenosis seemed to them advantageous, since it diminished the natural difference in size between the heart of an adult like Thomas and that of a girl like Kathleen. Dr. Nora, an immunologist at Texas Children's Hospital, carried out a crude tissue matching—to the extent that this was possible in the short time available. And while Operating Rooms 1 and 2 were being prepared, just in case, Cooley went to see Everett Thomas again and told him that chance had provided a donor. If Thomas gave a final consent, he would operate late that evening or night. But he would first determine whether a valve operation had any prospect of success. If not, he would implant a new heart. He found Helen sitting beside Thomas's bed, and so he was able to talk to both of them at once.

Helen Thomas's recollections, 1970:

"I was worried. I said to Dr. Cooley: 'I want you to tell me you'll do everything humanly possible to bring Everett through with the valve operation and not experiment with a transplant just for the sake of headlines.' . . . He told me: 'Certainly, I couldn't do that to another human being.' And I do believe that he found on the operating table that the valves could not be repaired and that a transplant was the only way to save his life."

Denton A. Cooley in World Book Encyclopedia Science Service, *August 1968:*

"I am apprehensive before any transplant operation, but of course, on the first one the burden was the heaviest. I had personal reservations because of subjecting the patient to something I was not sure of myself. It was a gamble."

Operation notes on the transplantation of Kathleen Martin's heart to Everett Claire Thomas:

MAY 2, 1968

11:00 P.M.   Transfer of donor to Room 2, of recipient to Room 1.

11:50 P.M.   Opening of Thomas's thorax reveals hopeless destruction of the heart.

11:55 P.M.   Donor's heart stops beating.

MAY 3, 1968

12:45 A.M.   Dr. Cooley and Dr. Hallman remove Thomas's heart. Dr. Bloodwell removes donor's heart.

12:55 A.M.   Donor heart taken to Room 1.

1:01 A.M.   Donor heart fitted and sutures placed by Dr. Cooley.

1:35 A.M.   Completion of last suture.

1:37 A.M.   Opening of aortic clamp. Wild, irregular heartbeats.

1:39 A.M.   A single electric shock suffices to induce rhythmic heartbeat.

Denton A. Cooley's recollections:

"There was a lot of tension in the operating room, of course. We tried to get everyone keyed up to their peak performance, just like going into an athletic contest. . . . It took about thirty minutes to make the transfer, whereas others have reported an hour and a half, two hours. . . . People ask me what was the biggest thrill I've had in my professional career. Well, I believe it was . . . to see this graft, which is from a sixteen-year-old girl, to see it take over and beat vigorously, you might even say courageously, in support of this adult man's whole body. It was just the most gratifying thing, the most thrilling thing—everyone in the operating room cheered."

In the early morning hours of May 3, Cooley strode beaming into the small hospital room where Helen Thomas had waited in the company of Armen D. Jorjorian, a hospital chaplain. Cooley told her that he had had to implant a new heart in her husband, but that happily the operation was over and the new heart beating as if it had never been born in another body. At that moment Helen Thomas lost some of her hard-won composure. But Cooley's optimism was contagious, and she nodded smilingly when he told her to go to sleep now. Then he hurried to Operating Room 6, which had been turned into a temporary isolation room where Thomas could spend the first days after the operation. As yet Cooley did not know that he had completed the first successful heart transplant in the United States. Nor could he anticipate that he had taken the first step along a path that within a few weeks would lead to his being both the speediest

heart transplanter in the world and the surgeon who had done more transplants than any other.

Denton A. Cooley's recollections:

"I spent the night with him. . . . We kept the tracheal tube in, so he
couldn't speak when he regained consciousness, but he would smile for
me, and the next day when we took his tracheal tube out he talked. He sat
on the side of the bed, and he was just marvelous. He was the happiest
man. I've forgotten what he said, but it was just what a real man's man
would say—something like: 'It looks like we've made it.' "

Perhaps the actual course of events was not quite so triumphant as it
later seemed in the glow of memory.

On the morning of May 4, when Helen, in sterile gown and accompanied by Dr. Hallman, was allowed to step up to Thomas's bed, the respirator was still working. And Thomas scribbled a note to ask Helen whether
he had new heart valves or a transplant. Somewhere, behind the barri-
cades of his simple faith and confidence, there must have been some small
dread of the unknown. But his face showed no shock when Helen told him
he now had a young girl's heart inside his chest.

Everett Thomas did, however, sit up for a short time on May 4. He was
given his first liquid meal and late that evening said to one of the nurses:
"My trust in God and Dr. Cooley has been rewarded. I know that God
stood behind him while he was operating on me."

The first reports of Cooley's operation and his patient's good condition
produced a sensation, since no other heart recipients in America had survived. The press, which hitherto had focused on Methodist Hospital and
DeBakey, now turned to St. Luke's and Cooley. Although there happened
to be a strike against Southwestern Bell Telephone at the time, management personnel kept the lines open especially to carry the tremendous
number of calls to St. Luke's—until the calls themselves ended by blocking the telephone lines.

Like everyone subjected to thoracic surgery, Thomas suffered a good
deal of pain. In addition, an abnormally high pressure in his pulmonary
circulation stubbornly resisted returning to normal. He also had unusually
high blood sugar levels. It almost seemed as if the operation had induced
diabetes. In addition to Imuran, hydrocortisone, prednisolone, digitalis,
and antilymphocyte serum—which he was the first heart transplant patient to receive—he also had to be given insulin. Nevertheless, he recovered swiftly, and was so sure he would regain his full health that he told
Helen and Mark to go back home as soon as possible. The operation was

bound to result in enormous hospital bills, and every dollar they could save counted.

Helen Thomas's recollections, 1970:

"The last thing he told me was: 'You will have to handle my part for me, as you've got to be home. My job is to be here in the hospital and get well. And I have the doctors here to help me.' He promised me that I would be notified immediately if anything went wrong, and, after all, we could keep in touch by telephone. Even then he would scold me about telephoning too much, and I only called when the suspense got unbearable."

Here was the plainest proof that Thomas was on the road to recovery —that five days after the operation he was already beginning to think in his usual prudent fashion about the financial problems of his family.

Meanwhile, Cooley was already engaged on his second heart transplant. The sensational news about Everett Thomas had seemingly driven two new heart recipients and one heart donor to Houston. A woman from Alexandria, Louisiana, had no sooner read of the operation on Thomas than she telephoned Cooley and implored him to save her husband, James Cobb, a man of forty-eight, who lay dying in Alexandria Hospital. Cooley consented to have the patient transferred to St. Luke's. Almost simultaneously another sufferer from severe heart disease arrived, a sixty-two-year-old hospital administrator, John Stuckwish, from Alpine, Texas. His last hope was also a transplant. And finally, on Sunday afternoon, Cooley received a call from Conroe, Texas. A fifteen-year-old boy named William Joseph Brannon had received a fatal brain injury in a traffic accident. His mother was calling to offer Cooley her son's heart because she wanted to think of it continuing to beat in some living person. Brannon was moved to Houston immediately, and Cooley had to decide whether to implant the heart in Cobb or Stuckwish. He decided in favor of Cobb because Cobb was younger and would probably withstand the effects of the operation better. When Cooley made his decision, he assumed that it was equivalent to a death sentence for Stuckwish. It seemed improbable that within so short a time a third heart donor would be available.

This time it took Cooley forty-two minutes to perform the transplant operation. St. Luke's was besieged by reporters, the hospital switchboard swamped by telephone calls.

On May 7, contrary to all expectations, a donor was found for Stuckwish also. On April 28 a workman, Clarence Nicks, got into a fight in a

Houston water-front bar. He was brought to St. Luke's Hospital with severe head injuries; he now lay dying, and his heart was available. Stuckwish's condition had by this time so deteriorated that he was brought to the operating table in a coma. Cooley began the operation in such haste that he had to skip the anesthesia. Stuckwish's heart action stopped, his brain currents faded, and only at the very last moment did the team get him attached to the heart-lung machine, pump blood back into the brain, and transplant Nicks's heart to him.

By next day, however, it became evident that Cooley was not to have an unbroken string of successes. Just fifty-eight hours after the operation James B. Cobb died from an unanticipated allergic reaction to the antilymphocyte serum. Only after his death was it discovered that twenty years before he had received tetanus antitoxin, which, like the antilymphocyte serum, was obtained from horses. The following day John Stuckwish's liver and kidneys failed. One leg became gangrenous. He died of acute jaundice, arteriosclerotic complications, and double pneumonia.

Yet the reports of these deaths had no more influence upon the wave of transplants than had Louis Washkansky's death on developments in Cape Town. For Everett Thomas was alive. He remained cut off from the world, knowing nothing of what was going on. But he seemed to be making a splendid recovery.

Summary of reports on Everett Thomas from May 15 to May 30, 1968:

May 15   Cooley says Thomas is well, happy, in good spirits.

May 16   Cooley says Thomas "is enjoying the whole adventure" and has remarked that if he had known how easy a heart transplant was he would have asked for one much earlier.

May 17   The Thomas family returns to Phoenix, since Thomas is no longer in danger. Thomas is getting up for considerable periods every day. He jokes with Barbara Hurn, the red-haired nurse who is in charge of the transplant patients.

May 18   The dose of antirejection drugs Thomas is receiving is daily reduced. The electrocardiogram monitor and all other regular tests show no rejection. Thomas, who is still unaware of the deaths of Cobb and Stuckwish, declares: "When I decided for the transplant, I made a positive decision. In the future, it will be important for every incurable heart patient to make this positive decision. Undoubtedly there will soon be a world in which sufferers from heart disease no longer exist."

May 19   Thomas feels so well that he complains about the scaffolding for the new building of the Texas Heart Institute. The wooden panels block the view from his window.

May 20 Construction workers, hearing of Thomas's complaint, remove the panels. From the scaffolding outside Everett's window they shout greetings to him. Thomas says: "I haven't felt so well for twenty-five years. When I leave this room I'd like to tour the whole country speaking in favor of heart transplants."

May 21 Dr. Cooley's fourth heart transplant. Louis Fierro, 54, used-car dealer from Elmont, New York, receives the heart of Hubert Brungardt, 17, of Pasadena, California. Two hours after coming out of the anesthesia Fierro sits up on the edge of his bed.

May 24 America's two living heart transplant recipients, Everett Thomas and Louis Fierro, are in fine fettle. Cooley declares that heart transplantation is no longer a matter of experiment, but a revolutionary therapeutic means for saving lives. St. Luke's Hospital plans to set up a special heart transplant unit.

May 26 Louis Fierro continues to recover in spite of diabetic symptoms, which are regarded as a side effect of the cortisone treatment. The antilymphocyte serum proves to be miraculously effective in his case also. Letters pour in from all over the world for Thomas and Fierro.

May 29 Thomas can move about freely and might soon be discharged. He declares: "My gratitude to Dr. Cooley and God are boundless. It imposes on me the obligation to devote my life to promoting heart transplantation."

May 30 A growing stream of heart patients is rushing to St. Luke's Hospital. A lack of donors delays Dr. Cooley's fifth transplant. But it is expected to take place any day.

It was difficult to describe Everett Thomas's condition in the early part of June, four weeks after he had received his new heart. The new heart still did not react to nerve stimuli. When he moved or performed his test exercises, it took the heart three minutes to increase its pumping action. Even then, the acceleration did not result from nervous stimuli, but from increased secretions of hormones in the blood. Thomas was only dimly aware of such limitations upon his physical abilities. The tremendous experience of living again strengthened his faith in "positive thinking." He had always liked communicating his thoughts to others. Now he was obsessed by the need to inform the world about his new experience.

As soon as he was able to take his first few steps outside his room, he became a familiar figure around St. Luke's Hospital. Tall, slow-moving, but erect, he strolled through the halls talking to everybody he met. He joked, even laughed, but he seldom forgot to put in a solemn word about the blessing of a new life or about Dr. Cooley, who had become a kind of divinity for him. When Fierro likewise left his room, a small, skinny, bespectacled man, and joined Thomas, the two were united in the feeling that they were symbols destined to promote heart transplantation. Fierro did not have Thomas's religious faith or sincere sense of mission. But he had spent the greater part of his life dealing with customers and praising the qualities of his cars. In much the same way he now praised his new heart. When the construction workers decided to make Thomas an honorary member of their team and presented him with a hard hat as a sign of his membership, Fierro was naturally included in the ceremony. Press photographers were invited, and so had their first look at the "Americans with the second hearts."

A few days later Thomas, again accompanied by Fierro, stood in the limelight of his first big press conference, which was held in the auditorium of St. Luke's Hospital. Neither he nor Fierro realized quite how frail they still looked. Both were determined to convince the audience that they were healthy once more, and they wore their hard hats with an expression of cheerful clowning. Asked how he felt, Fierro replied: "Like a millionaire." And Thomas interjected: "I'm the other millionaire." With boastful garrulity Fierro declared: "I never felt any pain. I didn't even know the operation was over. . . . I eat like the devil and enjoy everything. For exercise I hop; sometimes I dance. Before the transplant I couldn't even make four or five steps. Now I can't wait till I dance the peabody again. That used to be my favorite at the Roseland dance hall in New York."

But Everett Thomas was even more garrulous, especially when he was expressing his simple philosophy. "A heart," he said, "is simply a muscle pump . . . and mine has been replaced much as an automobile fuel pump. I was a rusty automobile. Now that I have a new fuel pump, I'm a new car." He announced that he was planning to visit hospitals and heart patients to urge more transplants. "For me heart transplantation is the greatest contribution to the preservation of human life, and the donation of a heart is the gift of gifts. We are going to be the Blaibergs of America and represent for our country what he represents: the advance guard of a new medicine."

That was on June 11. The following morning, news arrived in Houston that Philip Blaiberg had returned to Groote Schuur Hospital in Cape Town and was dangerously ill, battling with death again.

Intermezzo / Philip Blaiberg

Notes of an Italian correspondent in Cape Town, 1968:

"On June 10 I left Cape Town temporarily to visit my parents. By then certain ominous reports were already beginning to come in. It seemed that Blaiberg had been taken back to Groote Schuur Hospital with a case of hepatitis. Barnard, accompanied by Dr. Botha, was again on one of his world tours, and early in June had declared to enthusiastic students at Heidelberg: 'In a few years we will be able to perform several heart transplants on one and the same patient. Then patients whose first transplanted heart ceases to function will be able to receive a second or even a third heart, and go on living.'

"He went on to London, where reporters received him on June 10 by asking whether it was true that Blaiberg was sick again. Shortly afterward Groote Schuur called to tell him the bad news, and he flew back to South Africa on the first available plane.

"I myself arrived back in Cape Town at about the same time. I found it was no longer a vast encampment of journalists, as it had been at the beginning of the year. But there were enough of my colleagues from the press, radio, and television to keep a twenty-four-hour watch around the hospital. I was, of course, struck by the way the sources of publicity had nearly dried up in the intervening period. The hospital had learned from the past and from medical criticism of the publicity excesses; the staff now understood the techniques of closing doors and issuing noncommittal communiqués. Barnard put on his most optimistic expression whenever we caught sight of him, but otherwise he was very tight-lipped.

"My own attitude at the time was such that I probably did not want to probe too deeply, for fear of unpleasant surprises. The world did not want the Blaiberg myth destroyed. I was therefore gratified when I could report on June 14 that the bacteriologists at Groote Schuur had found a virus responsible for Blaiberg's hepatitis and were treating it accordingly. I also passed on Eileen Blaiberg's statements of June 15 and 16 that Blaiberg was again showing an active interest in his surroundings, was happy and talkative. On June 18 she declared that his condition was no longer critical and that she was certain he would recover completely. When, on June 26, Barnard flew to Amsterdam in order not to miss the ceremonies for the opening of a new university there, I assumed that the crisis was over. On July 6 there was another alarm, and from a hospital communiqué it was possible to deduce that Blaiberg's condition had worsened. At the same time rumors were heard that Barnard, who had returned to Cape Town, was planning a second heart transplant for Blaiberg. But these rumors were denied by Eileen Blaiberg, and two days later the hospital announced that Blaiberg had overcome the crisis. Tourists assembled in front of Blaiberg's home for prayers of thanksgiving.

"The real facts were that Barnard had come within a hair's-breadth of losing his patient. And Blaiberg had come within a hair's-breadth of losing his role as the first man to live any length of time with another's heart—a role he had been playing with a good deal of tragic and tragicomic zeal.

"After 'participation' in a rugby game on May 21—a piece of play-acting, but a highly effective bit of publicity—Blaiberg had complained of an unusual sense of heaviness in all his limbs. On May 24, his fifty-ninth birthday, he had been taken to Groote Schuur on the seemingly innocent pretext that he needed one of his regular checkups. A number of alarming symptoms came to light, but the question of whether his condition was due to rejection, incipient infection, or the toxic effect of the antirejection drugs could not be definitely answered. Meanwhile, he developed a severe case of jaundice. On June 4, Blaiberg was again placed in the sterile rooms in which he had spent the first months of the year. Examination of his heart showed various symptoms, but none that at this point was regarded as indicative of rejection. It was hard to tell whether the jaundice was a virus infection or a toxic condition due to the drugs. Around June 10, Blaiberg was in such desperate condition that he lost consciousness at times. It was then that Barnard was notified and returned from London.

"Since no definite indications of liver infection could be found, it was decided to discontinue the dosage of Imuran, which is particularly toxic to the liver, even though that meant increasing the danger of rejection. When the liver tests thereafter showed very rapid improvement, it seemed certain that Blaiberg had been suffering from Imuran poisoning. That meant excluding one of the most important of the antirejection drugs from Blaiberg's continuing treatment. It was hoped that rejection could be suppressed by increasing the doses of cortisone and actinomycin. But by the end of the month alarming changes in the heart were discovered. It enlarged, and the blood pressure dropped. Dropsical swellings appeared. Schrire and Barnard assumed that they were now confronting a massive attempt at rejection of the heart. Around July 6, Blaiberg developed a high fever and had increasingly long periods of unconsciousness, as had happened to Washkansky after his lungs became infected.

"Faced with the prospect that the most important symbol of his work might die before his eyes, Barnard resolved to take any risk. The only remaining course seemed to be replacement of the failing heart by another transplant. On July 6, Barnard got in touch with Eileen Blaiberg and explained that this was Blaiberg's sole chance. He asked her consent, and was given it. That same night preparations began. But since there was as yet no donor in sight, the team decided to try a serum that, as I later heard, Dr. Botha had received from Professor Brendel in Munich. So far as is known, neither Botha nor Barnard had hitherto used antilymphocyte serum, nor had they paid any special attention to the German serum, which was, in fact, based on the same principles as the American serum. Brendel believed, however, that the German serum had a higher degree of purity than the American serum; whereas the latter could be administered only by intramuscular injection, the German serum could be injected directly into a vein, and thus worked far faster and more effectively.

"During the desperate night and early-morning hours of July 6 and 7, the serum was tried. Aside from violent chills, Blaiberg showed no reaction for a while. On the afternoon of July 7, Eileen Blaiberg for the first time received permission to enter her husband's room; so far she had only been able to watch him through the window. This signified that the doctors had little hope and wanted to let her say good-bye to her husband. Blaiberg himself opened his eyes just for a moment and whispered: 'This is the end.' Thereafter he no longer reacted to her presence or to her pleas that he must hold out. Finally Eileen went home, prepared every moment to hear that he had breathed his last. Her surprise was all the greater when Barnard himself telephoned late that night, his relief easily heard in his voice. He told her he had wonderful news: Blaiberg was going to live. The German antilymphocyte serum had begun to take effect. The heart and lung symptoms were slowly disappearing, and the rejection was being overcome without Imuran.

"But, as I say, at the time I knew nothing about all this background. I merely heard that Blaiberg was enjoying his new life again."

Everett Thomas was never informed of the truth about Philip Blaiberg's second bout with death. The published news of Blaiberg's swift recovery confirmed him in his faith in the miracle of his new heart. Although he was now reading the newspapers again, he closed his mind to all reports about new heart transplants that ended in the deaths of the recipients. His confidence remained unshaken when Cooley operated on his fifth transplant patient on June 12—an insurance salesman named Sam Willoughby, who had come to Houston from Iowa. When Willoughby collapsed into a coma and no donor was available, Cooley made an intrepid attempt to implant a sheep's heart in his body. He did so in the hope of being able to keep Willoughby alive until a human heart could be found for him. But Willoughby died on the operating table shortly after the sheep's heart was implanted.

If in some recess of his mind this incident shook Thomas, he regained his confidence when Cooley undertook his sixth transplant and saved the life of a gravel pit proprietor named George Henry DeBord, from Helotes, near San Antonio. DeBord was dying when he came to Houston. He received the heart of a young gasoline station attendant, Maxie Anderson, whose mother consented gladly, telling the reporters: "It's wonderful that his death can help someone else. He was always such a helpful boy." Publicity was apparently winning the day for heart transplantation. Only a few days later there were pictures in the newspapers of DeBord holding a jar containing his own former heart.

A few days after the DeBord operation, Cooley met his model patient, Thomas, walking slowly but erect down a hospital corridor. The doctor informed him that he seemed in such good shape that there was no reason to keep him in St. Luke's any longer. However, he had better not return to Phoenix; for the time being he would have to remain in the vicinity of St. Luke's so that he could be examined every few days. It would not be long before Thomas would be able to go back to work, and no doubt a job could be found for him in Houston, Cooley added. What was more, since his courage and determination had contributed so much to the development of heart transplantation, St. Luke's and the Texas Heart Institute would bear all the hospital costs that were not covered by Thomas's own hospital insurance.*

That was the happiest day in Thomas's second life. Suddenly he was relieved of a tremendous burden, the fear that Helen would have to sell the house in Phoenix in order to pay for his rescue. Shortly afterward, he learned that William Harrell, president of the Medical Center National Bank, had offered him a job starting August 1 as a trust officer. The bank —a fairly new and imposing building mixing modern architecture with the traditional Greek style of banks—was on the other side of Fannin Street, only a short distance from St. Luke's. Thomas could see his future place of work from the hospital. The prospect of going back to work, of being able to support himself again, filled him with confidence. He had feared that he could never return to the time when he had directed and arranged his family's life. Now that time was coming back, and he had to make new arrangements.

He telephoned Helen in Phoenix. They agreed that they would have to look for a home in Houston so that the family could be together—with the exception of Mark, who would remain in Phoenix and go on with his studies. In Sharptown, not too far from St. Luke's, they located an apartment at a rent appropriate to the salary Thomas would be receiving from the Medical Center National Bank. Barbara Hurn, the head nurse in

* Total costs amounted to $38,179, of which Thomas's insurance covered $9,709.

charge of the transplant patients, lived in the same building. She made Thomas promise that he or Helen would call her at any time of the day or night if he did not feel well or needed help. Quietly, Cooley spread a protective net over his first patient, whose life was just as important to him as the life of Philip Blaiberg to Barnard.

Soon afterward Helen and the boys moved from Arizona to Sharptown. The day came when Dr. Leachman released Everett Thomas. He sent him out into the world with numerous admonitions and medicines. Leachman felt that if ever a patient would carry out every order with the greatest punctiliousness, that patient was Everett Thomas. Thomas henceforth had to come to Dr. Leachman and Dr. Nora three times a week for a checkup. The quantity of Imuran he took daily was governed by the results of their tests. Every third day he received an intramuscular injection of antilymphocyte serum. He had daily doses of prednisolone and once a week an especially high prednisolone "push." In addition, he received daily digitalis, circulatory drugs, drugs to reduce fluids, drugs to combat the bone damage caused by cortisone, antacids for the stomach, and insulin. But all this drug taking did not alter Everett Thomas's sense of being a new man, or affect in any way his veneration for Cooley. When he moved into his apartment, he told reporters: "When you shake Dr. Cooley's hand, it gives you faith. When he goes into that operating room, he is not alone. God's hand is on his shoulder." And he added: "I feel wonderful."

In his desire to fulfill the obligations of a "normal life," he would not let himself be driven to the hospital. On July 24 he took the wheel of his own car and drove to the St. Luke's parking lot. Several reporters instantly showed up, and he told them: "Sure, I drove the whole way. And from August 1 on I'll be driving to my new job every day, and walk from there to have my tests at the hospital." Asked whether walking tired him, he replied (although he knew he could not walk too far): "I can outwalk you any time."

On August 1 he took his place at a desk in the Medical Center National Bank. The desk stood on a mezzanine floor overlooking the lobby of the bank, so that he could be plainly seen from the lobby. He realized quite well that he had not been hired because the bank was in such urgent need of a trust officer. His name appeared in the newspapers almost every day, and the bank was willing to draw whatever publicity value went with that name. His duties were not onerous. Anyone who wanted to have a word with the first surviving American with another person's heart in his body was brought up to see him. Thomas was glad to talk to people. There was that task he had conceived on the day of his first press conference—to travel the length and breadth of America as a living testimonial to heart transplantation. For the present he would promote the good cause from right where he was. Whenever he went over to the St. Luke's cafeteria for a sugarless, low-salt, low-fat meal, he would sit bolt upright in his neat business suit, his face slowly broadening and taking on that moon-shaped cortisone look, but invariably friendly and willing to talk to anyone.

His statements, simple but coming straight from the heart, as it were, were reported to the millions. He preached his positive attitude toward the world: "I never had the slightest doubt the transplant would be a success . . . because I never make negative decisions. . . . When you come to a fork in the road you must decide positively to take one branch, not negatively to discard the other. When you come to a turning point in your life, you must decide positively which course to take and be convinced it is best for you." Or: "The transplant has deepened my faith in God and in my relationship with Him. It has made me love and appreciate my wife and family more. . . . When you are about to lose something you realize how much it means to you."

He remained unshaken by the reports of transplant deaths in the United States and in the rest of the world. In Houston, Fred Everman, a barber on whom Cooley had operated on July 20, and a lathe operator named Henry Jurgens, who had received his new heart on July 23, were still surviving. But Cooley's ninth patient, a housewife named Beth Brunk, who received an implanted heart on July 29, died fifty-five days later of intestinal hemorrhages and infections. And his next patient, Maria Giannaris, a five-year-old girl, met death even more quickly.

Maria had been sent to Houston from Johns Hopkins Hospital in Baltimore, where nothing could be done for her. Cooley implanted in her the heart of a boy named James Dudley Herron of Lafayette, Indiana, who had suffered a brain injury. Cooley's fame was now so great that an Air Force plane brought the boy, his brain dead but his heart still beating, 900 miles to Houston. When the operation was over, on August 19, Cooley called it an important medical break-through and added: "We now have the opportunity to observe the progress of the transplanted heart in an unmature recipient." Maria's father declared: "Dr. Cooley and his associates have a special gift from God." That same day Cooley was informed that the relatives of a dying woman were willing to place her heart at his disposal. He transplanted this heart into his eleventh patient, Carl van Bates. Van Bates survived the operation, but Maria Giannaris's heart beat for only seven days. Then her body rejected it in what could only be called a brutal fashion.

It seemed as though Thomas refused to acknowledge these alarming events. He read with satisfaction every press notice that considered Cooley's transplant series a major contribution to American medicine. He felt pained or uncomprehending whenever critical voices were raised. And during the month of August many were asking whether it was medically justifiable to go on performing transplants when the number of deaths far exceeded the number of successes. They asked whether it was right to spend $20,000 or more on a single heart transplant when for that sum many time-tested operations could be done, saving the lives of those who now died because they could not afford ordinary surgical procedures. They wanted to know why men like Cooley refused to see that a better solution to the rejection problem must be found before they went ahead with more and more such experiments, which benefited no one.

Everett Thomas's answer to such skeptics was: "Am I not living a useful life? In the history of medicine, people have always had to die so that the right course could be found. Dr. Cooley's wonderful work is lifesaving surgery. Am I not a living proof of that?"

Thomas drove out to Bolivar Point to go fishing and thereby demonstrate how good his new life was. He met Louis Fierro, who had meanwhile been discharged from St. Luke's. Fierro had taken a job with the used-car firm of Jacobe & Pearson, which like the Medical Center National Bank was happy to employ a "man with a new heart" as an attraction. His employers gave him a secondhand Chrysler Imperial and enough of a salary for him to stay at the Tidelands Motor Inn, where (contrary to all the rules for heart patients) he tanned himself at the swimming pool so that he would have a look of blooming health. Each time Fierro came to St. Luke's for a test, he would look in on the heart patients who were waiting for a transplant, in order to encourage them and show them what a life full of strength and health they might expect.

Toward the end of August, Everett Thomas decided that he ought to remain in Houston permanently. Nowhere else would he find so good a place for his work in the cause of transplantation. He had been allowed to take a booth at a medical congress; there he sat, equipped with pictures, diagrams, and a line of argument, to promote "new hearts." Many people there smiled at what seemed an exaggeration of naïve zeal. But he went on with his proselytizing, talking to clubs, schools, and groups of visitors from other states. When he had to take care of business affairs in Phoenix, including the possible sale of his house, he decided on the riskiest and most spectacular demonstration of his vitality. Alone, armed only with the bottles of drugs in his pockets, he took a scheduled airliner.

In Phoenix reporters of the local *Gazette* immediately tracked him down, and he repeated his profoundly convinced and convincing "I feel wonderful" and his remarks about God's hand on Cooley's shoulder. Then he flew back to Houston, returned to his desk at the bank, and shut his mind to such mounting evidence as the fact that Cooley had lost his twelfth patient, a two-month-old child in which he had implanted the heart and lungs of a day-old infant. He fended off the criticisms of Cooley's procedures which were beginning to be mingled with the tributes to the surgeon as the "uncontested champion heart transplanter in the world." On September 22, Thomas forcefully stated his doctrine to Jim Curran of the *Houston Chronicle:* "If God hadn't intended us to have them, he wouldn't have given man the knowledge to do them. I believe God and you are one and God and I are one. If two lines are parallel, then a line parallel with either is parallel to the other. If we are leading parallel lives with God, and we all are identifiable parts of one, made by God, even with different mothers, then why should not one's physical parts be transferable without reproach? . . . When the heart was removed from the donor, the soul already had gone and the heart was useless to the body. The body is only a taxi that carries the soul through life."

Denton A. Cooley's recollections:

"He treated me as if I was some form of deity. . . . He always treated me this way. It's obvious I didn't have time to spend with Mr. Thomas, being a busy practicing surgeon. Even though he was watched over meticulously by the immunologists and cardiologists, he saw me rather seldom. Even so, he related to me constantly as his doctor."

Early in October, Thomas drove to work at his bank as usual and talked to a reporter from Washington who was preparing an article on heart transplants and wanted to know in detail how Everett Thomas felt. The journalist had been in New York, Palo Alto, Richmond, and other cities, and had carefully looked into the heart transplant "industry" in Houston. Evidently he had come to some highly critical conclusions. He knew that of somewhat more than fifty patients with transplanted hearts, over thirty had died.

He wanted to ask Everett Thomas whether it was really worth while going through a heart transplantation. Thomas invited him to walk over to the St. Luke's cafeteria and see for himself how excellent his, Thomas's, health was. On the way he walked with exceptional vigor to prove his point to the stranger from Washington.

When he next reported for his usual examination in St. Luke's, he went at the exertion tests a bit more forcefully—almost as if the doubts of his last visitor were driving him to special achievements.

Denton A. Cooley's recollections:

"We had been studying him rather extensively, in a number of ways, for evidence of rejection, but we were also interested in the performance of this transplanted heart. . . . It was after one of these sessions, I believe, when he was doing some exercises with us, a test, that he manifested signs of heart failure. The signs would probably have manifested themselves anyway, within a few days, but it seemed to me that they were kind of precipitated at that moment by the studies. He was probably trying too hard to help us."

On October 9, Everett Thomas's desk on the mezzanine floor of the Medical Center National Bank remained empty. Thomas did not feel well. His pulse raced; he was attacked by violent nausea. He must have caught a cold, he decided. But when Leachman and Cooley heard of his symptoms, they felt a grim foreboding. The symptoms closely resembled those described in reports from Cape Town, Palo Alto, and New York, and those they had themselves observed, whenever a rejection "episode" became acute. Promptly, they had Thomas moved to the transplant department. By the time he arrived there he had changed greatly. His rounded cortisone face looked somewhat sunken. But he felt no doubt that Cooley would help him. When he realized that he was having a rejection reaction, he declared, with that amiable composure so typical of him: "You'll control it. I won't be dead until the coffin lid closes on me."

He was not told when only two days later Louis Fierro, his companion in the first weeks of triumph, suddenly suffered spells of vomiting and racing heart, and now lay in another room at St. Luke's. Fierro's face still showed the sun tan he had so carefully cultivated. On October 14, three days after he had re-entered the hospital, he was dead. Every effort to check the acute rejection of his heart by doses of antilymphocyte serum, cortisone, and actinomycin had failed. His heart simply stopped. The autopsy showed that the coronary vessels of the sound heart he was given had so degenerated within five months that they were like the vessels of a sclerotic old man. Meanwhile Everett Thomas fought on. In his case, too, all the drugs failed. The antilymphocyte serum proved ineffective. Still worse, Thomas seemed to have developed an allergy to this serum.

Cooley was deeply affected by the death of Fierro, the second of his long-term survivors. Of his transplant patients, Everman, DeBord, and van Bates were still living. But Thomas was his patient with the longest survival record, and Cooley fought hardest for him. He was able to prevent a sudden cardiac stoppage such as had killed Fierro, but the slow decline of the heart proceeded inexorably. Pulmonary edema led to shortness of breath, then to liver and kidney failure and dropsical swellings.

While Thomas was visibly dying, though he still believed otherwise, Cooley on October 25 operated on his thirteenth patient, Jerome Decker, an emaciated insurance salesman from Los Angeles who had lain for eight weeks in St. Luke's awaiting a new heart. Decker had sold his share in an insurance agency in order to pay the hospital bills. But it had proved impossible to find a donor. Was the period in which donors were readily reported and relatives happily gave their consent really over? Cooley issued appeals for donors. Like Thomas, he fought against believing that the most glorious phase of his life in surgery could end on a note of defeat. Only one day after the operation on Decker, who survived the operation but faced a highly uncertain convalescence, Carl van Bates died; he had lived only sixty-eight days with his new heart. He died from a virus infection that is ordinarily considered harmless and usually produces nothing more than lip sores after a cold: the herpes simplex virus. In van Bates's weakened body it became a brutal killer.

Meanwhile, Everett Thomas still fought on. In other rooms at St. Luke's many patients waited between hope and despair to see whether Thomas, who had so long embodied the success of Houston transplants, would live or die. On October 14, when the death of Louis Fierro was announced, some lost courage and returned home to die. Fierro had visited them so often to assure them that it was worth waiting for and risking the transplant operation. As late as October 10, thirty-five cardiac patients had been in the hospital, or in hotels and rooming houses in the vicinity, waiting for donors. And since there was not a single well-to-do person among them, they had used up most of their savings. Some of them, like Sidney Lebowitz, a Queens member of the New York City Council, refused to bow to fate and sent out desperate appeals on their own, asking the public to help, asking every family and every doctor who heard of a victim of an accident or murder to consider letting Dr. Cooley have the dead person's organs. On November 5 a donor for Lebowitz was found. Only four days after the operation, he was attacked by an infection and on November 12 he died. Another of those waiting was Andrew Perhacs, a fifty-five-year-old basketmaker. On November 9 a donor was found for him, but he, too, died quickly. On November 17, Lee Boyd, a Canadian railroad worker, received the heart of a woman who had died in childbirth. He was among Denton Cooley's last heart transplant patients; for in the meantime the life of Everett Thomas, the great beacon light of transplant surgery, came to an end.

By November 18 he was little more than a human wreck, poisoned by drugs, distorted by edema. Leachman knew that medical means had been exhausted, and so Cooley decided upon a surgical solution: the implantation of a second new heart. He was aware that Barnard had been ready to resort to this in the summer, but had never carried it out. Thus it would be a new thrust into unknown territory. He could not bear to let Thomas die, any more than Barnard had been able to give up on Blaiberg.

Denton A. Cooley's recollections:

"I talked to him and told him I'd like to try a second, and it had never been done, at that time, on a human being. . . . He was just so sick. He knew he was at the end of his tether. And it was possible that this new heart could give him another six months. . . . He'd gone a little over six months, close to seven months at that time. He thought he'd get another six months, and something else would come along, because Everett was convinced, as we were, that we were making some progress with the rejection problem. And that if he could just live long enough he could overcome some of these things."

That was Everett Thomas's last decision, and the last flicker of his faith in Providence's meaning well by him. He was scarcely able to form words. But he consented.

Cooley desperately tried to find a donor heart. Then he was struck by another heavy blow. On November 20 he received word that George DeBord, who had recently told newspapermen that he was going hunting again, had been attacked by the same symptoms as Thomas. DeBord was hastily brought from San Antonio to Houston. Cooley was forced to recognize that in this case, too, there was only one chance to prolong his life: a second transplant. On November 21 the heart of a twenty-seven-year-old woman became available. Cooley found himself with two dying patients, both of whom needed one heart.

Denton A. Cooley's recollections:

"This was one of the few times in our entire series of heart transplants where there really was a choice to be made. These two recipients were practically alike in most respects. . . . I made the decision. We were far more deeply indebted to Everett Thomas. He'd been so courageous and so co-operative. And so I made a decision to use this donor heart with Everett Thomas. . . . We went ahead with the second operation when he was virtually moribund; his blood pressure was almost unobtainable; he was a big, puffy fellow with a lot of edema. But we went ahead on the twenty-first of November and retransplanted at that time, put in a second transplant. The man was so sick at the time that it would have been a miracle if it could have brought him around."

It would indeed have been a miracle. Thomas was no longer aware of his second and last trip to the operating table. The operation took an unusually long time because Cooley encountered extensive cicatrization. He finished the last sutures at 5:45 P.M. But the new heart was reluctant to beat. Several electric shocks were needed before it took up its task. Cooley did not know that at the same time, in Stanford, Norman E. Shumway, in a similar act of desperation, had also implanted a second heart. His efforts to do a heart transplant in a pilot named Darrell Hammarley had failed after only six hours, and Shumway immediately repeated the experiment because a donor happened to be available.

Cooley was much too deeply absorbed in his struggle to save Thomas's life to glance at happenings in Stanford. But the struggle was hopeless. At four o'clock in the morning on November 23, Thomas's third heart beat feebly one last time. Then it stood still.

Denton A. Cooley's recollections:

"Actually I believe it [the cause of his death] was acute rejection of the second heart. These patients develop what we call preformed antibodies, and I think that maybe these preformed antibodies made that second heart reject faster than it would have under ordinary circumstances."

Thus Everett Thomas's life ended. The heart that could not save him would not have given George DeBord a second lease on life either. On November 28, DeBord died. In the meantime Thomas was buried in St. Francis Cemetery in Phoenix. Helen Thomas once more took over the responsibilities he had entrusted to her in April and then made his own again during the short period he served as a symbol of the future of heart transplantation.

From the taped notes of a medical journalist:

"I am certain that on the day of Thomas's death Denton Cooley sensed that the Houston heart transplant wave had subsided. But the plunge into the trough of that wave of hope was not just a Texan problem. It was a problem for the whole world.

"On November 24 I was in Paris to prepare a report on Father Boulogne, who had received a transplanted heart at the Broussais Hospital nine days after Thomas. The French doctors Dubost and Cahera, who had operated on the Dominican monk on May 12, had all along been far more reticent than Barnard or Cooley. Nevertheless, they regarded Boulogne, who by November 1968 had survived about as long as Everett Thomas, as their great triumph. Boulogne, who was now taking short walks in Paris, attracted a good deal of attention. When passers-by saw him in his black cloak and white habit, they would exclaim: 'There he is!' The medical sensation of the past year was not quite forgotten. But those who noticed Boulogne would scarcely have been ready to donate a heart or to contemplate a possible heart transplant for themselves, as they might have been eight months before. Among all the heart recipients I have known, Jean-Marie Boulogne was the only one whose superior intelligence simply would not let him give way to delusions of grandeur or tragic foolishness. He observed: 'I am their first case here. They don't want it to fail. . . . I am just playing the game.' And he would add: 'It is terrible to see how the instinct for survival generates illusions.'

"When the report of Thomas's death arrived, I happened to be talking to Des Broussais, a young immunologist whom I had known when we were both medical students. We were sitting in a café at the time; he glanced at the story and laid the newspaper quietly aside. 'He is the tenth to die this month,' he said. He did not tell me that on that very day Dubost was attempting another transplant—which ended in the rapid death of the recipient. But even if he did not yet know of this fresh failure, his fatalism was all too obvious.

"On November 24, in Lyons, Noel Moissonier died; he was the fourth heart transplant in France, and survived the operation by less than two weeks. In Toronto, Henry Taylor and Alfred Gagnier had recently died; their hearts had been implanted at the end of October and the middle of November. A few days later they were followed by Gaëtan Paris of Montreal, who at any rate had lived with his new heart a record five months. In Ankara and Istanbul, Maviz Karagoz and Ali Akgul died; in Valparaíso, Maria Penaloza. In Melbourne, George Whittler lived for only fourteen hours with a new heart. The Russians, who had entered the race somewhat belatedly on November 4, lost their first patient, a Leningrad woman, after two days. Darrell Hammarley, in whom Shumway had implanted two hearts at intervals of only six hours, died of a cerebral blood clot on December 13.

" 'Darkness is falling,' Des Broussais said to me. 'We may be able to keep Boulogne alive for a while. But even at that, we won't know precisely why he lived longer than the others. Once we believed, just as Shumway and Barnard did, that the heart would pose fewer immunological problems than the kidney. In fact, the problems are greater. Antilymphocyte serum has only limited effectiveness. Survival or nonsurvival is a question of favorable or unfavorable circumstances that remain mysteries. For us to count up the months, weeks, or days of Father Boulogne's survival throws no light on the question. Nor does it help Barnard that at the moment he can still point to Blaiberg and reckon that his patient has already lived eleven months, and therefore holds the survival record. Blaiberg will die, too, because surgical skill, no matter how great, is of little use as long as we cannot deal with rejection, and a number of other adjustment problems, without using drugs whose effects are so destructive.'"

Last Act / Philip Blaiberg

Notes of an Italian correspondent in Cape Town, 1968–1969:

"I can only plead ignorance as an excuse for what I reported in the spring and summer of 1968 about the supposedly excellent condition of Philip Blaiberg. But for my reports after his second discharge from Groote Schuur, on September 27, 1968, I must blame my optimism and, probably, my eagerness to have faith. The truth is that in spite of all those photographs of a smiling Blaiberg, the man's condition was desperate after he overcame, with the help of antilymphocyte serum, the nearly fatal crisis of May and June 1968.

"He was unable to walk. In August and September 1968 he relearned, for the second time, the simplest movements, and finally had recovered sufficiently so that Barnard or Bosman, or perhaps both (I am not sure), wanted to send him home. But he refused to leave. His conviction that he was the living symbol of successful heart transplantation forbade him to appear crippled in public. He wanted to be released on a note of triumph, as in March.

"But he could not make it. After many weeks of exercises, he was barely able to walk with a cane and was therefore taken home secretly. Not even his wife knew the date of his release. She was at a party on the evening of September 27 and learned that her husband was already home only when he telephoned. The press release reported it afterward, adding that Blaiberg still had to recuperate, but that he was essentially in perfect health. In reality, it was an event for him when he was able for the first time to dress himself again.

"Schrire, Marius Barnard, Bosman, and Botha, who were chiefly responsible for treating Blaiberg, fully realized that there was still no way of recognizing the rejection of an implanted heart in time. They even suspected that a constant creeping rejection was taking place, which had to be repressed continuously. They tried to keep this continuous repression going by intravenous injections of antilymphocyte serum three times a week. In addition, they kept up an intermittent bombardment with prednisone. Along with his basic daily dose of this drug, Blaiberg received at certain intervals massive 'pushes' of 200 milligrams of prednisone. This treatment (together with numerous other drugs, from digitalis to the dehydrating drug Lasix) sent Blaiberg into a state of euphoria such as is often induced by cortisone derivatives. He no longer saw the realities of his own situation and imagined he was making progress when the opposite was all too clear.

"I can only explain the optimism of the accounts that appeared in the world press during the winter (that is, the South African summer) of 1968–69 as based on this impression of euphoria. Blaiberg turned up at an occasional party, spoke cheerfully in occasional interviews, and appeared on the beach several times. In order to conceal the fact that he could not walk without help, he and Eileen played the loving couple, walking along in close embrace. At home he spent many hours signing autographs or letters.

"The preservation of his image as a man living normally with his new heart was undoubtedly a masterpiece of unconscious showmanship. The truth remained concealed behind the walls of the apartment in Wynberg —at least, until March 1969. In the meantime, invitations from European fans had led to preparations for a tour of Europe by Philip, Eileen, and Jill Blaiberg. But the Groote Schuur team realized that such a trip would end in disaster for Blaiberg. The frequent tests showed increasing damage to various organs of his body, partly due to the highly toxic drugs. In addition to kidney disturbances, there was damage to his skeletal structure. Even more ominous were indications of changes in the coronary vessels of his new heart. Like other heart transplant patients, Blaiberg felt no local symptoms because his new heart lacked nerve connections. But the doctors suspected that they were no longer confronted solely by rejection problems. Rather, they were facing another phenomenon: the young heart, transplanted in a healthy condition, was being attacked by the same disease that had brought Blaiberg to Barnard's operating table—coronary sclerosis.

"Since Barnard himself was again on his travels, one of his associates undertook the task of convincing Blaiberg that it would be better for him to give up the European tour for the present. As far as I know, he asked Blaiberg to do this as a personal favor to Barnard; Barnard would have many a sleepless night if Blaiberg went on the tour. Blaiberg consented; he stayed home in the apartment, cared for by his housekeeper, Katie, and the team of doctors while Eileen Blaiberg flew to Europe with her daughter. That was in April 1969. Eileen, with a skill partly natural, partly studied, presented the Blaiberg myth everywhere.

"The Barnard team used the interval to subject Blaiberg to many tests.

The results were virtually unequivocal: the changes in the coronary vessels were so pronounced that if the nerve connections had been present Blaiberg would have been suffering severe attacks of angina pectoris. When Eileen Blaiberg returned, she found her husband still euphoric, but physically going downhill rapidly. On May 17 he was taken to Groote Schuur. May 24 was his birthday, and since queries from the newspapers could be expected, he was taken back to his apartment as the day approached. But he had to be carried up the stairs and put to bed. He went through the birthday show and also the move to a new house of his own on Lady Anne Avenue, which Eileen Blaiberg had bought from the proceeds of the Blaiberg myth. This move seemed to me a confirmation that Blaiberg was 'indestructible'; he had now been living for some fifteen months with his new heart. In fact, the change of residence marked the beginning of the end. Whenever Blaiberg was able to get out of bed, he would take hours for such simple acts as shaving. He again began suffering from shortness of breath.

"At the end of May, oxygen bottles and a respirator were secretly brought to the house on Lady Anne Avenue. The tests showed clearly that the arteriosclerotic changes in Blaiberg's heart were not proceeding slowly, as had been hoped. Rather, they were developing with cruel speed. Barnard had to face the inescapable fact that his symbol, the patient upon whom his fame and much of his argument for the continuance of heart transplants were based, was dying. As in June 1968, he saw only one chance to save Blaiberg: a second heart transplant.

"He confessed the hopelessness of the situation to Eileen Blaiberg and asked her consent. This time she hesitated. Whatever her motives, whether because she herself was exhausted or because she realized that Blaiberg's survival could be bought only at the price of more suffering and would scarcely be a real life, she postponed decision. The world suspected nothing, but a nurse took over the care of Blaiberg. On Sunday night, August 10, he became so short of breath that he had to be given oxygen almost continually. Barnard was notified.

"Barnard kept on insisting that the patient could be saved only by another transplant. But Eileen Blaiberg could not come to a decision. Finally she discussed the matter with Katie, the colored girl who had cared for the patient so long and whose human feelings were uncorrupted by personal or medical interests, by the desire for fame or gain. According to Eileen Blaiberg's own testimony in the *Daily Sketch* (April 6, 1970), Katie replied that the doctors had had enough out of him. Eileen Blaiberg rejected Barnard's proposal.

"On Tuesday, August 12, Blaiberg was quietly transferred back to Groote Schuur. At last the public learned how sick he was. He spent the following five days more or less dozing and receiving oxygen—just as if, by way of a detour through a borrowed and often painful life, he had come back to where he had already been, facing death. On Sunday, August 17, he died. When Barnard and the pathologist of Groote Schuur Hospital examined his second heart, they found confirmation of the tests of the past half year. In nineteen months the new, healthy heart had not only been subject to chronic rejection attacks. It had also succumbed to the same arteriosclerotic process that over a lifetime had destroyed Blaiberg's own heart."

Did it have a meaning?

From a letter by Dr. Manfred Kyber-Visconti, 1971:

"Two years have now passed since Dr. Philip Blaiberg died in Cape Town. He took with him into the grave the hopes of millions who wanted to believe that heart transplantation would be more than a momentary sensation. In 1968 no fewer than ninety-nine heart transplants were performed throughout the world. In 1969 there were still forty-eight, in 1970 seventeen, and in 1971 only nine. Of the fifty-eight heart transplant teams that were competing all over the world, fifty-six stopped work. All in all, we have witnessed the longest and most sensational test of a new operation in the history of medicine. And we are confronted with the question: did it have a meaning? Did all the fuss merely provide a few persons with a brief prolongation of their lives and raise them from obscurity to a dubious prominence? Only a few of those fifty-eight teams of surgeons were qualified for scientific work of this nature and could derive any real knowledge from their experiments. And too many patients died to satisfy nationalistic aspirations or dreams of personal glory. But those patients— both the dead and those who survived for shorter or longer periods—who went through the adventure of a new heart in scientific centers did provide experience. And no experience on this earth, whether it is negative or positive, is without meaning."

Norman E. Shumway et al., in California Medicine, *August 1970:*

"The initial enthusiasm, approaching hysteria, which greeted the first clinical cardiac transplants now seems to have been replaced by a generally pessimistic outlook. Both reactions are probably inappropriate. The journalists' 'medical break-through' rarely results in a radical change in patient care. It is, rather, the cautious clinical application of information gained in the laboratory that results in the gradual development of new therapeutic methods. At this point we believe cardiac transplantation remains within the realm of clinical investigation."

Dr. Herberg Thom in a letter from Palo Alto, 1971:

"Perhaps there is an element of irony in the situation. Today, four years after the beginning of the world-shaking wave of heart transplants, there is only a single place in all of America where heart transplantation—without headlines and all the other noisy attributes of that wave—is still being done. Moreover, it happens to be the very place where for many years the fundamentals of heart transplantation were being worked out, likewise without headlines and sensationalism. That is Stanford University, and the leader there is Norman E. Shumway. He has never given up, even now that the straw fires have gone out.

"If we except Cape Town, where Barnard now and then still makes an effort to keep alight the torch that brightened his life, Shumway's hospital and laboratories are actually the only places in the entire world where hearts are still being transplanted. But it is being done so quietly, with such scientific stringency, that no one outside a very narrow group knows about it. Of the twenty-three persons who received new hearts there, eight are living at the moment, and Shumway's patient Carl P. Sheaffer is among the four persons in this world who have survived for three years after a heart transplant. Each of the four knows he must expect no miracles and that his survival may end any day. But he also knows that he represents part of the quiet effort to break the barrier that still blocks the way to real success—the barrier of rejection with all its mysteries."

4 / Tommy Gorence

I

"New York, November 21, 1964

"Dear Harold:

"Forgive me for not getting around to that report I should have sent you immediately after the meeting of the Society of University Surgeons. I think the title you suggested—'Liver Transplantation: A Letter from America'—is a good one.

"It seems that up to the present there have been no serious attempts at liver transplantation in Europe, aside from Great Britain. What experimentation there has been is largely American. There are two centers here. One is Peter Bent Brigham Hospital in Boston, the other the Medical Center of the University of Colorado in Denver. The leader in the field in Boston is Francis Daniels Moore, chief of the surgical department at Peter Bent Brigham, who is now fifty. In Denver it is Thomas E. Starzl, a younger surgeon who moved from kidney transplants to liver transplantation.

"The number of patients in the United States suffering from incurable liver diseases is considerable. The list of diseases is headed by cirrhosis of the liver, primary cancer of the liver, and gall duct atresia, that malformation in which children are born without an opening from the gall duct, or without a gall duct, and so are condemned to death. In all these cases the only possible recourse is complete replacement of the destroyed or no longer functioning organ.

"Moore and Starzl are well aware that they are venturing into an area fraught with far more difficulties than kidney transplantation. Surgically, the problems are considerable. I shall have to discuss some of them, at the risk of repeating common medical knowledge. In kidney transplantation it is possible to place the organ in any part of the pelvic cavity where it can conveniently be connected with an artery and vein. The structure of the liver excludes such a procedure. It is connected to the circulation in too many ways: (1) with the portal vein, into which various veins from the intestines and stomach flow, bringing materials obtained from the digestive process to the liver for further breakdown; (2) with the hepatic artery, which supplies the liver with oxygenated blood; (3) with the vena

325

cava, into which the liver returns the material it has processed; (4) with the bile duct, through which the liver sends gall, a by-product of its chemical processing of the blood, into the duodenum to help with digestion. Implanting a new liver requires re-establishing all these connections.

"Moore and Starzl were fully conscious of the technical as well as the physiological complexities. The liver seems to have innumerable functions; we know today of some 500. For successful transplanting, the fact that the liver stores carbohydrates, proteins, and vitamins, or changes lactose into glucose, is not so important. But its function in regulating blood clotting is crucial. It is obvious that in the course of a liver transplant there can be dangerous surprises, in the form of hemorrhages if the blood's ability to coagulate is reduced, or blood clots if coagulability is increased. When we consider how toxic Imuran and the other immunosuppressive drugs are, and what high demands their toxicity imposes upon the detoxicating functions of the liver, a further problem appears. Liver medicine is still largely a matter of groping in the dark.

"December 2, 1964

"I must apologize again for not keeping my word; something came up that kept me from finishing this letter. But perhaps it was all for the best. On the return flight from a biologists' convention in Los Angeles, I stopped over in Denver for a few days and had an opportunity for an interesting conversation. But first let me continue where I stopped in November.

"Between 1958 and 1960, Francis D. Moore and Thomas E. Starzl undertook their first liver transplant experiments on animals. Moore and his people experimented on thirty-one animals in all. Eighteen died after twenty-four hours. Eight lived four days, and a few six, eight, or twelve days. Starzl actually tried transplanting eighty times. But none of his animals lived longer than four days.

"At any rate, the researchers discovered that there are far more problems in keeping a donor liver alive up to the moment of implantation than there are for a kidney. Twenty minutes away from the body and a liver is fatally damaged. Yet it can take six hours and more to implant a liver because of the many anastomoses, or connections. At the same time, there are all sorts of circulatory problems. During the liver exchange, for example, the vena cava of the recipient must be clamped off and severed above and below the recipient's liver. In order to continue the venous circulation until the end of the operation, Starzl had to connect posterior veins of the animal's body with anterior veins by means of a plastic tube.

"Between 1960 and 1963 a way was found to rinse the donor liver while still in the donor's body with dextrose solution chilled to 15 degrees centigrade, and to continue this rinsing during transfer to the body of the recipient. In this way the activity of the liver was prolonged for the time needed to carry out the implantation.

"In the course of the experiments, the survival time of the animals was increased from days to weeks. Thus the period was reached within which rejection normally begins—and it did indeed begin. After Imuran had proved its effectiveness in kidney transplants, Moore and Starzl applied the drug in their liver experiments. The results seemed so promising that last year, at the beginning of 1963, Starzl believed he had reached the point where he might attempt a transplant on a human being. This first human experiment took place in Colorado General Hospital on March 1, 1963. The patient was a three-year-old child dying because of gall duct atresia. After high (as we now know, too high) doses of Imuran, Starzl transplanted the liver of a girl who had died during an operation for a brain tumor. The recipient bled to death on the operating table. When her liver was severed from its connections, the blood-clotting mechanism failed.

"Two months later Starzl tried a second time on William Grigsby, a black suffering from cancer of the liver. The donor had been an alcoholic; consequently, his liver was not in the best shape. But no other donor could be found. The rinsing of the liver worked well until the last suture was placed and the opening of the clamps permitted Grigsby's own blood to pour into the new liver. Grigsby received oxygen, and although he suffered from dyspnea during the first forty-eight hours, he seemed to be recovering. Then he was struck by a violent inflammation of the veins with high fever. On May 17, twenty-two days after the operation, he died. The autopsy showed many blood clots in his lungs, in the liver, and in the vena cava. One of the clots was more than an inch and a half long and half an inch thick.

"On June 10, Starzl made his third attempt, this time on a man of sixty-six, both of whose legs had earlier been amputated and who was now suffering from cancer of the liver. But while the patient's liver was being exposed for the transplant, the donor, who had been expected to die, recovered. Fourteen days passed before a new donor was found. Then the transplantation proceeded without incident. But seventy-two hours later the patient began to suffer severe dyspnea. With artificial respiration he lived another four and a half days. Then he died; the autopsy revealed intestinal hemorrhages and blood clots in the lungs.

"Nevertheless, Francis D. Moore and his assistant, Nathan P. Couch, also shifted, three months later, from experiments on animals to their first attempt at human liver transplantation. In Peter Bent Brigham Hospital, Joseph J. Bingel, an elderly construction worker, was in the last stages of liver cancer. On September 14 a policeman named Callahan was shot in a Boston suburb during the holdup of a supermarket. He died two days later, and Moore and Couch transplanted his liver to Bingel. For the first few days, functional tests showed that the liver, after a brief pause, was beginning to work normally. But shortly afterward Bingel developed jaundice, accompanied by high fever and signs of a rejection crisis. Neither Imuran nor cortisone checked the crisis, and on September 22, Bingel drew his last breath.

"Moore thereupon renounced any further liver transplants in human beings. Starzl, on the other hand, continued to try. He operated on a woman of twenty-nine, Jeanine Goodfellow, whose liver was so enormously enlarged by a carcinoma that it weighed twenty pounds. The operation lasted two hours. Jeanine Goodfellow was the first patient to survive three weeks, and even to leave her bed. Then she, too, had a sudden rejection crisis and died on the twenty-third postoperative day. She had, at any rate, survived longest of all the patients. Starzl was sufficiently encouraged to continue his experiments. He tried three more liver transplants. But when all of them ended in the rapid death of the recipients, he gave up.

"At the meeting of University Surgeons that I mentioned at the beginning of my letter, Starzl told me that he would attempt no more human liver transplants until further animal experiments offered some prospect of overcoming the principal causes of the failures: blood-clotting disturbances and rejection.

"Since then, there has been silence. But that does not mean the subject of liver transplantation is closed. In Boston, Moore and his associates are continuing to experiment on animals. And, as I found out in Denver, Starzl, too, has no intention of giving up. New experiments on dogs appear to show that it would not have been necessary to establish an artificial plastic connection between the veins; rather, the vena cava can be clamped off at the liver for a considerable time without danger. Since the plastic tubes may have contributed to the formation of blood clots in the deceased patients, this discovery is important. At the same time, the Denver team is trying to manufacture an antilymphocyte preparation from equine serum that will combat liver rejection more effectively than Imuran, and without that drug's toxicity.

"If anything new develops in liver transplantation, you will hear from me. That is a promise. But the group in Denver does not think there will be anything significant to report for three or four, possibly even five, years.

"Yours,

"O."

II

Early in 1968, Tommy Gorence wrote two letters to his mother, Joan Gorence, in Oneonta, New York. The first:

Dear Momsie,

How's it been? Good I hope. We didn't have parade, thank goodness. . . . Would have slept right through it.

The care package needs a refill. Hint, hint. And would you send up a picture of me, before I came up here for summer school. You know, when I had the long hair. . . . How's Auggie [Tommy's dog]? And of course how are you? . . . I got two warnings, but I'm sure I can pull them back up. I'll be going to help classes and stuff like that, easy. Well, that's about it.

Love,
Tom

P.S. I haven't smoked them all, but I can still collect cigarettes (and matches). (hint, hint)

His second letter:

Dear Mother darling,

Would you send up a care package which consists of
1. Cookies
2. Candie
3. Magazines, "Mad," etc.
4. Little money
5. White shirts, 15½", 31" they still don't have them.
6. bread, peanut butter, and jelly knife
7. matches
8.

thank you.

How's Aug? Tell him when I get home this thanks giving I'll take him hunting maybe. . . . Everything all okay up here.

Love,
Tom

Thomas B. Gorence, called Tommy, had just turned sixteen at the time he wrote these letters. For several months he had been a cadet at the military academy in Manlius, east of Syracuse, New York. In his dark blue, red-trimmed tunic with the light blue trousers and visored cap, he looked like the healthiest young man in the world. More than six feet tall and weighing 200 pounds, he was broad-shouldered and muscular, with a long, good-natured, boyish face. Strictly speaking, he was still somewhat childish, as his letters show, but a fairly good pupil, co-operative, contented, occasionally given to pranks, a more or less secret smoker, and a noisy player on the electric guitar. On the whole he was a well-bred boy, polite and still unaffected by the trend of youthful rebellion against standard American ideals, against the military, the police, and such institutions as the hundred-year-old Manlius School. Tommy wanted to be a military pilot, or at least to join the state police someday—like his father, Johnny Gorence, who had died in a plane accident in 1966.

Tommy Gorence's whole life changed on Saturday, February 17, 1968, when he and a bunch of his buddies went over to the gym. They were in high spirits, in spite of the cold. As far as health went, they were a select group. Tommy could not recall ever having been seriously ill, aside from being bitten by a rabid dog once, and having a tonsillectomy. On the physical examination given to new arrivals at the academy he had been rated A-1. He was proud of the trophy he had won when he was twelve and a star player on Oneonta's Little League team. He was proud of his first few flying hours, for he had already started taking lessons. In basketball he was one of the toughest players on the team. Now the team members marched into the lofty gym and donned their gym clothes with the word "Manlius" and a big number on the sweat shirts. Tommy was number 30, and he was soon in the thick of the game.

Suddenly he tumbled to the floor. One of the other players had accidentally jabbed him in the vicinity of the liver. Tommy turned pale, but soon picked himself up and went on playing. Shortly afterward he received a second blow. This time he stood leaning forward, both hands pressed against his abdomen. He was no sissy, and gestured to the others that he would soon be all right. His friends, however, became worried, seeing him standing there in agony. They helped him dress. Tommy was feeling so bad that he made no protest. They led him to C Company's building and down the bare green corridor on the ground floor to Room 315. There they placed him in the lower bunk. Then they remembered that eight or ten days before he had complained about stomach pains and gone to the infirmary. But the doctor had found nothing wrong. His friends thought he had probably eaten something that disagreed with him. Now, too, they thought the pain would go away. But it did not; it grew worse. Tommy's face turned livid. The doctor was called. When he saw Tommy Gorence and felt his abdomen, he began to suspect some internal injury. He informed Leibert Sedgwick, the dean of the school, and then called Syracuse University Hospital. Sedgwick drove Tommy to Syracuse.

*Dr. Bruce E. Chamberlain, surgeon of University Hospital, Syracuse,
in a letter about Tommy Gorence dated February 26, 1968:*

"At the time I saw him in the hospital he appeared to have a stable
blood pressure, but his pulse was a little fast and he appeared pale, as
though he had lost some blood. Diagnostic studies disclosed blood in the
peritoneal cavity. I felt that he should be operated on because of the question of rupture of either liver or spleen."

Joan Gorence was an energetic woman in her forties. Since becoming a
widow, and with Tommy off at Manlius (her elder son, Bill, was in the
army and stationed in Arizona), she had been preparing to take her final
examination so that she could qualify as a teacher. She was going to be
married soon to Francis B. Knapp, a friend of her late husband's, but she
was not the kind of woman to be content solely with the role of housewife.

She was sitting over her books, the dog, Auggie, dozing on the floor
beside her, when the telephone rang. A woman's voice informed her that a
doctor at the University Hospital in Syracuse wished to speak to her. Then
a man's voice came on the line. After asking whether she was the mother
of Tommy Gorence, the man said: "Your son has had an accident while
playing basketball. He received a blow in the vicinity of the liver and has
been brought to the hospital here. He is suffering from an internal hemorrhage and we must operate to stop it. We are therefore asking your permission. It may be that the spleen has also been injured. In that case we
would have to remove the spleen."

Resolute and self-sufficient though Joan Gorence was, this news so
stunned her that she could not answer at once. The voice at the other end
of the line persisted. "Are you still there? Don't be alarmed. The spleen is
not an organ essential to life, and removing it will not involve any danger
to your son."

At last Joan Gorence brought herself to speak. "I'll leave for Syracuse
immediately. I want to see him."

The voice countered: "It's a hundred-mile drive. We cannot wait that
long; there's the risk of his bleeding to death internally. We must operate
at once."

Joan hesitated for a moment longer. Then she said: "All right, you
have my permission—you'll do everything in your power to make him
well . . ."

"Of course. We'll be expecting you here as soon as you can make it."

Joan Gorence now proceeded to act in her usual clearheaded, resolute
way. While dressing, she telephoned the Red Cross and asked that Bill in

Arizona be notified and granted a special leave to come to Oneonta. Then she phoned Francis Knapp, whom she called Fran, and her neighbors, to ask them to take care of Auggie. Shortly afterward she drove out into the wintry day, hoping fervently that the roads would not be blocked by snow.

As she drove, her thoughts returned to that September 26, 1965, when she had similarly driven to a hospital to see her husband after the plane crash. That time she had not driven northwest, but southwest, to Binghamton, and she had not been alone. Two state-police officers, friends of her husband, had taken her, and on the way had tried to spare her feelings by telling her only half the truth. But comforting lies had not spared her the reality she encountered in Binghamton: a paralyzed human body, incapable of speech, that in no way resembled the man she had met twenty years before, when she was a seventeen-year-old girl, at a vacation camp in Cooperstown.

Cooperstown lay to the northeast of the highway she was now racing along between wintry hills. John M. Gorence had then been a discharged soldier without a high school diploma and without a trade. The old farmhouse near Cooperstown into which they had moved after their marriage in 1948 probably still stood there. They had carried water from a spring, had built their own furniture. In Cooperstown, Bill had been born, and three years later Tommy. After four years of trying, Johnny had been unable to find any regular work in Cooperstown, and so they had eventually packed their possessions into an old car, and Joan and the children had moved into her parents' home. Johnny went to California to look for a job. But California had not been the promised land either. Johnny had returned, still jobless, and finally found work in a cabinetmaker's shop in New York City. But she had loved him.

Joan Gorence knew no more about medicine than most people. She understood the dangers of an internal hemorrhage, but she did not know how important the spleen was and whether it really was superfluous, or whether the doctor in Syracuse had only told her a half-truth—as Johnny's friends had done when Johnny lay with a broken back and they had told her he might recover, although everyone knew he no longer had a chance. She knew for certain, however, that she would wish no one the kind of dying he had undergone. It had taken eight indescribable months. Every day she had driven sixty miles from Oneonta to Binghamton to sit beside the bed in which a living corpse lay. When Johnny, after many weeks, was able to stammer a few words, he had begged her: "Help me die." She had been forced to face the fact that if he survived at all, he would survive only in this condition; she would have to work to keep the family going. And so she had decided to be a teacher and had begun her studies—torn between her work and the shattered man who could not die.

To his own relief (and, in all honesty, to hers), John M. Gorence died on a day she had planned to visit him but arrived too late. And she had learned, forever, that life no longer means life when one is helpless and without hope—though doctors may still call it life.

Dr. Bruce E. Chamberlain in a letter about Tommy Gorence, February 26, 1968:

"I was amazed to find that . . . he had a huge centrally located tumor of the liver with the bleeding source from one of the necrotic nodules and also from a small tear. . . . With considerable difficulty the bleeding was controlled and the procedure was completed at this point. It appeared impossible to resect any part of this tumor. Since operation the pathology has been returned as a . . . carcinoma."

When Leibert Sedgwick, the dean of the Manlius School, approached her, Joan Gorence felt that something unusual must have happened. Sedgwick, a quiet, solid man with close-cropped hair and large glasses, was obviously having difficulty keeping his composure. For a moment she thought that she had come too late, that Tommy had died. With a tremendous effort she managed to ask whether the operation had gone all right.

Sedgwick assured her that Tommy was alive and that the doctor himself wanted to speak to her. He led her into a small office and introduced her to Dr. Chamberlain.

"Mrs. Gorence," the doctor said, "it was a difficult operation, because the bleeding was from the liver, and the liver cannot be removed like the spleen. We had to sew up a bleeding tear. But Tommy is now out of any immediate danger."

She caught the word "immediate," but waited.

Chamberlain resumed: "What I have to tell you now came as a complete surprise to me. Tommy is so robust that it never occurred to me until we exposed the liver. What we discovered is really extremely rare in a boy Tommy's age. We found a large tumor in Tommy's liver. . . . I'm sorry, but it's cancer."

Before Chamberlain uttered the terrible word, Joan had been thinking of some internal injury that might affect Tommy's future. It seemed inconceivable that Tommy could have cancer. He was sixteen years old. And hadn't he been examined when he entered Manlius, and hadn't they found that he was in perfect health?

Unfortunately, Chamberlain replied, there was no doubt about it. What Tommy had was a hepatoma, a primary cancer. Many liver cancers developed from metastases, the original cancer cells migrating from other organs; but in Tommy's case the tumor had begun in the liver itself.

Joan reasoned that since Tommy had noticed nothing until the time of the accident, and since nothing had been detected in him before now, the condition must be a case of early cancer. And the newspapers were always saying that if cancer were discovered early enough, it could be cured by operation.

That was true in many cases, Chamberlain replied, but unfortunately not in the case of a primary liver cancer. If the cancer were secondary, only parts of the liver would be involved and it might be possible to remove such parts successfully. But the primary cancer had already infected all parts of the liver. The entire liver would have to be extirpated. And nobody could live longer than thirty-six hours without a liver.

"What about radiation?" Joan Gorence asked desperately.

The doctor replied that Tommy's tumor was so widely distributed over the entire liver that radiation would not help. But he did not want her to rely on his opinion alone. In a week or two Tommy could be transferred to the Fox Memorial Hospital in Oneonta, and the doctors there would advise her further.

"How long can he live?" Joan asked. "How long can he live if nothing is done?"

Perhaps six months, perhaps somewhat longer, Dr. Chamberlain replied.

Joan Gorence realized at that moment that she would have to fight for Tommy's life, although she had no idea how. But first she wanted to know what sort of immediate future he faced. She could not bear the thought of an end like her husband's being repeated, so soon, and by a sixteen-year-old boy.

The doctor told her that Tommy, thanks to his otherwise sound constitution, would recover and would be without complaints for a while; but that the tumor would continue to grow inexorably and would ultimately form metastases in other organs.

So that was what Tommy faced, what she faced. Once more a long period of waiting for death. She could not go through that again. But she pulled herself together and assented to Tommy's being sent to Fox Memorial Hospital as soon as possible.

Dr. Bruce E. Chamberlain to Dr. Richard Haines, Oneonta:

"Following the emergency surgery his general course has been good except for some prolonged, slowly recurring fever. I believe the fever partly is due to the necrosis created by the liver sutures to control bleeding. . . . He does have some rather purulent-appearing drainage from the wound. However in spite of this his fever is resolving and his general condition has improved a great deal.

"He received a total of ten pints of blood at the time of the operation, and has received two pints for general support since. I have made arrangements for the transfer to your service at the Oneonta hospital on Monday, February 26."

The Tommy who arrived in Oneonta looked very different from the boy who had been hospitalized in Syracuse. He had lost a good deal of weight in the nine days. Pale, with a drain in the abdominal incision, he lay on the stretcher and was carried into the ocher yellow building of Fox Memorial Hospital, only a few hundred yards from his mother's home.

The sudden operation, the fever, and a feeling of weakness he had never known before confused Tommy, as it would have any healthy young boy who suddenly realizes that health is not something to be taken for granted. Some of the treatments he had experienced in Syracuse—especially being packed in ice bags to lower the fever—had left him with a kind of shock. He began recovering only when his brother, Bill, a few of his school friends from Oneonta, and, in particular, pretty Karen visited him. Karen, who was one of the first to find out about Tommy's real condition, had lost her own mother to cancer. Up to the end, no one had told Karen that her mother's condition was hopeless. Although Karen had been very young at the time, she had often reflected on how much more happiness she could have given her mother in those last months if she had known the truth. Now she had the feeling that she could somewhat make up for this failure with Tommy, and so she visited him nearly every day. Since he knew nothing about his real condition and imagined he would soon be returning to Manlius, his youthful optimism slowly returned.

Meanwhile Joan Gorence had begun her fight for her son's life. She called on Dr. Richard Haines, and when he confirmed Dr. Chamberlain's diagnosis, she appealed to all her friends, acquaintances, and relatives, asking them whether they had heard of any possible cure for Tommy's condition. She herself began to search; she read everything she could find about cancer in magazines and newspapers. A few days after Tommy had been moved to Oneonta, she came upon a paperback entitled *Laetrile: Control for Cancer*. She bought the book and read about Laetrile, a novel drug which, the claim was, if regularly injected could check cancer. The book spoke of institutions with such impressive names as the John Beard Memorial Foundation in San Francisco or the McNaughton Foundation in Montreal, which had promoted the development of this drug since 1963. Scientists with reputable titles were quoted, such as Professor R. N. Bouziane, biochemist at the University of Montreal, dean of the American College of Bio-Analysts and specialist in chemotherapy at Jeanne d'Arc Hospital. By the time Joan Gorence had finished the book, she believed she had found a way that might save Tommy. She took the book to the hospital and asked Dr. Haines to read it, be convinced, and try Laetrile on Tommy before it was too late.

Joan never found out whether Dr. Haines had read the book, but in any case he had no intention of trying the drug and counseled her to bow to the inevitable. She herself then tried to buy Laetrile. But she found that its sale in the United States was forbidden by the Food and Drug Administration. One pharmacist actually told her that the drug consisted simply of ground apricot pits. But Joan Gorence would not relinquish the one salvation she believed she had found. On March 4 she telephoned the Food and Drug Administration in Washington and asked whether it was really true that she could not buy the drug that might save her child's life. The authorities in Washington promised to answer in writing, and by March 8 she had a letter from them.

The letter pointed out that the Canadian Medical Association had made a careful study of Laetrile in 1965. Its conclusion was that even the composition of the drug that had been offered for sale as Laetrile in the United States did not correspond to the Canadian Laetrile, and that in any case neither of these drugs was effective against cancer. Laetrile, the letter from Washington continued, had also been tried out in extensive experiments on animals by the National Cancer Institute. The letter concluded by expressing sympathy for the victims of cancer and their families, but pointing out that unfortuntely many so-called cancer remedies were constantly being touted without any proof of their scientific value, and that Laetrile belonged in this category.

Joan Gorence was bitterly disappointed. But she had often read that people were cured by drugs that official medicine condemned. And was not Professor Bouziane a genuine scientist with all the titles and honors of one? She therefore decided to telephone Montreal and ask Bouziane in person for help for Tommy.

After some difficulty Joan reached Dr. Bouziane in Montreal. He confirmed the fact that he had worked with Laetrile. He also informed her that the McNaughton Foundation in Canada was still in existence, that its president was the son of General McNaughton, who had commanded the Canadian armed forces during the war, and that the foundation treated many Americans with Laetrile. But Bouziane did not suggest that she bring Tommy to Montreal. Instead he told her of cancer clinics in Tijuana, Mexico, which specialized in the use of Laetrile and whose patients were almost exclusively Americans who could not be treated in their own country because of the existing ban.

After this conversation Joan Gorence felt close to despair. She had never been in Mexico. But she had read that Tijuana was hot and dirty, a town of quick divorces, bullfights, brothels, naked dancers, marijuana peddlers, and abortionists. And what she could find out during the next few days about the cancer clinics in Tijuana seemed calculated to destroy her hopes. The magazine *Parade* described the cancer clinics and a Dr. Ernesto Contreras who treated Americans for $10 a day in his Good Samaritan clinic, with an extra charge of $3 to $6 for every Laetrile injection. *Parade* also described another clinic, the Bio-Medical Center, run by a former American nurse who offered cancer cures at the blanket price of $500, using another drug, Hoxsey, that was likewise banned in America.

The more she found out, the worse it all looked. By now Tommy was back home, still ignorant of his true condition, and she was granting his every wish to make him happy. Although Dr. Haines advised against it, she bought Tommy the motorcycle he had long been wanting. But while Tommy, toward the end of March, was zooming unsuspectingly through the streets with Karen and his friends, his mother was agonizing over the merits of taking him to Tijuana. Everyone she consulted said it was madness to take a deathly ill boy to this city of prostitutes and abortionists, only to have to watch him die there. And she herself shrank from the trip and the sordidness of the setup, even though she had resolved to act at any cost.

On March 31 she married Fran Knapp. But her thoughts dwelt on her son, who was once again in school, although taking a limited program. He had even planned to go down to Manlius on his motorcycle and show it off to his friends there. Then in April he began complaining about pain in the vicinity of the liver. By the beginning of May the pain became so bad that she had to give Tommy analgesics that Dr. Haines prescribed. For a while Tommy had high fever and felt gravely ill. But he recovered and was soon back on his motorcycle. Joan thought she had been granted a new reprieve, and at the same time hope revived when someone sent her a newspaper clipping about a newly developed cancer drug called asparaginase. She decided to show the clipping to Dr. Haines and ask him to treat Tommy with the new drug.

Joan Gorence Knapp in a letter to her mother, May 29, 1968:

"Dr. Haines . . . said something about 'They are working on drugs all the time, but there is nothing that can help Tommy at this moment. This happens often in medicine and it just has to be accepted.' I said that I wouldn't and couldn't—that if it were his child he would take any chance. That I wasn't going to just plan a 'nice funeral' and let it go at that! . . . Somehow I reached him. He said that if I really had to try one of the new drugs he would send me up to a Dr. John Olsen in Cooperstown who was working on cancer research."

.   .   .

On May 17, Joan set out with Tommy for the city where he had been born. She told Tommy that Dr. Haines wanted Dr. Olsen to examine him; Dr. Haines thought Tommy's pain might come from pleuritis and Dr. Olsen was a specialist in that.

Joan Knapp in the letter to her mother:

"He didn't offer much hope, repeating all that Dr. Chamberlain and Dr. Haines had said. He mentioned in passing, however, that 'What Tommy needs is a new liver.' "

Joan, overwhelmed by disappointment, took these last words as just a phrase to underline the doctor's helplessness. She did not give the matter any further thought. But a few days later she learned that he was hinting at an operation she had never heard of: a liver transplant.

III

"Boston, April 26, 1968
"Dear Harold:
"This time I mean to be better about keeping you posted. Once again there's quite a bit to tell you on the subject of liver transplantation.
"At the meeting of the American Surgical Association here in Boston, which ended yesterday, Thomas E. Starzl of Denver, Colorado, announced that the mood of 1963–64 has been changing and that he and his colleagues have launched a new attack on the problems of liver transplantation. He made the following points: 'Until last year the kidney was the only organ that had been transplanted with subsequent significant prolongation of life. There had been nine reported attempts at orthotopic liver transplantation, seven in Denver and one each in Boston and Paris. Two of these patients had succumbed within a few hours after operation, and none had lived for longer than twenty-three days. This dismal picture has changed within the last nine months, inasmuch as seven consecutive patients treated with orthotopic liver transplantation from July 23, 1967, to March 17, 1968, all passed through this previous lethal operative and post-operative period. Three of the recipients are still alive after 9, 2⅔, and 1 months; the others died after 2, 3½, 4⅓, and 6 months.'
"A layman might think that these results were hardly impressive enough to warrant Starzl's optimism. But those who know how many break-throughs in medicine have begun by counting days and hours of

survival rather than months will see it differently. In any case, Starzl has made certain experiments that seem to have a significant future.

"At the beginning of last year a child named Julie Cherie Rodriguez was brought to the pediatrics department of Denver General Hospital from Pueblo, Colorado. Although only thirteen months old, the child was suffering from primary cancer of the liver. The mother, Mrs. John Rodriguez, was informed that there was no hope for her daughter.

"Starzl meanwhile had been attempting to improve the methods of liver transplantation. He was refining a technique that avoided the use of the plastic shunt (see my letter of December 1964) and looking for an alternative to Imuran, which specifically burdens the liver. He had had good results in dog experiments with antilymphocyte serum.

"When the case of Julie Cherie Rodriguez was brought to Starzl's attention, he decided to resume his transplant series on human patients, which he had discontinued four years earlier. Aside from Julie, who was now a year and a half old, there were several other children in the ward, most of them suffering from gall duct atresia. Among these were Paula Kay Hansen, a child of almost two, from Texas; Kerri Lynn Brown, fourteen months, from Long Beach, California; and Carol Lynne MacCourt, likewise fourteen months, from Salt Lake City. The parents, who saw no other way to save their children, were ready to say yes to any experiment. Starzl persuaded the U.S. Public Health Service of the justification for a new experimental program to develop liver transplantation and was given a grant enabling him to operate on most of the patients without charge and to treat them for an indefinite period of time.

"Since the patients were mostly children, a special sterile section was set up in the children's department of the hospital. Facilities were provided so that the mothers would be able to live near their children during treatment. Special nurses were picked for each child; however, they would not be in attendance whenever the children had to undergo painful treatment. The object was to keep the little patients from developing a negative psychological reaction toward their nurses. In particular, Starzl was thinking of the antilymphocyte serum, the injection of which can be very painful.

"Julie Rodriguez underwent surgery on July 23, 1967. Starzl removed the cancerous liver and discovered no metastases in the surrounding organs. He then replaced the morbid organ with the liver of an eighteen-month-old child who had died of pneumonia. The operation on Paula Hansen followed on August 1, Kerri Brown on September 5, and Carol MacCourt on October 8. Subsequently Starzl undertook three more transplants; one of the patients was Randall Wayne Bennett, a two-year-old boy from Texas who suffered from gall duct atresia. Along with minute quantities of Imuran, these children received antilymphocyte serum. In addition, Julie Rodriguez was subjected to radiation. After operation the children were placed in the sterile rooms and regularly tested.

"The detailed case histories depict the physicians' struggle to preserve the transplanted livers in babies who could not express themselves, did not know what was happening to them, and could not describe their feelings, but only smile or cry. For ten weeks Julie Rodriguez suffered from paralysis of the right side of her diaphragm, which had been squeezed during the operation. This mishap taught Starzl how to avoid such accidents in the future. He also learned that the chief danger from disturbances of the blood-clotting mechanism arose during the first twenty-four hours after the operation. Later the new liver recovered its regulatory powers.

"Starzl administered antilymphocyte serum to the children daily at first, then several times a week. In the course of time he discovered that the serum could not be omitted even once without risking a rejection reaction; for the liver subsequently ceased to respond to the drug. For the rest, he waged the usual two-front war against rejection on the one hand and infection on the other. He treated Julie with every imaginable antibiotic, from methicillin to chloramphenicol. When fungus infections appeared, he had no choice but to turn to amphotericin B, which is toxic to the kidneys. When kidney damage became evident, he had to resort to still untried drugs not so harmful to the kidneys, such as fluorocytosine.

"But by August, four weeks after the operation, cancer metastases had appeared in the right lobe of Julie's lung. Thus their apparent absence during the operation had been illusory. These metastases were removed in another operation. Shortly thereafter cancerous tumors also developed in the abdominal cavity. They blocked the large intestine and later the ureter. After desperate attempts to check their growth by supposedly tumor-inhibiting drugs like oncovin had failed, Starzl had to operate twice more to remove these tumors, in October 1967 and March 1968. Finally, indurations appeared in the new liver, but fortunately these proved not to be cancerous.

"It turned out that the difference in size between the original and the new liver, and thus between the old and new blood vessels of the liver, led to circulatory disturbances in some portions of the liver. These disturbances resulted in the death of those parts. Bacteria accumulated in the necrotic tissue, producing abscesses which could not be relieved by drainage and daily rinsings. At the time Starzl delivered his talk in Boston, little Julie Rodriguez still had open drainage wounds from which bacteria entered her blood stream, causing bouts of fever. Yet at this writing the child has been *living* for nine months with her new liver, and all tests seem to show that this liver is continuing to function normally in a cancer-riddled little body heavily dosed by toxic drugs.

"Although the other small patients have not lived as long as Julie Rodriguez, they have exceeded the longest survival time of 1963—twenty-three days—without the fatal hemorrhages, thromboses, or rejection reactions which followed the operations of that year. Carol MacCourt died on December 7, 1967, only two months after her operation; Paula Hansen four and a half months after the transplant, on December 12, 1967; Kerri Brown six months after the operation, on March 9, about six weeks ago. Aside from little Julie, two patients are still alive at the moment, Eddie Miller and Randall Wayne Bennett—the latter afflicted by jaundice after a severe rejection reaction following a hiatus in the treatment with antilymphocyte serum.

"Carol MacCourt was the victim of an infection by an unknown fungus. After her death fungoid abscesses were found even in her cerebellum. Two months after the transplant Paula Hansen showed signs of slow liver failure. Her liver, like that of Julie Rodriguez, fell prey to infarcts resulting from circulatory disturbances. The kidneys ceased to function and Paula had to be treated by peritoneal dialysis. Cardiac massage helped her over a temporary heart stoppage. Blood clots entered the intestinal blood vessels and destroyed parts of the duodenum. Twenty-four hours after an emergency operation on the abdominal cavity, the little girl died. The autopsy showed the full extent of the infarct destruction in her liver. Kerri Brown died similarly of liver infarcts, her death accelerated by pneumonia from an unknown virus. Starzl believes, however, that such deaths can be avoided in the future by more careful selection of the donor livers.

"In short, for the first time there is an optimistic tone in the reports from Denver.

"During the discussion that followed his lecture, Starzl declared: 'The results have established that the actual operative procedure can be done in man with relative safety and that subsequent survival is possible for at least as long as nine months.' Francis D. Moore commented: 'Dr. Starzl's work in this field is absolutely outstanding, and for those of us interested in liver transplantation this is a banner day when we can contemplate four [sic] patients alive and well with lethal liver disease removed and a new liver in place.'

"On the strength of all this, I think it highly likely that Moore himself will once more venture a human transplant, if a suitable patient comes his way. The results are bound to be interesting.

"Yours,

"O."

IV

Joan Gorence Knapp had never heard of Francis Daniels Moore. And although the newspapers a while back had been full of accounts of heart transplants, she had never read of a liver transplant. But on May 20 she received a letter from her mother, Elsie Boyd, who lived in Florida. Enclosed was a clipping from the *Sunday Telegraph* reporting a first "liver transplant" by a British surgeon named Roy Calne in Cambridge. Joan read the article with bated breath. Suddenly she recalled Dr. Olsen's remark about a "new liver," which she had taken as a mere phrase.

Between one moment and the next she decided what she must do. She would go back to Dr. Olsen in Cooperstown, show him the clipping, and seek some way to give Tommy a new liver, even if it meant taking him to England. Since a letter had also come from Bill, in Arizona, asking her to obtain a birth certificate for him from Cooperstown, she used this as a pretext to set out next day.

She did not know that surgeons in Cooperstown had begun experimenting years ago in transplanting various organs between animals, and that they had succeeded as far back as 1963 in keeping dogs with transplanted lungs alive for two months. Nor was she aware that Dr. John Olsen and Dr. Francis D. Moore had long been in close touch. She drove to Cooperstown expecting a bitter struggle with Dr. Olsen, of the sort she had waged when she had tried to get the doctors to use new drugs. She could only cling to the recollection that the doctor himself had spoken of a "new liver." It did not occur to her that Dr. Olsen might actually have considered her son Tommy a suitable case for Dr. Moore and for a new attempt at human liver transplantation.

She was enormously relieved when Olsen told her that work on this operation had been going on in America since 1963, and that in 1967 alone seven liver transplants had taken place. She also learned that three of the American patients who had received a new liver were still living, including two children—and that one had lived for more than ten months. Moreover, this child had been stricken by the same disease as Tommy's—cancer of the liver.

Joan Gorence Knapp in a letter to her mother, May 29, 1968:

"Dr. Olsen said that he had been in touch with . . . a Dr. Moore in Boston. . . . He talked for over an hour with me—discussing the merits of different hospitals. . . . He seemed to think, all things considered, Peter Bent Brigham Hospital, in Boston, would be the closest and the best.

He knows Dr. Moore personally, and Dr. Moore had been at Cooperstown Hospital, and most important, Dr. Moore was interested in the case.

"He explained to me that left alone, the tumor would continue to grow, and since the rest of Tom's body was extremely healthy, it would grow slowly and painfully, with no hope. . . . If the operation fails it will be relatively quick and painless. If the body rejects the transplant, or the liver fails, it will still be relatively painless. BUT IF IT WORKS TOM WILL BE WELL.

"In other words, the operation should be done as soon as possible while Tommy is as strong as possible. But this may mean shortening his life. I saw enough in the seven months that Johnny lived to realize that just living isn't worth anything—when it only means waiting for the drugs to put you to sleep for a little relief from the pain or, as in Johnny's case, from the helplessness, when it only means praying for death with no hope at all of getting even a little better.

"Dr. Olsen told me to go home and think it over and if I decided to go ahead to tell Tommy that he did have Cancer . . . and to tell him what we proposed. Then we were to come up and see him on Friday, May 24. . . .

"I told Tommy the next day—so he would have a little time to think and decide, also to think of any questions he might want to ask the doctor. . . . He had no idea that he might have Cancer! I don't remember exactly what I said. . . . I said something like: 'I want you to have another operation. You have a Cancer of the Liver and the Doctors want to do a liver transplant.' I kept on talking so he wouldn't have too much of a chance to think about the Cancer, itself, but would concentrate on the hope that was being offered. I . . . filled him in on what had happened since . . . February. . . . He was pretty upset at first, but said he wanted the operation. He was awfully brave. He said he could easily stand the postoperative pain, which they say will be about like what he went through the first time, and the tubes—he's hoping that they won't have to use the ice blanket. . . . It must be like lying on a cake of ice for hours.

"We talked for a long time. He was astounded to learn that everybody knew about it except him. . . . He laughed about how easy it was for him to get the motorcycle. . . ."

Next day, May 24, Joan and Tommy drove to Cooperstown once more. Throughout the drive Joan talked a great deal; if she kept up her chatter, Tommy would have less chance to brood.

Joan Gorence Knapp in the letter to her mother:

"Dr. Olsen talked with us for about an hour. Tommy had lots of questions and the doctor answered them as frankly as possible, I believe. He said that we would have to go down for tests and that then we would come home to wait for the donor liver. . . . Tommy will stay in the hospital for about three months—then we will have to go back for periodic checkups. Tommy asked if he would ever be able to join the Army, Air Force or the Troopers as he had planned. Dr. Olsen said he was pretty sure the Army wouldn't take anyone who had any type of cancer, even skin cancer—but that within five years Tom should be able to take any civilian job that he wanted."

Dr. Olsen promised to make all the necessary arrangements in Boston. Actually, Joan and Tommy had to wait only a week. At the end of May, Joan heard that Peter Bent Brigham Hospital was ready to take Tommy on June 3. Dr. Francis D. Moore himself would operate, and probably they would not have to pay for the operation because it would be serving the cause of science.

On June 2, Joan prepared to take her son to Boston. She arranged for Bill to receive another special leave, and even chartered a small plane. On the morning of June 3, Tommy breakfasted in the kitchen of the house on Hudson Street for the last time, while Auggie lay at his feet. Bill then drove them to Cooperstown, and an hour and a half later the three landed in Boston.

Joan learned that there were rooms for rent in the vicinity of the hospital. She began looking for one at once, while Tommy waited in the cab. Now that they were so close to the destination, he was becoming more and more silent; he was scared and complained of pains in his stomach.

Joan finally found a small room in the home of an old lady on Sachem Street. Tommy had to lie down on the bed for a while until he recovered his strength. Then they walked up the long hill to the hospital. Tommy felt less frightened after they arrived and he was in his hospital bed. Joan made sure he had a television set and played cards with him for a few hours.

Joan Knapp in a letter to her mother, July 3, 1968:

"We met Dr. Alan Birtch, Tommy's chief doctor, the next day, and Dr. Francis Moore, the Chief of Surgery. . . . There is also a battery of doctors—pathologists, radiologists, anesthesiologists, hematologists, bacteriol-

ogists, and many, many more—I couldn't spell them even if I could remember them! They finally decided that they wanted to SEE what they
were up against and scheduled exploratory surgery for Friday, June 7.
. . . The operation stressed the need—these doctors described the cancer as 'gigantic'—but also made them confident that the transplant would
succeed."

Francis D. Moore was a tall, lean, impressive-looking man with regular, clear-cut features and brown hair graying at the temples. His public
manner, his swift, sure step and terse, firm speech, were those of a man
conscious of his position as Surgeon-in-Chief at Peter Bent Brigham,
Moseley Professor of Surgery at the Harvard Medical School, and director
of many medical research programs. In the thirties he had decided to become a surgeon, although his sundry artistic gifts might have taken him in
many other directions. He was a man given to direct action and found his
fulfillment in surgery. Still, he was not a "simple" practicing surgeon, but a
thoughtful scientist who published papers on such questions as the effect
of surgical procedures on human metabolism, the immunity reaction in
transplants, or the ethics of experimenting on human beings. On this matter, he had arrived at an unqualified affirmation. "Without the experimental method," he wrote, "medicine would become traditional, since it could
not move ahead on the basis of established observations and experience."
Also: "To those who have never dealt with such desperate patients, it may
come as a surprise to witness the enthusiasm with which the patient with
late cancer or the families of children with severe heart disease approach
an entirely new and untried procedure." He gave weight to the psychological factor: "When we move . . . to such desperate measures as kidney or
liver transplantation for fatal disease, it is evident that the hopes of the
surgeon, the fears of the patient, and the inborn optimism of youthful
science combine to push the patient onward."

Few of the experiments and advances at Peter Bent Brigham in the
field of kidney transplantation would have been possible without Moore.
He was the guiding spirit behind the so-called Bartlett Unit, the special
intensive-care and research section in which Melbourne Doucette had
spent the last months of his life; an endowment by his wife's parents,
whose name it bore, had helped create it. In his book *Give and Take*,
published in 1964, he had shown the wide range of his interests. But transplantation of the liver had especially fascinated him.

Thomas E. Starzl's new campaign of liver transplantation of children
had come at a timely moment. Moore's own research on animals had
yielded many of the same conclusions. Then Tommy Gorence had turned
up, accompanied by his remarkably resolute mother. Here were the fac-

tors that built a bridge between human destinies and the scientific urge to know.

When it developed that the necessary tests would take considerably longer than the three days mentioned in Cooperstown, Joan returned to Oneonta to collect the things she would need for a longer stay. She came back to Boston by bus—a trip of ten hours. Then she looked for living quarters again. She was directed to 1627–29 Tremont Street, a house belonging to Francis L. Fabiano, an American of Italian descent who offered rooms to relatives of patients at Peter Bent Brigham who came from a distance. There she would be only a stone's throw from the hospital entrance. Fabiano gave her permission to use a hot plate in her room. When it became clear that Tommy would not be returning to Oneonta, as had originally been planned, but would wait in Boston for his new liver, Joan sent a want list home. Soon Francis Knapp came to Boston, his car loaded with kitchenware, an iron, pictures, a vacuum cleaner, and even a rug. Joan was setting up house so that she could be close to Tommy for months on end, both before and after the operation.

Fabiano had rarely had a more reliable tenant. Mrs. Knapp was so different from most of his roomers that he was to remember her vividly later on. The gloomy stories he had been hearing through the years had convinced him that medicine failed more often than it succeeded, and rendered him highly skeptical of the "money-making medical gods next door." But here was Joan Knapp, ready to entrust her boy entirely to those medicos. From what she told him about the forthcoming operation, he would say it had one chance in a hundred of working out, yet Mrs. Knapp was waiting impatiently for it.

Joan did not know that Moore and Birtch were just as impatient as she, for medical reasons. Tommy's tumor of the liver, because of its size, was exerting strong pressure on the blood vessels; if it continued to grow, attaching a donor liver to these vessels would be extremely difficult. All the hospitals connected with the Harvard Medical School had been asked to keep watch for a suitable donor. On June 14, Moore was informed that a twelve-year-old boy, the victim of an auto accident, was dying in the Children's Hospital and that his parents would consent to transplantation of his liver.

Joan Knapp in a letter to her mother, June 26, 1968:

"They told us around three, June 17, that they were ready. . . . They took Tommy down to the operating room at 3:45 P.M. and showed me to a quiet waiting room. . . . Dr. Francis Moore was in charge, with Dr. Birtch assisting. . . . Several of the interns and younger doctors stopped by to see me during the long wait—and said that things were going well. I later learned that the cancer had put extra pressure on the artery supplying the liver . . . so they had to remove one of Tommy's kidneys to use that vessel to ensure a good blood supply."

Moore and Birtch were not unprepared when they found that the hepatic artery had been so weakened by pressure from the cancer that it could not adequately supply blood to the new liver. The child from whom the liver was taken had weighed 80 pounds, whereas Tommy Gorence, in spite of his illness, still weighed 180 pounds. Connecting the vessels from the donor liver to Tommy's blood vessels was difficult enough in any case. The weakening of the hepatic artery complicated the problem. The best possible solution lay in attaching the liver to a different artery, and only the right renal artery was available. This meant removing the patient's right kidney. Aside from the complex technique of this novel connection, removing the kidney was in itself not without risks. Tommy's left kidney was healthy enough. But during the postoperative treatment the boy would have to bear the assault of drugs upon his system with only one kidney. Such a prospect naturally aroused concern. Yet Moore and Birtch had no choice; they could only hope that Tommy Gorence's youth would help his body bear this burden.

Instead of the six hours that similar operations had taken, more than eight hours were required in Tommy's case. When the time came to attach the gall duct of the new liver to the duodenum, Moore renounced a time-consuming and complicated method and simply sewed an opening in the new gall bladder to an opening in the duodenum. It was past midnight before Tommy Gorence was at last wheeled to the intensive-care unit.

Joan Knapp in a letter to her mother, June 26, 1968:

"Dr. Alan Birtch came by at 12:45 to say that everything was fine. . . . He said Tom was in the recovery room and suggested that I go home and get some sleep."

Now that Tommy had survived the operation, Joan counted on his living—like the little girl in Denver. Even if it was only ten months or a year—she had gained some time. Doctors could make new discoveries, and perhaps she, too, would find new approaches, as she had found this chance in Boston because she had determined to find it. She did not realize that the fight for Tommy's life was only now beginning—with anti-rejection drugs, antilymphocyte serum, antibiotics, infusions, punctures, and injections.

For Joan, the following days, during which Tommy lay in a room in the Bartlett Unit and she was allowed to see him only briefly, in sterile clothing, passed like a dream. She saw that Tommy was fed artificially and lived under a respirator—and she also saw that he was in pain. But he was alive and knew that he had to endure all this in order to return to real life. Her faith and her optimism knew no bounds.

And Tommy recovered rapidly.

Joan Knapp in a letter to her mother, July 3, 1968:

"Except for a bland diet Tommy has been taken off all restrictions. He can go outside the hospital on the several sun porches or to the lovely little garden at the Children's Hospital next door. So far, his air-conditioned room is more appealing than hot and humid Boston. . . . We no longer need to wear the gowns, masks and plastic gloves when we visit him and everything looks wonderful! The doctors and nurses go around with great big smiles—outshone only by Tommy's and mine.

"The Hospital released the news to the papers today. . . . Tommy was identified as 'a sixteen year old Basketball player from Oneonta, New York,' which tickled Tom. He said, 'Wait till the kids at Manlius hear that!' I'm sure he would rather have been called a Motorcyclist."

She saw everything in a rosy light. But even Moore and Birtch took an optimistic line when they spoke to newspapermen.

Dr. Birtch in the Oneonta Star, *July 5, 1968:*

"Convalescence is not a simple matter. But he has done very well so far. . . . Experience is not sufficient to allow [us to say] what the critical period is. But he is doing as well as could be expected."

Dr. Moore in the Binghamton Press, *July 6, 1968:*

"He is up and around, feeling good, eating well and reading newspapers."

This recovery continued until July 8 or 9. It seemed as if the optimism, even after this most complicated of all the liver transplants to date, would prove justified. Tommy Gorence had been in a vigorous state before the operation, and he also had the natural resilience of youth. Perhaps that had contributed to success. Perhaps the troubles Starzl had encountered with his patients—the hemorrhages, circulatory disturbances, and infarcts of the liver, the subsequent infections—were not inevitable. After all, the operation had been performed with extraordinary care, and the postoperative treatment had also been of the best.

On July 9, Tommy suddenly developed fever. The doctors, baffled as to the cause, decided to reopen the operation incision. This sudden reverse shook the boy's confidence in his recovery, and he plunged into doubts and fears when he heard that more surgery was in the offing. But his mother was sure that if Dr. Moore said it was necessary, it was; she implored Tommy to keep up the fight and to accept this additional operation. And so he underwent surgery again on July 10. A liver abscess was found, reminiscent of the case histories of Starzl's patients. But such an abscess did not have to be fatal. An abscess had also developed in Julie Rodriguez's liver, and she was still alive.

Then, in the course of the following days, the same kind of complications appeared that had brought death to Kerri Lynn Brown and Carol Lynne MacCourt—infections, kidney failure, and finally failure of the lungs.

Joan Knapp could hardly believe it. She had fastened all her hopes on the new liver. She had been so certain that Tommy would live. When she could no longer close her eyes to the facts, she still clung to her determination not to capitulate and not to admit that Tommy himself was giving up. Only her landlord, Fabiano, recognized the look on her face when she came back from the hospital in the evening. It was that look of weariness and ebbing faith with which he was so familiar. He was tempted to tell her what he thought about the "gods next door." But he forbore. And each morning she left the house and walked over to the hospital with fresh hope.

Joan Gorence Knapp to Lothar Reinbacher, 1970:

"Several times, when Tommy was feeling bad, he said: 'Mother, let me die.' Each time I answered: 'Tommy, we have to go on fighting.' His poor body was stuck full of needles and tubes all the time. He was on artificial respiration and on the artificial kidney. The whole room was so full of apparatus I could hardly get to his bedside, and I didn't want to disturb the doctors in their efforts or be in their way. . . . His last words were: 'I love you.' Then he dropped into a coma. . . . He died on July 31."

She was not in his room when he died, and she did not see him again after his death. She wanted to keep in her memory a picture of him alive, even if at the end he had been only a wraith of the strapping Tommy of old. In despair she might be, but she was not weak. She accused no one, neither Dr. Moore nor Dr. Birtch nor Dr. Olsen nor herself. She had lost Tommy. But at least he had not died helplessly like his father; he had fought to the end. And although he had died in pain, it had not been a prolonged torment, an agony that never seemed to end.

She and Fran and Bill buried Tommy's ashes on Saturday, August 3, 1968, in Hartwick Cemetery, where his father had been buried some two years before.

"New York, October 20, 1968

"Dear Harold:

"It's more or less a law óf medicine that genuine advances rarely take place in the form of a single glorious break-through. Usually they are accompanied by suffering and death, and result from a long alternation between insight, disappointment, fresh insights, errors, new knowledge, setbacks, the acquisition of further knowledge, and so on.

"Nothing has borne out this law more than the development of liver transplantation as I have observed it since my last report in April. I wrote you then about Thomas E. Starzl's promising experiences with seven patients, and about Francis Moore's praise for Starzl and his plans to resume human liver transplantation. Today, six months later, the experiment has entered a phase of setbacks, and the doctors are by no means so sanguine. The turning point came when Moore, in June, performed a liver transplant on a boy named Thomas B. Gorence. Moore applied all the real or supposed conclusions of Starzl, as well as the results of his own research. But the boy died after six weeks, shattering all the hopes associated with his survival. On August 26, four weeks after Gorence's death, little Julie Rodriguez also died. The most depressing aspect of her death was that cancer metastases were found not only in her brain, but also in her newly implanted liver; in other words, the transplant was attacked by the very disease for which Julie's own liver had been removed on July 23, 1967.

"Yesterday Starzl addressed the most recent congress of the American College of Surgeons. He used the word 'discouraging.' He raised a question that had been haunting him: could it be that the antirejection drugs, the Imuran or antilymphocyte serum, without which a transplant is impossible, might stimulate the spread of cancer? After the discussion, however, Starzl and Moore indicated that they did not mean to give up, and that they were going to continue working until the riddles are finally cleared up—for at present new ones arise as soon as a few of the old ones appear to be solved.

"There is really no other way to go about it, unless the whole idea of liver transplantation is to be abandoned. When the liver is incurably diseased there is no possible substitute for it, as there is for the kidney or the heart. Even the most fervid believers in progress do not imagine that there will ever be an artificial liver. The natural organ is a magnificent and inimitable masterpiece.

"Yours,

"O.

"P.S. I have just heard from England that several liver transplantation teams have been forming there. There is one under Professor Roy Calne in Cambridge, another under Robert Williams in London. In France, Garnier and, in Germany, Gutgemann are apparently preparing to enter the field. All this strikes me as another indication that there is no turning back. Once conceived, a scientific idea exerts an irresistible lure."

Mechanical Spare Parts

1 / Marcel DeRudder

Gerald Leach in The Biocrats: Ethics and the New Medicine:

"The human heart is an extraordinary organ. The size of a man's fist, weighing 10 ounces, it pulses 40 million times a year to drive nearly a million gallons of blood through 60,000 miles of tubing. It generates roughly 20 watts to do this, and makes this energy itself. It can rapidly alter its beat between 60 and 200 strokes a minute, its output from 2 to 12 liters a minute. . . . The plan to replace this pump with a totally implanted machine is one of the most daunting challenges that technology has ever set itself."

Houston Chronicle, *April 21, 1966:*

"An artificial heart was implanted today in a 65-year-old man during a six hour and 45 minute operation at Methodist Hospital.

"The artificial heart attached to Marcel DeRudder of Westville, Illinois, was functioning well. . . . Dr. Michael DeBakey and a team of surgeons implanted the artificial heart while replacing one of the patient's own heart valves."

The telephone calls came one March evening in 1966. The callers were friends of the DeRudders in the town of Westville on the eastern border of Illinois. Westville was a small place of 2,500 inhabitants.

"Edna," the callers said, "you ought to tune in at nine o'clock. They're having a TV program on a genuine heart valve operation by Dr. DeBakey, the fellow who operated on the Duke of Windsor last year—there's been a lot in the newspapers about him. Maybe he can do something for Marcel."

Marcel and Edna DeRudder had lived for many years in a modest frame house on the southern edge of Westville, where the town ran out into a seemingly endless stretch of cornfields. By now Marcel DeRudder was sixty-five, a stocky man with a rather florid face under gray, close-cropped hair. All that icy Illinois winter he had kept to his bed because of his heart weakness and a blood clot in his left leg.

Marcel's childhood had been spent in Cuesmes, Belgium. But he had grown up not far from Westville, in a town to which the immigrant miners had given the name "Belgium" in memory of their homeland. Marcel had also become a miner, proud of being in an occupation that called for tough men, proud also of his reputation as a dancer at the Franco-Belgian Club. In 1923 he had married Edna, and for twenty-five years had stuck to his heavy work in the mine shafts of Georgetown, until one day he was brought home sick and the doctors told him his heart was done for.

The young people of Westville knew only from hearsay about the kind of life Marcel DeRudder had experienced in the early years of the century. When miners and their families fell ill in those days, they lived or died mostly without calling in a doctor. Marcel had survived rheumatic fever, but no one had wasted a thought on the possibility that his heart valves might have been affected and that work in the damp mines might be fatal for him. So he had spent another twenty years working underground, while his mitral valve slowly scarified and calcified. When the collapse finally came, around 1940, his heart valve sounds indicated such severe damage that the mineworkers' union doctor prescribed digitalis and gave him only a few years to live at best.

Shortly afterward he was relegated to retirement on a $54-a-month disability pension. Ever since, he and Edna had lived in their white-painted, gray-roofed house with its patch of lawn and scattering of trees. And since they had never had children, who might have helped them, Edna worked as a cashier in the IGA store, on Main Street. With what she earned, they were able to make out.

A citizen of Westville, Illinois, 1970:

"Ours is a pretty small town. Maybe everybody doesn't know everybody else, but almost everybody does. DeRudder used to walk slowly down Main Street past the Ford agency, the branch of the John Deere factory, and the feed store as far as the IGA. He'd sit in the veterans' bar across the street playing cards and waiting till Edna's day was over and she could go home with him. Because he was a husky-looking fellow and his complexion was a good color, some people thought he was an imaginary invalid who was collecting his pension and letting his wife work for him. But they were unfair, and all wrong."

In the years since he had had to stop working in the mine, Marcel DeRudder had repeatedly tried to find a job. For a while he had been a guard in the Illinois State Museum in Springfield, about 150 miles from Westville. Every Monday morning he rode the bus to Springfield, stayed in a cheap rooming house until Friday, and returned exhausted to spend the weekend at home. When he no longer had the strength for that, he'd begun doing upholstery work in his garage. A few other retired persons would stop by from time to time and lift or turn the article of furniture he was working on, for he himself could not do it. Finally, when he couldn't even stretch cloth or tighten a seam, he had to occupy himself puttering around the house, doing a bit of housework, and sitting outside the door in a work shirt and felt hat waiting for Edna to come home.

A friend of Marcel DeRudder's, 1970:

"He felt that some people thought he was a good-for-nothing, and that hurt him. He wanted nothing more fervently than to be well again and to be able to work the way he used to in the past. And so for many years he clung like a bulldog to the hope that the doctors would be able to restore him to health."

In the past ten or fifteen years DeRudder's friends had often shaken their heads over the way Marcel looked at every TV show involving medicine and read every newspaper article (though he had never been much of a reader) that had anything to do with heart diseases. As soon as he thought he had found out something about a new medicine or a new operation, he would drive to Champaign, fifty miles west, to consult Dr. Ensrud, the United Mine Workers doctor; as a UMW member, DeRudder was entitled to free medical service. He would ply Dr. Ensrud with his newspaper articles and ask him to prescribe the new medicine or send him to the distant specialist he had read about. From the time the *Chicago News* ran its first articles on heart valve operations and open-heart surgery, Marcel had accumulated a great deal of knowledge about developments in this field in Boston, Philadelphia, Baltimore, and Portland. He did not understand everything he read, but he had acquired an unshakable faith that sooner or later he would be cured. It was only a matter of finding the right doctors. And he had managed to persuade Dr. Ensrud to send him to such sites of heart surgery as Rochester, Chicago, Boston, and Baltimore. Since the UMW would pay for treatment but not for the trips, he had traveled by bus or been driven by helpful relatives, even as far as Boston or New York. The trips took a great deal out of him, yet he went on trying.

Usually he returned dead tired and bitterly disappointed. Everywhere he was told about the great advances in surgery for heart valve defects, and about the implanting of wonderful artificial valves. But he was also told that after all these years of illness his own heart was too weak to withstand an operation. Even if the valve defect could be repaired, he would die on the operating table.

Nevertheless, each time Marcel read something new about medicines or specialists, his hopes revived and he again set out for Champaign. Edna suspected that Dr. Ensrud had made several appointments with remote specialists only to be rid of Marcel for a while.

A friend of Marcel DeRudder's, 1970:

"In recent years, since he could no longer command self-respect or the respect of others by manliness, strength, or hard work, his sickness acquired a new meaning for him. In a way he saw it as a symbol of manly toughness. Hadn't the doctors given him up twenty-five years ago? But he was still alive because he was so tough, and all the famous specialists who couldn't do anything for him assured him that his survival was a miracle. Anyhow, in recent years he'd talk to everyone he met—on the street or on Sunday after church, or in the bar where many of the oldsters played pool—talk about his illness and his trips to famous hospitals and famous doctors, and he'd always emphasize that the doctors thought him an extraordinary case."

Edna would have been more sympathetic toward Marcel's recent loquaciousness and his desperate attempts to find some improvement if he hadn't begun to go to purveyors of miracle cures. Since Dr. Ensrud refused to send him to any of these dubious practitioners, Marcel had paid the fees himself, spending their sorely needed household money. Finally he had gone as far as St. Louis to be treated by a chiropractor, and after his return had believed for a short time that he was feeling better. But then the terrible winter had begun with a thrombus in his leg and an almost total collapse of his heart, and he had stopped hoping for cure or improvement.

Shortly before nine o'clock, in response to the telephone calls from his friends, Marcel DeRudder, tired, taciturn, sat down in his chair in front of the television set.

Edna DeRudder to Jerry LeBlanc, 1970:

"It was such a long struggle. He had been everywhere, to the Mayo Clinic, to the ones in Maryland, Boston, Chicago, St. Louis, and there was never much encouragement. No one ever operated on him. He had just about given up hope that he'd ever be well. . . . He felt he was a burden, just useless, and he wanted more than that. . . . One night we saw Dr.

DeBakey perform open-heart surgery on television. Some friends had called us about it."

The surgical technique that the short, hook-nosed man in the rumpled green surgeon's smock demonstrated before the television cameras that night was sheer routine for him—one of thousands of heart operations he had been doing for years. The commentator spoke of DeBakey's virtuosity. He mentioned that hundreds of thousands of Americans died every year from heart diseases and that the nation should be allocating more funds to research on such diseases. But he said nothing about any novel surgical plans DeBakey might have for treating these diseases, and the watchers that night had no notion of the ideas that were in the mind of the man from Houston while the cameras were focused on him.

Years before James D. Hardy made his first attempt at a human heart transplant and Christiaan Barnard gave the signal for the frenzied heart transplant race, DeBakey had been considering another approach to the problem of the incurably sick heart. He wanted to devise an artificial, mechanical heart, a machine that would be a masterpiece of medical engineering. DeBakey himself was not the author of this idea. As early as 1937 the Soviet scientist Vladimir Petrovich Demikhov had attempted to replace the hearts of living animals with a metal pump. Its power came from an electric motor and was fed into the animal's thoracic cavity by a steel arbor. After the Second World War, Demikhov had carried on more experiments; but the animals had never lived through the ordeal.

Other surgeons and technicians had taken up the idea, among them Willem Kolff. During his last years in Kampen, after the initial success of his artificial kidney, he had designed a primitive heart pump and taken it with him to Cleveland. Between 1950 and 1960 he had built new pumps, with the aid of the engineers of Thompson Ramo Wooldridge, Inc. He intended these to be implanted in the chests of animals, and later human beings, to replace the heart and function without outside sources of power.

For a while Kolff had attempted to build plastic models of the right and left ventricles. In order to imitate the natural contraction, expansion, and renewed contraction of the heart, he had made his ventricles out of flexible Silastic contained within a heart-shaped rigid plastic housing. The space between the flexible Silastic and the rigid outer layer was filled with oil. Small electromagnets pushed cylinders into the oil at the pace of a normal heartbeat; in compressing the oil, the cylinders squeezed the Silastic ventricles. As the cylinders moved out again, the ventricles expanded. Kolff had implanted this device in animals already attached to heart-lung machines. He had removed the animals' hearts except for the atria and their valve systems. In some cases, he had connected the plastic ventricles with these atria; in other cases, he had attached the artificial ventricles directly to the blood vessels with plastic valves and tubes. But the instantaneous deaths of all his animals had taught him that there were some fearful realities that stood in the way of his dreams of a mechanical heart.

Later he had experimented with small electric motors that moved like pendulums between the right and left artificial ventricles, compressing each chamber in turn. At this point he was relinquishing the vision of a fully implantable artificial heart, for the motors needed cable connections with a source of electricity outside the body. The motors, too, proved inadequate—they were either too heavy or too weak. Moreover, they generated tissue-destroying heat; and Kolff's efforts to use the blood stream itself for cooling the motors ended in disappointment. He advanced somewhat, however, when engineers of NASA—the National Aeronautics and Space Administration—proposed that he use compressed gas as his motive power. At first even Kolff, receptive though he was to the boldest fantasies of the future, shrank from the vision of people someday walking about with tubes protruding from their chests to connect their artificial hearts with bottles of compressed gas. Nevertheless, he went ahead and built ventricles in which the space between the elastic inner and the rigid outer wall was filled with gas. The gas pouring in and out created the pumping action. A thin tube connected the ventricles with a gas generator, and an electronic device regulated the pumping action so that it corresponded to a definite heartbeat. After innumerable failures Kolff succeeded in 1960 in keeping dogs alive with his mechanical pump for several hours.

This success proved deceptive. The animals did not die from failure of the pumps, but because even with heparin treatment quantities of clots formed in their blood. Moreover, the red blood corpuscles were so shattered that other organs, above all the kidneys, collapsed. The very same problems that had marked the initial use of the heart-lung machine and of artificial heart valves came to the fore—and in highly aggravated form. It seemed that as soon as the blood moved through plastic ventricles for any length of time, it underwent clotting and breakdown. Kolff's great struggle had been to offset this effect, and now he was once more engaged with it.

In the meantime other surgeons and engineers had taken up the idea of building artificial hearts. Richard Parks in Pennsylvania, K. E. Woodward of the Harry Diamond Laboratories in Washington, Adrian Kantrowitz of Maimonides Hospital in New York, and Michael DeBakey were among those who were working on the project. DeBakey, with his characteristic élan, ambition, faith in progress, and fascination with the use of plastics in surgery, had set up a development team at Baylor University in Houston. Among its members was a young Argentine surgeon named Domingo Liotta who had worked under Kolff in Cleveland, as well as under Dr. William Akers of nearby Rice University. Unlike Kolff, DeBakey had not tried to go all the way at once. He had set his team a limited task whose solution seemed urgent for his surgical work.

Like other heart surgeons, DeBakey had found that he could successfully replace one or several defective valves. But the heart, especially the left ventricle, was often so weakened that after the operation all efforts to restart it failed. On the other hand, such a heart would recover if it were given time. In order to permit this, DeBakey had sometimes kept the patient on the heart-lung machine for a few hours after the operation until the heart had recovered enough to beat on its own. The trouble was that a few hours usually did not suffice. A longer period of assistance for the heart might have led to success; but that was not yet possible. There were still distinct limits to the time the heart-lung machine could be used; after a few hours the destruction of red blood corpuscles began to assume fatal proportions.

DeBakey's assignment to his team, therefore, had been to construct auxiliary pumps which could be implanted in the thoracic cavity of a patient who had undergone heart surgery for a considerable length of time— days, and perhaps weeks. They were not intended to replace the entire heart, but to take over the work of the left ventricle until it was able to bear the burden by itself. Once this was achieved, the pump would be removed. DeBakey hoped to get the same wonderful effect with the pump as he did by using Dacron patches in arterial operations. The Dacron became coated with a layer of natural fibrin which, being a product of the blood itself, held the formation of clots and the destruction of the red blood corpuscles within narrow limits.

By 1963, Akers, Liotta, and other DeBakey associates had developed an initial pump. They called it the "left ventricular by-pass." The pump, shaped like a small banana, was made of Dacron and Silastic. At both ends on the inside of the "banana" were artificial heart valves. The outside was connected by a tube to a gas pressure valve system; gas admitted and withdrawn at regular intervals caused the inner sac to pulse like a pump. In order to relieve the burden on the left ventricle of their animals, Akers and Liotta attached the upper end of the pump to the left atrium and sewed the lower end into the aorta. As soon as they started the pump, it sucked fresh, oxygenated blood from the atrium and pumped it directly into the aorta, by-passing the left ventricle. The rhythm of the pumping movements was regulated by a relay connected to an electrocardiograph that registered the cardiac activity of the animals.

After nearly one hundred experiments on animals, Akers and Liotta believed they no longer need fear blood clots or destruction of the red blood cells, because the inner walls of their pump became coated with a layer of fibrin, just like DeBakey's arterial substitutes.

In the middle of 1963, DeBakey decided to apply the pump to a man for the first time, as soon as opportunity afforded. The moment came in July 1963 when a fatally ill forty-two-year-old black with a totally crippled aortic valve was brought into Methodist Hospital. On July 18, DeBakey replaced the aortic valve and succeeded in restoring the heart action. A day later the man's heart stopped. In an emergency operation DeBakey opened the thoracic cavity again and restored the heartbeat by massage. But the patient remained unconscious. His reflexes faded and his kidney activity stopped. Accumulations of fluid in the lungs threatened to suffocate him, and it was apparent that the heart might cease beating at any moment. In this desperate juncture DeBakey decided, on July 19, to try out the pump. For the third time within a few days the patient's heart was exposed; he was attached to the heart-lung machine and the pump implanted in the manner that Liotta and Akers had devised in their animal experiments. When the heart-lung machine was switched off and the whitish plastic pump, with a low hissing of gases and clicking of valves, took up the work, even DeBakey—who had implanted so many plastic prostheses in human bodies—was gripped by a sense of awe. Before him, for the first time in history, lay a human being whose life persisted only because a stream of gas entering through a tube was moving a machine inside his chest.

The enlarged left ventricle reacted almost immediately to the lessening of its burden and began to shrink. DeBakey had closed the wall of the thoracic cavity except for the point at which the gas tube emerged. The electrocardiograms showed distinct improvement, and X rays indicated that the pulmonary edema was also receding. But initial satisfaction was followed by profound disappointment. The kidneys did not resume their function and on July 20 the patient fell into a complete coma. On July 21 he ceased to react to any stimuli. He presented an aspect that no doctor had ever seen before. Deep inside his chest the pump was working, forcing the blood through his body, although the body was nothing but a lifeless shell. However, the hemoglobin content in the blood serum rose strikingly, showing that even in the Dacron pump the red blood corpuscles were disintegrating. The loss of reflexes suggested that blood clots were forming and with each beat of the pump were driving new thromboses into the cerebral arteries. On July 22 the patient died, while the pump continued to suck and click inside his chest until Akers, the engineer, pressed the switch that stopped it. The autopsy confirmed the damage to the blood and exposed blood clots and infarcts throughout the brain. The deposit of fibrin on the Dacron walls of the pump had not sufficed to prevent coagulation and destruction of the blood. Apparently what held good for immobile bits of tubing did not apply to a pump whose walls and valves were in constant motion.

But DeBakey did not give up. The fact that the pump had worked and relieved the heart for a while confirmed his faith in the solubility of all technical problems. Akers and Liotta were told to go on with their project, to build better pumps and find new materials that would not damage the blood. At the same time DeBakey used his prestige, his political connections, and his acquaintanceship with Lyndon Johnson, fellow Texan and future President (who himself had suffered a heart attack), to obtain funds for an extensive artificial-heart development program.

Michael DeBakey in Time, *May 28, 1965:*

"It is deficiencies in materials . . . that are holding us up. The materials we have, good as they are, still damage the blood to some extent. . . . I am confident that if $50 million were made available today for just this kind of research, an artificial heart, or the vital parts of one, could be ready for permanent implantation within three to five years."

In 1964, DeBakey had prevailed on the National Heart Institute in Maryland to make $8 million available for research into artificial hearts; his own team received $2 million. By the beginning of 1966, Akers and Liotta had developed more than sixty new pumps. The last, Number 66, had what they considered to be two decisive changes. They had designed it so that the pump no longer had to be implanted in the thoracic cavity itself, but only in the chest wall. Shaped like a small grapefruit, the pump was connected to the left atrium of the heart and to the aorta by two plastic tubes. Its functioning could now be observed directly; if anything went wrong it would not be necessary to reopen the thoracic cavity. Moreover, it could be removed without a major operation as soon as its work was done and the heart could continue functioning without support. The most critical advance, however, consisted in the use of a new plastic. Akers and Liotta had coated all the interior parts of the pump with a Dacron weave so soft that it was given the name "Dacron velour." Even in prolonged animal experiments there had been no significant blood clotting and no serious damage to the red blood corpuscles.

DeBakey, who spent every free minute he had in the laboratories, grew more confident from week to week. In February 1966 news came from New York that Adrian Kantrowitz of Maimonides Hospital had developed a by-pass pump closely resembling DeBakey's unsuccessful 1963 model. On February 4, Kantrowitz implanted his pump in a thirty-three-year-old cardiac patient. But violent hemorrhages caused by blood damage soon began. Shortly afterward, in spite of the support from the pump, the patient's heart began to race inexplicably, and twenty hours after the operation the man died. This incident only strengthened DeBakey's resolve to try the latest model of his own pump and to prove that the by-pass idea, in spite of Kantrowitz's failure, was just as valid as the fundamental conception of the artificial heart.

At the end of February, DeBakey issued orders to have a pump kept in a constant state of readiness, so that it could be implanted within half an hour in case it became evident during an operation that a patient's heart would stop without mechanical support. DeBakey's conviction that heart pumps would succeed was by now so deep that he was actually considering something no physician had ever dared to do before. He wanted to publicize his next attempt to keep a human being alive by supporting his heart with an artificial pump. He was ready to admit television cameramen and newspapermen to his operating theater so that the whole American public would see and grasp the importance of what was going on in Houston—and approve the cost of such work.

This was the thinking behind DeBakey's unusual action in going before the television cameras. And the broadcast from Houston found its way to Westville, Illinois, and into Marcel DeRudder's living room.

A friend of Marcel DeRudder's:

"Later there were all sorts of stories about it in the newspapers. It was said that after the television broadcast Edna DeRudder sat down and wrote to Dr. DeBakey, asking him to help Marcel. But that's hardly likely. She wouldn't have dared write a letter to a big doctor like him. As far as I recall, it was different. Edna had never seen a heart operation, and the fact that Dr. DeBakey could fix someone up that way made a great impression on her. When it was over, she asked Marcel whether he wouldn't like to make one more try. He had tried in so many places, but he had never thought of Dr. DeBakey. Maybe this doctor really could do more than all the others. This time Marcel was not so eager. He had pretty well given up. But Edna kept urging him. Maybe she was afraid she would soon be helplessly watching him die. Who knows? In any case, a few days later they went to see Dr. Ensrud once more. Marcel talked to him about DeBakey. This time he didn't insist on it, the way he used to in the past. Nevertheless, Ensrud promised to write to DeBakey.

"Four or five weeks passed without any reaction from Houston. Marcel would only wave his hand wearily when I inquired. I imagine he thought

Dr. DeBakey was by now so famous that he could no longer bother about ordinary people.

"But then, in April, there suddenly came a letter from Houston. If I remember rightly, it was from Dr. DeBakey's office. Marcel was invited to present himself in Houston on April 14. Formerly Marcel would have been all excited at something of this sort. And maybe for a moment he thought: Now do you see how serious my case is, if a big doctor like DeBakey invites me to come to Texas? But this time he was quietly thoughtful. He said to me: 'I don't think they can help me down there either. But maybe, when they open me up, they can learn something that they can apply to others. If that's the case, I'll be doing some good, and people will realize I haven't been just a useless invalid.'

"On April 14, Edna and her sister, Catherine, drove him to the airport, and he climbed heavily into the plane for Chicago, from where he would fly on to Houston. Maybe you wonder why they let him fly alone in his condition. I think the flight was being paid for by the union, or by one of Dr. DeBakey's research funds. But Marcel didn't want Edna to come along for fear she'd lose her job in Al Davis's IGA store. She was sixty by now, and you don't find a new job at that age. That's how it is when you're poor. Before he got into the plane he looked around once more, and somebody who was there later told me he looked as if he meant: I won't be coming back."

April 14, 1966, was a Thursday. Marcel DeRudder had seen a good many big cities in his search for health, so the sprawling city did not scare him. But he found the hot southern air hard to breathe. A cab dropped him in front of the nine-story, windowless façade of the Methodist Hospital. For a moment he looked at the orange-toned mural above the entrance; it showed Christ with arms protectively upraised above twelve mosaics representing great physicians such as Hippocrates, Galen, Vesalius, and Harvey—intended to symbolize the progress of medicine. Marcel DeRudder did not know anything about Galen and Vesalius. But before he went through the door he looked up into the face of Christ.

He was familiar with the way great medical institutions took in patients and processed them. A name bracelet was put on his wrist. Then he was shown to a room on one of the upper floors. He undressed and got into bed. Exhausted, he answered a nurse's questions. He looked up at the ceiling and waited for the interns who, he knew from experience, would do the preliminary work. Marcel DeRudder knew little about artificial hearts and by-pass pumps. But he knew that this time he did not want to be sent home with nothing accomplished, as so often before. He was going to insist on an operation, even if he was told it meant certain death.

Michael DeBakey to Jerry LeBlanc, 1970:

"It was the case that Mr. DeRudder's condition and the process of developing the pump coincided to the extent that we were ready to try and so was he."

A former doctor at Methodist Hospital, 1970:

"It would probably be wrong to say that from the start—that is, after examining the letters from Dr. Ensrud—Dr. DeBakey thought of Marcel DeRudder as a candidate for the first implantation of By-pass Model 66. On the other hand, the letters from the doctor in Champaign had indicated that DeRudder was one of those cases of mitral valve destruction that would almost surely end with death on the operating table, so that the by-pass represented his only chance to survive. Possibly this was the reason DeBakey let DeRudder come to Houston at all. From April 15 to 20, DeRudder was subjected to tests by the cardiologists, among others Dr. Lancaster, so we could obtain a clear diagnostic picture. The results revealed a condition so grave that we all marveled how this man had possessed the vitality to live so long. It began to seem dubious that he would arrive at the operating table alive."

Later the nurses could not recall having had a calmer or more composed patient that whole year than DeRudder.

Silently, without complaint, he put up with everything—all the tests he had been through so often, and others he had never had before. He stared at the ceiling when he was rolled to the X-ray room and when blood samples were taken from him. Now and then he turned his gaze away from the ceiling to the mostly dark blue smocks—in contrast to the green-clad surgeons—of the cardiologists and internists who examined him. He answered their questions about his medical history with far less emotion than in the past. He asked whether he would undergo surgery and looked up at the ceiling again when it was suggested that he be patient. He remained unmoved when he was informed that on Monday, April 18, the doctors would carry out an angiography, an operation dreaded by so many other patients. In a letter to Edna he wrote that on Monday probes would be pushed into his heart and that then the doctors would make their decision. On Monday a nurse wheeled him down the corridors of the second floor. He said nothing when a masked doctor opened an artery in his arm and inserted the cardiac catheter. He did not utter a sound when the X-ray–opaque dye went racing through his body from head to foot, causing the wave of heat that so terrified other patients. He showed some excitement for the first time on Tuesday when a nurse waked him from a doze and called to the other patients: "He's coming." And then DeBakey, accompanied by a team of respectful doctors, stood beside his bed.

The visit was brief. Dr. DeBakey held out his scrubbed hand with its pelt of black hair and said: "I am Dr. DeBakey. I'm glad you are here. We'll do everything we can for you. We plan to operate in a few days, but I want to have a talk with you before we do."

DeBakey returned the following evening and carefully explained to DeRudder the nature of the by-pass pump. He had originally intended to use the pump only if there was danger of the heart's stopping during an operation, he said. But the tests had shown DeRudder's condition to be so serious that the pump appeared to provide his only chance for survival, and if DeRudder consented he would therefore use it at once.

Michael DeBakey to Ronald Bailey and Alix Kerr, 1966:

"There was no doubt in this man's mind he wanted the by-pass."

After the talk with the doctor, Marcel DeRudder seemed immensely relieved. When he was asked whether his family should be informed that he was to be operated on the next day, he shook his head. No, he said, he did not want to upset Edna. Best for her not to know until it was all over. Then he submitted to the routine of surgical preparations: the extensive shaving, the enema, the visit from the anesthetist. Just as calmly, on the morning of April 21 he let himself be wheeled down to the operating wing on the second floor. Other waiting patients lay beside him, and one out of sheer nervousness talked urgently at him. But DeRudder lay silent, observing the bustle around him and, as the moment for the operation approached, looking up at the ceiling with an air of tranquillity.

At 7:30 A.M. on April 21, Operating Room 3 was set to be the stage for a historic event. On a raised platform above the seemingly confused medley of doctors, nurses, tables, machines, and instruments, Ralph Morse, a *Life* photographer, waited to take color shots of this first implantation of a new heart pump. Nearby, sitting on a metal rail, surgical hood and mask covering his face, a movie cameraman aimed his camera at the operating table and at the only part of DeRudder's body not concealed under sterile sheets—his chest. The soft music that sounded from a stereo set—as always in DeBakey's operating rooms—in no way modified the mute tension gripping everyone present.

At 7:30, DeBakey made the first incision. Dr. Jimmy Frank Howell assisted him, and Dr. William Akers, in charge of By-pass Number 66, waited for the crucial moment. By 7:50, DeRudder's chest had been opened. The heart-lung machine took over the work of his heart. The exposed heart was a swollen, discolored, painfully twitching organ, which almost immediately stopped beating as the heart-lung machine superseded it. An incision into the left ventricle revealed the mitral valve. It was mercilessly crippled by calcium deposits and blood clots—few of the innumerable heart valves that DeBakey had seen had been as bad as this one. He removed the clots and the valve tissue, reached out for the Starr-Edwards ball valve that a nurse was holding in readiness, fitted it in, knotted the threads that henceforth would attach it to its new surroundings, and closed the ventricle, with the certainty that it would never beat again on its own without help from the pump.

Almost three hours had passed when, at 10:14 A.M., DeBakey called: "Pump." Akers occupied the spot opposite DeBakey and held in readiness the first plastic tube, which was to connect the pump chamber with De-Rudder's aorta. DeBakey opened the aorta above the place where it left the heart and fitted the lower end of the plastic tube into the opening. Then came the next incision, opening the left atrium of the heart. De-Bakey reached for the second pump tube and connected it to the atrium. It was nearly eleven o'clock when he finished the suture. Akers produced the pump chamber, with its curved, light-colored lid, dark rim, and larger white lower part with protruding stubs for the tubes. DeBakey removed a part of DeRudder's fourth right rib, attached the pump to the tubes, and fitted the pump into the gap between the ribs. By 11:14 it was in its place —a round plastic pot growing from DeRudder's chest, a piece of smoothly polished, cold technology in living flesh.

Akers fastened the compressed-gas tube to the pump and turned his attention to the motor and the switching mechanism which would start the pump going and regulate the tempo of its beats. Seconds later DeBakey removed the connections to the heart-lung machine, and at the same moment Akers switched on the pump, setting the tempo at forty beats per minute. A low hiss was heard; then the pump sucked blood from the atrium. It showed darkly through the plastic lid, and with the first compression stroke was squeezed into the aorta. At the same time DeRudder's heart began to beat—including his distorted and exhausted left ventricle.

It was now 11:18 A.M.—and the pump functioned. DeRudder's heart functioned. His blood pressure rose. His blood streamed through his body.

No one said a word. Morse's camera clicked and clicked and clicked— he wanted to miss nothing of this scene, which the whole world must hail as the fulfillment of an almost too audacious dream.

DeBakey waited. His hand lay lightly on DeRudder's beating heart.

Akers reported that the pump had now taken over 60 per cent of the work of the left ventricle, and that DeRudder's left ventricle had strength enough for the remaining 40 per cent. By 11:34, DeBakey felt sure that the pump was doing the work he had expected of it. He was about to begin closing DeRudder's thoracic cavity.

At that very moment Akers exclaimed through his mask: "I'm not getting any blood." He stared at the lid of the pump. At the same instant DeBakey's hand felt the patient's right ventricle beginning to swell, filling with such a large quantity of blood that it threatened to stop. DeRudder's blood pressure dropped abruptly. The jagged peaks of the electrocardiogram flattened out. DeBakey's hand, trained by innumerable struggles with failing hearts, reacted automatically. It began massaging the heart and forcibly emptying the swollen right ventricle. "Did you see what happened?" he called to the anesthetist, who replied, his face livid: "I don't know. It was so sudden."

Dr. William Akers on May 1, 1966:

"What probably caused this trouble was his right ventricle was so deteriorated and thus not able to handle this increase in blood flow."

Ronald Bailey and Alix Kerr in an eyewitness report,
May 6, 1966:

"DeBakey faced two critical decisions: whether to shut off the by-pass, which might then become unusable if the blood in it started to clot, and whether to take the unusual step of reconnecting the heart-lung machine, which had been dismantled. . . . DeBakey decided instantly and barked out his orders: slow down the pumping rate of the by-pass, but leave it connected; hook up the heart-lung machine. In less than three minutes the machine was in operation again and the patient's blood was being pumped by three different power sources—his own heart, the machine, and the by-pass."

Dr. William Akers on May 1, 1966:

"In all our research in prior months on animals, we had always worked with a healthy heart. In this case . . . we were working with a marginal functioning heart. It emphasized the necessity to be in communication with the total body needs all the time. When the patient's heart weakened a bit thereafter, we took over the load. Any change in his organs we were aware of and adjusted blood flow. . . . You can't automate all this, else you would have an artificial man."

As soon as balance was restored, DeRudder's blood pressure returned to normal, and the electrocardiogram presented its usual jagged appearance. DeBakey let one of the nurses wipe the sweat from his brow and now waited a longer time, after having the heart-lung machine switched off again, until Akers could adjust the pump so that it pumped no more blood than the right ventricle could accommodate. Only then did he close the thoracic cavity.

The incident had done something to the spirits of the team. The mood was muted as DeRudder was wheeled into a room in the intensive-care unit. He was alive and breathing. From an open seam in the long incision the lid of the pump and the gas tube protruded. Under the lid the blood swirled with each beat of the pump, and beside DeRudder stood the apparatus with the twenty-five-pound motor that drove the gas into the pump. Nevertheless—the sense of a historic event and the expectation of a convincing triumph had suffered a blow. A second blow was soon to follow.

DeRudder did not come out of the sleep induced by the anesthesia. Hours passed, but he remained unconscious. He reacted to no stimuli. There seemed little doubt that he had suffered some kind of brain damage.

A friend of Marcel DeRudder's, 1970:

"Edna DeRudder did not hear about the operation until noon on April 21—not from Houston, but from a reporter on the *Chicago News,* who telephoned her. Edna reacted with characteristic fortitude. She said Marcel must have had good reasons for not letting her know, and she was sure he would call her if he needed her. But a few hours later several reporters had tracked her down, and from the way they acted you'd think artificial hearts would soon be on sale in a Houston supermarket."

Edna DeRudder, 1970:

"The phone never stopped ringing after that, and the front of the house was packed with cars. There was never so much excitement around here."

A friend of Marcel DeRudder's, 1970:

"The reporters wanted to find out everything they could about Marcel, the first human being with an artificial heart. They questioned people all over town, and all of a sudden everybody was pitching in and saying what a marvelous person Marcel had been. The newspapers tried to persuade Edna to fly to Houston at their expense and in return give an exclusive account of what was going on at Marcel's bedside. They all expected a triumphant victory for the mechanical pump. The *News* won the race, and on April 22, Edna flew to Chicago and from there to Texas. At the airport she was interviewed and told the reporters what Marcel had last said to her. Then she flew on to Houston, moved into a motel, and went to the hospital.

"Dr. DeBakey had his hands full just keeping Marcel alive. From what I've heard, he didn't go home at all, but spent the night at the hospital to be near Marcel. It's easy to see why. He had staked everything on a success with Marcel. The newspapers were sounding as though thousands of persons would soon be having artificial hearts. And in reality Marcel had not even regained consciousness. Nevertheless, Dr. DeBakey himself brought Edna to Marcel's bed and told her that he would not even be alive but for the pump. Her husband's appearance was a shock to Edna. He lay unconscious in a snarl of tubes and wires. His face was swollen; and there was that plastic potlid protruding from his chest. But in spite of the shock Edna thought that Marcel was breathing easier than in the past. And she believed DeBakey's assurances that now Marcel at least had a chance of a new life.

"That was on April 22. She stayed four or five days, often sitting for hours beside Marcel's bed, although he never once opened his eyes. She had conceived a great admiration for Dr. DeBakey, and in the hospital chapel she prayed for him as well as for Marcel. She told reporters how firmly DeBakey believed that Marcel would recover his health."

A former doctor at Methodist Hospital:

"They were all desperately hoping to bring him around. They removed spinal fluid in order to reduce the pressure on DeRudder's brain. Sometimes that had been effective when heart operations resulted in cerebral damage. But this time it did not help. It was all too likely that during the operation a blood clot had become established in DeRudder's brain—which would mean that the new pump afforded no security against blood clots. DeRudder's kidneys stopped functioning. One of the doctors pointed out that until the operation DeRudder had had high blood pressure. His kidneys might have adjusted to this blood pressure and would not work when the blood pressure was lowered. The pump was run more vigorously to increase the pressure, and the kidneys actually began excreting. The man's body was like a machine that could be regulated by pressing a button. But that was not enough.

"Something must have happened—perhaps changes in the blood of which we were ignorant. So many of the factors reminded us of the death of the Negro three years earlier. The only thing that really functioned was the by-pass pump. Probably it was well that DeRudder could feel nothing. Otherwise he would have had nasty pain, for the thoracic wall is very sensitive and the pump was fairly big. It ran and ran—and was watched continually. Every detectable change in DeRudder's circulation had to be taken into account in regulating the pump.

"That was how it went on April 23, 24, and 25, while the press releases tried to bring out whatever provided the slightest ground for optimism. Then on April 25 hemorrhages in DeRudder's thoracic cavity began. Possibly that, too, was caused by unknown changes in the blood produced by the pump. In any case, there was severe pulmonary blockage, and DeRudder was in danger of suffocation. A tracheotomy was performed and oxygen administered. But on the night of April 25 there was a sudden rupture in the left lung, which had also been damaged by his long illness. The oxygen poured into the thoracic cavity, compressing the right lung, so that it could not take in any more oxygen either, and DeRudder suffocated in seconds. He died at 3:04 A.M. The ghostly part of it was that as DeBakey, utterly exhausted, turned away from the dead man, the pump itself—after 111 hours and 44 minutes—was still running and pumping blood—until Akers switched it off."

A friend of Marcel DeRudder's, 1970:

"Edna heard about Marcel's death in her motel. The Methodist minister from the hospital brought her the news and took her to see her husband for the last time. A few hours later she wrote a letter to Dr. DeBakey thanking him for all his efforts. She told us he said to her that her letter meant more to him than the letters he had received from President Johnson. I don't know whether that was the truth—but anyhow it comforted Edna."

On Wednesday, April 27, Edna DeRudder took her dead husband home. Reporters followed her and the coffin to the airport, and others were waiting in Chicago. To the reporters she repeated what she had said before: "He wanted to be a guinea pig because he didn't want to go on living the way he had to. He wanted to help others." Then she added: "I feel sorry for Dr. DeBakey. He tried so very hard. They all worked so hard."

On Thursday and Friday, while DeRudder lay in Cyril Urbas's funeral home, some 2,000 of the curious came to see him. When the coffin was moved to Trinity United Church, six officers of the Illinois State Police were called in to direct the traffic. Akers came from Houston to represent DeBakey at the funeral. He sat at Edna DeRudder's side while the Reverend Joseph E. Seiler delivered the funeral sermon. Seiler spoke on the theme from the Gospel of John: "Greater love has no man than this—that he lay down his life for a friend." In the past few days, he said, the world had forgotten hatred and prejudice between nations and races to listen to the latest reports from Houston. The prayers that the patient might awaken from his unconsciousness had not been granted by God. But, like DeRudder, Jesus Christ had also laid down his life. God alone knows the meaning of His holy will. Raising his voice, the minister continued: "We meet today in grateful memory of a man who gave his life that others might benefit and enjoy a healthier one than he knew. He gave all so that others might live. . . . He gave up his life that medical science might someday save ours. . . . All that is left is to offer thanks for his life and friendship to God and continue to pray for this dedicated team of surgeons. This death was not in vain. Its legacy means more than money or material goods, for it gives hope to thousands."

Hundreds followed the hearse to Georgetown Cemetery. In death Marcel DeRudder was accorded what he had lacked in life: the recognition and respect of his fellow citizens of Westville; even if it was only for a few months or years, it was as long as man's short memory lasts.

2 / Esperanza del Valle Vásquez

I

A Czechoslovakian surgeon at a convention of East European physiologists, April 27, 1966:

"I had to shudder as I read the last issue of *Life* with its unusual color-photo reportage on the unsuccessful application of an 'artificial heart pump.' The fact that so great a magazine devotes so many pages to the Houston experiment shows the readiness of an anxiety-ridden audience to rush toward everything that promises even the spark of an illusion of longer life. But it also shows with particular clarity the influence of technology upon medicine. . . . For my part, I do not believe for a second that it will ever be possible to replace the human heart, with all its complex physiological connections, by technical apparatus. But born engineer-surgeons like Kolff and DeBakey will not soon abandon the path they have set out on."

Houston Chronicle, *April 27, 1966:*

"The artificial heart pump which aided Marcel DeRudder for more than four and one-half days will be modified and may be used again 'in several weeks,' Dr. Michael DeBakey says. 'I think we have gained considerable knowledge of the pump and established that it was successful. . . . We are proceeding to make modifications [to the pump] as rapidly as possible. . . .' "

Newsweek, *May 30, 1966:*

"In Houston an operation was also performed by a team headed by Dr. Michael E. DeBakey. . . . This time the LVB [left ventricular by-pass] operation aided the failing heart of Walter L. McCans, a 61-year-old retired Navy CPO, for 27 hours. . . . McCans was reported 'awake and responsive' 3½ hours after the operation. The next day, however, physicians detected lung complications and the patient was wheeled back into surgery. The surgeons removed both the LVB and the fluid that was accumulating in McCans's chest. . . . On Friday morning McCans died."

From a letter by Dr. P.M. after a visit to Houston, June 1966:

"DeBakey seems to be having a run of hard luck in his artificial-heart project. His second patient, McCans, died of uncontrollable hemorrhages in the thoracic cavity. For a while it looked as though the first successful by-pass operation would be credited to Adrian Kantrowitz in New York. Kantrowitz's by-pass consists of a simple plastic arc at the aorta, with a pumping membrane that is kept in motion through a tube leading outside. On May 18 he implanted the by-pass in Louise Ceraso, a heart patient who had been bedridden for years, and kept her alive for eleven days. He had hoped that her heart would recover sufficiently so that he could disconnect her from the source of compressed air and—with the by-pass still implanted—send her home; then, if she suffered from cardiac weakness again, she could once more be attached to the source of compressed air and the by-pass reactivated. But Louise Ceraso died three days ago of a blood clot that probably arose in the by-pass.

"DeBakey's team, financed by federal funds (now said to amount to $2 or $3 million), is working at high pressure on improvements. I visited Dr. Liotta, an obsessed engineer-surgeon who to my mind has become so involved in the pump mechanism that he has almost forgotten the problems of human physiology. I also saw Dr. Akers, Dr. Hellums, and the engineer O'Bannon, who is engaged on the pump relay and its regulator. The latest model of the by-pass is no longer to be installed inside the thoracic wall; the pump chambers will now be left outside the chest. Only a Dacron tube leads to the left atrium of the heart. The second tube is introduced into the right subclavian artery. At the same time, efforts are being made to produce an even finer Dacron velour for the inner side, so as to avoid the blood damage that occurred in spite of everything in the cases of DeRudder and McCans."

Newsweek, *August 29, 1966:*

"Last week the Houston surgical team, led by Dr. Michael E. De-Bakey, seemed to have achieved its first success. The patient: a 37-year-old victim of rheumatic heart disease named Esperanza del Valle Vásquez."

II

Her first impressions of America, as Esperanza later said, were of a murder and a horrid large brown cockroach. The roach was on the seat of the cab that took Esperanza and her sister Rosa María from Houston airport to the Methodist Hospital late in the evening of July 18, 1966.

Esperanza del Valle Vásquez came from Mexico City. She was a frail little thing. With her rather angular Indian face marked by prominent cheekbones, her black eyes and black hair, she had once been an exotic-looking girl. In her youth she had been strong-willed, full of naïve Catholic faith mingled with Indian superstitions, with an inflammable imagination and a great capacity for emotion and enthusiasm. Now, though only thirty-seven, she was an emaciated, asthmatic, withered woman, holding her sister's arm for support, terrified by the foreignness of everything around her. Only her emotionality and a spark of her will to live were left to her.

Since she had never left Mexico before and knew not a word of English, the flight to Texas alone had been an ordeal. She had screwed up her courage for it only because the doctor had explained that she must either die of her heart ailment or go for treatment to the Methodist Hospital in Houston. But just as she was leaving she saw the Mexican newspapers with their accounts of a terrible crime in America. Impressionable as she was, the story terrified her and made her think all the more that she was plunging into a hazardous adventure.

What the newspapers described was the brutal killing of eight young women, all nurses in training in Chicago. A sailor named Richard Speck had broken into their apartment. Armed with a revolver and a butcher knife, he had slaughtered one girl after another and escaped. This led Esperanza to imagine that America was full of murderers who skulked about after nurses. One might very well break into the Methodist Hospital where she was going. It was with this very real fear in her mind that she had set out for Houston accompanied by Rosa María, the second oldest of her seven still-living sisters and brothers. Esperanza's mother, Herlinda, had charged Rosa María with caring for Esperanza. For years now the family had known that Esperanza did not have long to live; they felt that nothing on earth could help her unless God performed a miracle. This trip to Texas was a kind of last desperate pilgrimage in quest of such a miracle. For mingled with their religious faith was a faith in modern medicine natural to a family whose members were almost all schoolteachers. And Rosa María was a capable companion toughened by life. At the age of sixteen she had walked miles every day to teach in a neighboring village. Having no books or materials to work with, she had used pebbles to teach the children numbers, and twigs for them to inscribe their letters on the bare earth.

Esperanza del Valle Vásquez's recollections:

"We went into the hospital at midnight and there was no one there. Then I heard something move, like moving furniture, and I was wondering if anybody was stealing something, maybe the patients. Finally we found someone who could tell us where the office was. They asked all the questions and it took a long time. . . . Then they fastened a plastic bracelet to my wrist, with my name on it. I felt that this was my pass to the operation, and I felt sure. I can't describe the sensation I felt when they put the bracelet on me. It was awfully confusing. I was taken to a room on the ninth floor. It was pretty, modern, and very, very clean. . . . My sister had no hotel reservation and the poor thing slept the first night in the television room on a couch."

The first night seemed endless. The hospital room was finer than any Esperanza had ever seen. It was huge, with its own bath, and a bed that could be moved to all sorts of positions by pressing buttons. There was also a speaker system so that she could talk directly to the nurses in their office. She could not understand why she had been placed in such an elegant room, for she knew that she did not have the money to pay for it. Dr. Cesarman, her doctor in Mexico City, had in some miraculous way arranged that Dr. DeBakey would operate on her for nothing and that the hospital would take her without charge.

No one had explained to her that she was being assigned to a new part of the hospital, called the Moody Research Unit because a deceased millionaire named Moody had donated the funds for the establishment of this unit. The rooms were intended exclusively for the care of interesting cases that were to be investigated or on whom novel methods of treatment were to be tried. The reward for the patients who were willing to help advance medical science was free treatment.

Although Esperanza had been given tranquilizers and was by now totally exhausted, she remained restlessly wakeful, listening to the sounds of the hospital or of her own body. From time to time her thoughts drifted to the Chicago murders—she kept looking at the door of her room as though something terrible might enter at any moment. Then again she would feel the irregular beat of her heart, which she had known for so many years—years during which it had seemed to beat with more and more difficulty, until she could barely stand, barely breathe, and went about her work in a beauty parlor with feelings of overwhelming weakness.

At last she hid her face under the blanket like a child and listened to the planes passing overhead—perhaps one or another was flying to

Mexico. Her thoughts drifted back home, to her mother, her sisters, and her son, "Pepe"—José Mineles—who was seven. Then her thoughts leaped back to her own childhood thirty years before in Texcoco, twenty-five miles north of Mexico City. In Texcoco she had been a healthy, happy child—in spite of the tragedy that struck the entire family when she was about eight. Until then they had lived decently, though sparsely, for her mother had another baby almost every year. But her father, Odilon, had always worked hard, and they had not lacked essentials. Her father had been a simple man from a poor family, and her mother's father and brothers, wealthy people with a big house, had never become reconciled to Herlinda's marrying a poor man. After many years of enmity they had finally hired a murderer who killed Esperanza's father.

It had done her mother no good that her brothers were sentenced to twenty years' imprisonment for this crime. Henceforth she had to care for her nine children alone. Esperanza remembered nights when her mother worked and worked at the sewing machine while she and her sisters tried to stay awake in order to keep Mother company, until at last they fell asleep around the machine. She also remembered that they had been too poor to buy school notebooks and had fashioned them out of wrapping paper, or had practiced writing on stones with sticks of wood dipped in mud. It had been a long way to school; often they had arrived soaked to the skin from heavy rains. Yet she had stayed healthy for twelve years, had never even had a cold—until the rheumatic fever struck.

Esperanza herself no longer remembered it, but Rosa María could recall that it had happened in 1941. Esperanza herself remembered only the terrible pain of it—so intense that she had to be carried to the doctor on a blanket. But after a while she had recovered and begun working at the age of fourteen. She had taken the bus from Texcoco to Mexico City, had learned the beautician's trade, and had worked for many years before she found out that the rheumatic fever had crippled her heart and that she would die young.

For many years Esperanza had tried to find help, first resorting to ordinary practitioners and then to the specialists at the *Instituto Nacional de Cardiología*. There Dr. Patricio Benavides had operated on her in January 1956. But she did not even know the nature of the heart operation. All she knew was that it had been a rapid operation—rapid and useless. The effort involved in the simplest actions had increased steadily with the years, and it had been a wonder that she gave birth to Pepe without dying. Then, one day, she had done the hair of an elegant lady who came into the beauty parlor where she worked. The lady turned out to be the wife of Dr. Teodoro Cesarman. After Esperanza had attended to her several times and been unable to conceal her weakness, Señora Cesarman took her to her husband. Seven or eight years had passed since then—that day on which she entered a different world and consulted a doctor who was, she was firmly convinced, the most careful and kindest medical man in the world. For all through these years he had cared for her, had supplied her with expensive new drugs, and had charged virtually nothing. Years ago he had predicted that only a new operation could help her and that she must wait until the right method was found; when the time was ripe, he would tell her.

At first she had been disbelieving, because the first operation had not helped at all. But after three years he told her that the time had come—in the United States doctors were treating her disease with a new kind of operation and she should not wait any longer, for his drugs would not help her indefinitely. But Esperanza was afraid of surgery; she had prayed and prayed that it would not be necessary. Dr. Cesarman understood her feelings and did not give her any ultimatum about going to America. Instead, he told her that the operation could not succeed unless she were convinced in her own mind that it would help, unless she were ready for it. And on the day a few weeks ago when her weight went down to seventy pounds and she was so weak she could barely comb her hair, she had told herself: Yes, I'll do it. I must do it.

She had felt so happy and relieved by her own decision that she went to Dr. Cesarman at once. Then she learned to her horror that the operation in Houston would cost $3,000, which she did not have, and that Dr. Cesarman would first have to see if there were some way to send her to Dr. DeBakey anyhow. Pretty soon he had let her know that she could go to Houston—at no cost.

Dr. Teodoro Cesarman:

"When Esperanza came to me she was a patient with a heart condition that originated from rheumatic fever. . . . A condition like hers depends on scars which the disease leaves on the heart valve. In Esperanza's case the sickness was severe, and she would already have needed an operation when she was eighteen years old. However, at the time facilities for such an operation were not quite adequate enough. She was operated on January 9, 1956, at the *Instituto Nacional de Cardiología*. Soon thereafter her condition worsened again and continued to do so to a point where she did not any more respond to medicine. Her state of health became very poor. She was not sent for another operation right away because . . . she needed more than one valve replaced. Only the new technical invention and experiment offered a possibility for her. When this became available, Esperanza was prepared for the operation. The reason I sent her to Dr. De-

Bakey is not that I feel that only he could do it, but that Dr. DeBakey at this time was the only doctor who was using the heart pump. It was also the only way she could survive the operation. The pump offered possibilities for survival where a person like Esperanza had, in the long run, absolutely no possibility to survive."

Dr. Michael E. DeBakey to Jerry LeBlanc, 1970:

"Mrs. Esperanza Vásquez's case fell into the same category as that of Mr. DeRudder. She had very poor heart function; that is, she was in failure all the time, you couldn't get her out of failure. . . . Her doctor in Mexico City had contacted me and explained the details of the case."

Dr. Michael E. DeBakey in Gazzetta Sanitaria, 1968:

"The cardiac catheter confirmed the diagnosis of grave mitral insufficiency and aortic stenosis, and indicated the necessity of replacing both the aortic and mitral valves. In consideration of the grave operative risk, it was decided to use a left ventricular by-pass with pump."

A former doctor at Methodist Hospital, 1970:

"When Esperanza came to Houston, she was so reduced by cardiac weakness that from the start she was a case for the pump. It was hoped that her relative youth would give her advantages as against DeRudder and McCans and that the pump might therefore succeed in her case.

"DeBakey waited until the beginning of August to give her an opportunity to get used to the foreign surroundings. After the initial failures he was very conscious of how essential it was to achieve a tangible success at last. He was anxious to take every possible precaution. Spanish-speaking nurses cared for Esperanza. DeBakey's wife, who likewise spoke Spanish and who frequently came to the hospital (the only way for her to see a bit of her husband), visited Esperanza several times. The patient's sister, Rosa María, was allowed unrestricted entry to cheer her when she was overcome by homesickness. The one thing that was denied her was a radio on which she could hear Mexican broadcasts. The idea was that after the operation the hospital might have to issue bulletins, and we did not want her hearing reports on her own condition.

"Dr. DeBakey had his usual effect on the patient after his first brief visit. She soon came to regard him, like her Mexican doctor, as a human representative of Divine Providence. Together, they were going to save her. In spite of that faith, however, there were several crises. There was considerable opposition in the medical school and in the hospital itself to further experiments with the by-pass. That opposition came from highly reputable physicians. Against so towering a personality as DeBakey's it hardly emerged openly; but it was there nonetheless. Shortly after Esperanza's arrival in Houston her sister talked with a doctor and for the first time heard details about the by-pass procedure. Frightened by the description, Rosa María asked what he would do in her position. To her surprise, the doctor replied: 'Do you want me to tell you the truth? If it were my sister, I'd pack her up at once and take her back home.' Mrs. del Valle Vásquez likewise received such warnings, but disregarded them; Rosa María thought, probably rightly, that Esperanza had staked too much on this and that to be taken home without anything being done would kill her. But even Esperanza herself, surely expecting an encouraging reply, once asked two doctors what her chances were and received the shattering answer: 'One to ninety-nine.' I imagine that it was only her belief in DeBakey or the influence of her sister that overcame the shock.

"Perhaps some of it was still there when, at the beginning of August, we obtained the usual written permission from the patient for the operation. We tried to explain to her the kind of risky operation it was, and that DeRudder and McCans had died after it. But she wanted to hear no detailed explanation. She showed signs of an almost panicky defense reaction. I am certain that she signed without understanding the by-pass problem—simply because she felt that the more she knew, the more she would think and doubt, and she wanted only to believe."

Esperanza del Valle Vásquez:

"I signed and my sister signed the paper. But when I signed I felt empty inside and was completely overwhelmed. People were still speaking to me, but I didn't hear them any more. I cried and cried. I asked my sister to get a priest for me and to ask him to bring me a crucifix or a holy medal. I wanted to communicate with God. And I also wanted to talk to Dr. Cesarman in Mexico City. I placed a call to him, but he could not be found."

She did not know that Dr. Cesarman refused to take the call because he wanted to avoid any conversations that might stir new doubts and scruples in her after she had signed. In the meantime Rosa María had found the priest of the Church of St. Vincent de Paul, Antonio Morales, a plump, bespectacled man who had come to Houston from Spain only four months before and could talk to Esperanza in her mother tongue.

Esperanza del Valle Vásquez:

"But the priest came empty-handed, and I asked him: 'Where is the crucifix? Where are the medals?' And he said: 'My hands are empty. You don't need any crucifix, you need the faith which you have within you. Nothing else. You will be strong, and it is all in your heart.' And I said: 'Father, but I feel so alone in my heart; I feel so cold in my soul.' He promised to stay with me. . . . And after a while peace came over me, I felt no more pain, and I knew then that I would come back."

A former doctor at Methodist Hospital, 1970:

"The influence of Morales was all the more important because of some unforeseen incidents before the operation. Esperanza was twice fully prepared for the operation and twice taken back to her room. The first time the anesthesia had already been begun and then she was reawakened. The second time she was wheeled back to the ninth floor before the anesthesia had been started. That was the only time her sister lost her self-control and exclaimed: 'Are the rich given first turn at the operating room and the poor have to wait as usual?' As far as I can recall, the reasons were some technical difficulties with the pump at the last moment, which simply couldn't be explained to the patient. The actual operation began on August 8, 1966."

The operation started at 9:30 A.M. that August 8. Although a cameraman was present, the impending operation was kept secret up to the last moment. The film was intended not for the public, but for strictly scientific use.

As in the case of Marcel DeRudder, replacement of the defective heart valves proceeded without incident. The first tube of the new type of pump was implanted in the left atrium of the heart and the second tube connected to the subclavian artery. Finally the pump, which was fastened in a special bandage outside the chest, was connected to the plastic tubes. When the pump was set for about 80 per cent of the desired heart function and began functioning around 12:10 P.M., Esperanza's own heart also began to work. DeBakey switched off the heart-lung machine. That marked the beginning of the period in which the first disaster had taken place in the case of Marcel DeRudder. But nothing untoward happened. The pump and heart worked smoothly together, and the heart continued to beat regularly when DeBakey cautiously reduced the pump performance to 60 per cent, thereby increasing the demands on Esperanza's heart.

After a period of observation, he closed the thoracic wall except for a small incision from which the atrial tube protruded. By 1:00 P.M. the operation was completed.

The first suspense ebbed away, to be followed by a second anxious moment. No one had forgotten the vain attempts to bring Marcel DeRudder back to consciousness. Graciella, a Spanish-speaking nurse, called to the patient to move her hands. Tensely, DeBakey and his entire team stared at the thin, almost transparent hands at the sides of the operating table. Only a few seconds passed; then the fingers moved. Graciella asked the patient to nod—and Esperanza nodded. Fate had been kinder to her than to DeRudder. Her brain centers had suffered no damage.

When, shortly afterward, Esperanza del Valle Vásquez was wheeled into the intensive-care unit and, still dozing, lifted into a bed, she thought she heard a voice close to her ear: "Esperanza, it's me, Graciella." And she thought with an effort: "Oh, God, again they haven't operated." Somewhere deep inside her she had gone into the operation remembering DeRudder's fate and fearing that she would not wake up. Since she was awake now, she thought she had been taken back to her room for the third time without undergoing the operation. But then she heard Graciella say more loudly: "Esperanza, the operation is over."

At that she awoke more fully. She felt tubes in her mouth and in her arms, and something beating in her chest. She could not talk because of the tubes, could not ask what she really wanted to: "Tell me I'm alive. Tell me I haven't died." Instead, she fell asleep again, and awoke for the second time a few hours later. She noticed this time that she was in a room full of machines making odd noises. There were no windows, only artificial light, and many doctors were standing around her, looking down at her or doing something with a piece of apparatus that had many wires leading to her head. Esperanza was sure now that she was alive. Silently she prayed and made a vow: "Dear God, I offer you my pain. All my pain. And I vow I'll not complain about anything no matter how much I suffer. I'll endure it all until I'm well." Then the figures around her changed into distorted shapes and she fell into a deep sleep.

DE BAKEY TEAM IMPLANTS THIRD MECHANICAL HEART.
DE BAKEY TRIES ARTIFICIAL HEART. MEXICAN WOMAN IS PATIENT.
—Houston, August 9, 1966

It had not proved possible to keep the operation secret, even though special guards took care that no unauthorized person approached the part of the intensive-care unit in which Esperanza del Valle Vásquez lay. From the morning of August 9 on, the intriguing words "artificial heart" swept through the headlines and were carried on the radio waves like a noisy messenger from a glorious future world of technology. This time, however, the reports did not distort the reality.

Esperanza suffered the characteristic pain of those who undergo heart operations: the pain of the incision in the thorax, the pain of the tubes, drains, and catheters, of the endless blood samplings, measurements, and injections. Every cough hurt furiously, and somewhere inside her artificial valves clicked and the stream of her blood moved through an equally artificial machine. She suffered from the sunless, electronically controlled atmosphere of the intensive-care unit, which DeBakey's own doctors often called "hell" and which patients who spent long periods there referred to as "the snake pit." But she did not forget her vow and endured without complaint whatever was imposed on her. And that was a great deal. This time the by-pass was obviously doing its duty, as DeBakey had hoped. On August 9 he ventured to reduce its aid first to 50 and then to 40 per cent. On August 10 blood tests showed no blood damage. X rays indicated that her heart, unnaturally enlarged before the operation, was beginning to shrink. Most of the tubes were removed. Esperanza was able to speak and take nourishment on her own. On Thursday, August 11, her heart performance seemed so good that she was allowed to sit up and dangle her feet over the edge of the bed. Shortly afterward she stood up for the first time and was led to a chair.

Tiny, with stooped, bony shoulders, the pump at her chest, her face contracted from the effort and streaming perspiration, she moved foot by foot, while the tube of the pump kept her connected to the compressor and the regulating machinery beside her bed. At that moment half of torment and half of triumph she did not realize that she was the first human being to walk on her own feet while a cable connected her to a machine that kept her heart beating. For a few minutes she sat breathing rapidly, her black eyes looking up at the doctors as if to ask: "Have I done well? Will I live?"

After she had returned to her bed and recovered, DeBakey decided to throttle down the pump still more so that it was performing only 30 per cent of the heart's work. All the tests showed favorable levels. Even the kidney functioning remained normal; there was no sign of the disturbances that had given rise to the suspicion in the cases of both DeRudder and McCans that the pump in some still unexplained manner had been responsible for the loss of kidney activity.

By the afternoon of the fourth postoperative day it seemed that DeBakey's idea of supporting a badly damaged left ventricle with a by-pass pump and slowly returning the natural heart to its normal function was valid.

Houston Chronicle, *August 13, 1966:*

"At 3:45 A.M. today Mrs. Esperanza del Valle Vásquez of Mexico City slept peacefully in her Methodist Hospital bed in Houston unaware that she had made medical history. Beside her, a revolutionary heart pump quietly continued its work."

Then, on the evening of that same day, the picture changed within a few hours. Suddenly Esperanza's blood pressure began to drop, and shortly afterward her kidney excretion diminished. DeBakey, who had kept close to the hospital, was immediately alerted. Here was that mysterious, deadly threat of kidney damage again.

As soon as the trouble appeared, the patient was administered Hydro-Diuril to stimulate kidney activity. But the drug showed no effect. Five hours later, during the night, blood pressure dropped once more, while the pressure in the left ventricle rose, showing that this chamber of the heart, which had seemed virtually recovered, was losing strength. The kidneys almost ceased to function.

Esperanza, waking from a doze, was alarmed to see all the white, blue, and green-clad figures standing around her. She could not say a word. DeBakey's first reaction was to step up the pump performance again, once more trying to normalize the functions of the heart and thus stimulate kidney function. The pumping action was doubled; within a few minutes the by-pass was pumping 800 cubic centimeters of blood per minute instead of 400. Esperanza had a dim inkling that something bad must have happened. But what followed took place with such remarkable speed that she never fully realized how alarmed DeBakey had been and how keenly reminded of the failures with DeRudder and McCans. Only moments passed after the pump had been switched higher before the unnaturally high ventricular pressure dropped, while the blood pressure rose to normal. And just as abruptly the excretion of urine began. The kidneys had resumed their work.

A former doctor at Methodist Hospital, 1970:

"When I think back on this day, it seems to me that for the artificial-heart team it was the happiest and at the same time the most deceptive day since the beginning of their work. When by simply turning a switch you can decide the degree of functioning of a human heart and kidneys—isn't that proof of the possibilities of technological medicine? What was more, apparently the pump itself was not responsible, in some mysterious way, for damage to the kidneys. It was only a matter of adjusting its performance correctly."

The crisis actually passed so quickly and the effectiveness of the pump was proved so unequivocally that everyone involved could not but feel a sense of triumph, albeit mixed with caution. It did not seem necessary to make more than casual mention of the incident in the bulletins issued to the press. By next day the pump performance was slowly reduced again. Esperanza's heart had overcome its weakness and with temporary additional aid from the pump was now once more on the road to recovery.

Houston Post, *August 14, 1966:*

"Mrs. Vásquez . . . surpassed a record here at 3:10 A.M. Saturday when she passed her 111th hour since receiving the device at 12:10 P.M. Monday."

On August 15, Esperanza's recovery apparently continued. She sat up in bed again and for the first time ate roast beef and vegetables. Then, only a few hours later, DeBakey was again alerted—and this time the situation was even more alarming. When he arrived he found Esperanza dramatically changed. She was struggling for breath. A hacking cough threw up reddish masses of mucus. From her sunken chest came rattling noises. The pump shook each time she coughed. Esperanza was only half conscious. Her dark eyes looked around, pleading for help.

Esperanza del Valle Vásquez:

"I had the feeling I was dying. Far away I heard a doctor's voice saying to me: 'Give me your hand, Esperanza, and don't be afraid.' But I couldn't see what they were doing."

Dr. Michael E. DeBakey to Jerry LeBlanc, 1970:

"One night . . . Mrs. Vásquez went into complete pulmonary edema, heart failure, and was ready to die. You see, we didn't have a lot of experience with the left ventricular pump and we didn't know just how much pumping it did, because we were watching her pressure and we were trying to come off the pump slowly. Well, we just raised the pump from 450 cubic centimers to 1,400 cubic centimeters per minute, more than tripled it, and within ten or fifteen minutes she was completely out of failure, and the lung cleared."

A former doctor at Methodist Hospital, 1970:

"Really, it all continued to seem miraculous. Who had ever before been able to pull a patient out of total heart failure with pulmonary edema within a few minutes, just by turning up a machine? Of course, the question remained how often such spells of heart weakness would occur and whether Esperanza's heart would recover, because of the valve repair and the support of the pump, to the point that the pump could be removed again, as planned. But one thing was sure: without the pump she would have died."

Dr. Michael DeBakey in Gazzetta Sanitaria, *1968:*

"The patient's condition improved rapidly. On the ninth day the flow across the pump of the left ventricular by-pass was reduced to 350 cubic centimeters per minute. . . . Progressive reduction of the flow across the pump produced no further rise in the cardiac pressure."

A former doctor at Methodist Hospital, 1970:

"It was as if the heart after the powerful impetus from the pump once and for all became accustomed to the easier working environment that had resulted from the valve operation. On the afternoon of August 18 the pump flow was reduced almost to zero for five hours. Since this had no unfavorable consequences, DeBakey decided to end the pump's support and remove the apparatus. This was done under local anesthesia within barely twenty minutes. The atrial tube remained in the chest so that in an emergency the pump could be connected again. The skin was closed around it. The tube to the subclavian artery and the pump itself were removed, and the patient was taken from the intensive-care unit back to her room. There she was kept under constant observation, so that the first signs of heart failure would be observed."

The day Esperanza returned to her room on the ninth floor, she formed the firm conviction that God had blessed DeBakey's hands. She was still in pain and was ultimately so punctured by injections that not a usable vein could be found in her body. After having kept her vow for so long and never complained, now that the worst seemed over she broke down for the first time and cried. Ashamed that she had broken her vow, she begged the nurses to leave her alone. She wept for a long time. After she had at last composed herself, and while she was still alone, she discovered the switch to the radio set at her bedside. When she pressed a button, she happened to hear her name and a few sentences she did not quite understand. But she gathered that something had been said about a new artificial heart and a miracle that had been performed on her.

Now she knew that out in the world people were talking about her. That was a new and wonderful feeling. The feeling intensified when a nurse told her that DeBakey had slept every night near her room, and that Queen Elizabeth of England had asked for daily reports on her condition.

On August 20, Esperanza got up twice. She ate everything that was given her, though she was pining for Mexican food. On August 22 she walked around her bed without help for the first time. And on that day she discovered directly how famous she actually was and learned that there were many Mexicans in other departments of the hospital waiting eagerly to see her because they hoped to have some share in her miracle and be cured themselves.

Esperanza del Valle Vásquez's recollections:

"The nurse that was sitting beside my bed said: 'Would you mind if I left you for one second? I am so hungry. I would like to get something to eat.' The nurse went out and suddenly the door opened and a man came in whom I'd never seen before. He said to me in Spanish: 'You are a miracle. I am happy I could see you and I am happy I could talk to you.' He ran out again and I never found out who he was.

"After I was allowed to have visitors, people would come in and ask if they could touch me, to see if I was real. Once somebody came in and said: 'Just write a word or two on this piece of paper for my father. He is very ill and I know that if you write something on it, it will give him faith in his recovery, because you are a miracle.' "

On August 23 she wheeled herself in a wheel chair to the X-ray laboratory. As she passed, patients were waiting to hand her flowers. On August 27 she got up by herself and walked about, and a hairdresser came to do her hair. When she looked at herself in the mirror, she saw that she had become a different person—she looked years younger. Two days later she was told that she could leave the hospital on September 6 and return home. She was now so famous that Rómulo O'Farrill, the millionaire publisher of the Mexican newspaper chain *Novedades,* who likewise lay ill in Methodist Hospital, had offered to have her and Rosa María flown back to Mexico City in his private plane. His son would pilot the plane.

Esperanza del Valle Vásquez's recollections:

"I was so happy. I placed a phone call to home and said: 'Mother, I can hear you and I am well and healthy again!' . . . And I ran from room to room in the hospital and I told everyone: 'I am leaving, I am leaving!'"

On the morning of September 6 she put on street clothes for the first time—a cherry-red suit that Rosa María had bought for her. Looking into the mirror, she once again noted how much she had changed. Before she and her sister could get into the car that was to take them to the airport, she was surrounded by reporters. This was her first experience with a press conference. As she tried to answer the reporters' questions, she clasped tightly the hospital's plastic bracelet with her name on it. She wore it like a talisman and said: "I'm always going to wear it. It means more to me than the most expensive diamond bracelet in the world." At the airport, too, she could not escape the reporters. She finally fled to the protection of Antonio Morales, the priest, who had come to see her off. He gave her and Rosa María his blessing, and then Esperanza tripped up the steps to the plane—a few weeks before, two or three steps would have been all she could manage.

Houston Chronicle, September 6, 1966:

"Mrs. Esperanza del Valle Vásquez, who, as far as medical historians know, is the first patient to survive the use of a mechanical heart, flew home to Mexico City today feeling 'very well and very happy.'"

Dr. Michael E. DeBakey:

"With the creation of the left ventricular by-pass we have demonstrated that it is possible to pump blood mechanically for days and weeks, so that the heart is relieved of half of its work. And if the artificial pump can do its work satisfactorily for days, we must be able to prolong its functioning for weeks, months, and eventually years."

The triumph was not limited to Houston. At home Esperanza del Valle Vásquez was given a glorious reception. At times she had the feeling that she had won a world soccer championship for Mexico. Reporters embraced her and told her how proud they were that a Mexican woman had been the first to survive an operation with a mechanical heart. For a while American and Mexican journalists trailed her every footstep. The newspapers carried accounts of her pilgrimage in September to the Church of the Holy Virgin of Guadalupe in Tepayac; of her gains in weight from seventy to ninety and finally to a hundred pounds; of her taking a three-block walk with her son, Pepe, and visiting the market; of her saying: "I feel as if I were born anew," or: "People who haven't passed through a grave illness don't know what life really means," or: "People who suffer understand their fellow men. If everyone suffered a little the world would be in a better state. To me every bit of life, even the smallest, is wonderful."

Twice a week she went to see Dr. Cesarman on the Avenida Hamburgo, not for medical checkups, but simply to see the man who had sent her to Houston. Esperanza began working again; in partnership with her sister Guadalupe she opened a beauty parlor called "Chata."

Esperanza's example inspired other heart patients to seek out De-Bakey. On October 19, one of them, Benjamin Flores, a twenty-six-year-old farmer from the Mexican state of Sonora, was operated on by Dr. DeBakey for a defective aortic valve. Flores was the first person after Esperanza to receive the left ventricular by-pass that had saved her life. Esperanza wept grievously when news came that Flores had died the day after the operation, of kidney failure.

On February 7, 1967, Esperanza returned to Methodist Hospital, again accompanied by Rosa María, for an examination—a full half year had passed since her operation. She was still wearing the hospital bracelet she had been given on July 18, 1966, and would not accept a new one because the old one was the symbol of her second life. She threw her arms around Dr. DeBakey as soon as she saw him. He found that her heart with its new valves and the remaining part of the pump was operating faultlessly.

But on the very day Esperanza left Methodist Hospital again, Arces Héctor Fernández, a thirty-eight-year-old Mexican, also received the by-pass—the second patient after Esperanza—and died with symptoms similar to those of Flores four months before. Of all the six persons who had received the by-pass in one form or another, Esperanza remained the sole survivor.

And she continued to survive. Her life was not one of carefree normality, but the life of a person with two artificial heart valves, undergoing regular checks, having to be constantly concerned about blood clots and red cell damage, under a continuous regimen of drugs with all their side effects. Yet she lived and worked; and after the threat she had lived with so long, her present existence seemed pure happiness.

III

From a letter by Dr. P.M. after a second visit to Houston,
late December 1967:

"The happy survival of Esperanza del Valle Vásquez continues to spur further development of the left ventricular by-pass here. This one undeniable success blots out the fact that the two subsequent by-pass operations ended fatally. Extensive animal experiments, which DeBakey conducted after these two deaths, have cast some light on the probable cause of the fatal kidney failure. The model of the pump that served Esperanza so well has also revealed defects. Fibrin accumulations of irregular thickness occur on the inside, disturbing the flow of blood. In July 1967, therefore, a new by-pass was tested, and on October 26 was implanted in a girl named Marta Acman, from a village in the vicinity of Ljubljana, Yugoslavia. She was suffering from such severe heart valve defects that no one in Europe dared to attempt a valve repair. DeBakey's operation, as he himself put it, 'went beautifully.' This new success of the by-pass has been taken as further encouragement to forge on with the work."

From a letter by Dr. P.M. after a third visit to Houston,
spring 1969:

"In every field of science a single great success can lead to dangerous illusions—that is well known. Unfortunately, this familiar experience has again been repeated.

"I wrote to you in 1967 about the impact that the cases of Esperanza del Valle Vásquez and Marta Acman had upon DeBakey's development of an artificial heart.

"What seemed like success in the case of Marta Acman has meanwhile turned into a sobering disappointment. After a favorable initial phase severe kidney damage appeared. She had to remain hospitalized for some six months. Further reports from Yugoslavia indicate that the kidney disturbances have persisted. She is given only a short time to live. This means that she, too, has been struck by a side effect of the heart pump which was first observed in the case of DeRudder and which has affected all the other patients with the exception of Esperanza. To add to the failures, in March 1968, a few months after the Acman operation, DeBakey's next by-pass patient, a businessman from Pennsylvania, Ralph Thiers, died of liver and kidney failure. The by-pass had kept him going for only thirteen days.

"The fact that out of seven patients undergoing surgery with the assistance of the by-pass only one—Esperanza del Valle Vásquez—has survived has, of course, jolted DeBakey. He now believes that the consistent kidney failures as well as some still obscure blood damage must be attributed to the pump. It would also seem that questions have arisen about the fundamental idea of healing severely damaged hearts by providing temporary pump support for the left ventricle. In such hearts the right ventricle is usually affected also, so that support of the left side alone does not suffice.

"DeBakey has now decided not to undertake any further experiments with artificial heart pumps until the problem of blood damage has been solved. Furthermore, he is creating a new two-chambered pump, thus approaching closer to the ventricular structure of the human heart. At the Baylor Rice Laboratories work is continuing on a whole-heart pump, which, while it will still have to be driven by compressed gas from outside the body, is to be implanted in the chest in place of the natural heart.

"The team has already built the first series of whole-heart pumps of Silastic and Dacron. These pumps consist of two separate chambers, in which a membrane moved by gas pressure does the pumping work. Each chamber terminates at the upper end in a plastic tube and two plastic funnels. Artificial heart valves are placed both at the opening into the tube and in the funnels. In experimental animals this whole-heart pump functions as follows: The animal's heart is removed in such a way that two stems of the atrium along with the ends of the vena cava and the pulmonary veins are left intact. Then the aorta and pulmonary artery are severed. The funnels of the pump are sutured to the stems of the atria and the tubes to the aorta and the pulmonary artery. The familiar compressed-air tubes already used in the by-pass connect the artificial-heart chambers to a compressor outside the animal's body. The speed of the pump can be regulated by a special governor. The inner walls of the pump chambers are coated with Dacron velour, the best material so far discovered for combating blood damage. All in all, the pumps imitate the natural heart's functioning, though still in a relatively crude manner.

"DeBakey now feels that it will be a long time before practical application of the whole-heart pump to human beings becomes a reality. Since his excessive haste in the case of DeRudder, he has more and more adhered to step-by-step advances and eschewed spectacular experiments. He is counting on many years, perhaps a decade, of animal experimentation before enough is known to eliminate all danger of blood clotting, blood damage, and other physiological disturbances. In addition, the technical problems of long-term functioning must be completely solved. Only then, he has said, will experiments on incurable cardiac patients be justified.

"I have the impression, however, that this conservative view is not shared by some of the technicians in his own artificial-heart team. Their feeling is that after the setbacks DeBakey has lost interest, élan, and daring. Ambitious, youthful, and impatient, with the technician's tendency to make light of man's biological complexity, they probably think that De-Bakey has given up on the problem. That is especially true of Liotta. At the end of January he submitted a paper—without DeBakey's knowledge, gossip has it—to the chairman of the American Society for Artificial Internal Organs, hoping to present it at the April meeting of the society in Atlantic City. The paper, entitled 'Orthotopic Cardiac Prosthesis,' described his experiments on ten calves in which whole-heart or double ventricular pumps were implanted for from twenty-four to forty-four hours and then removed from the dead animals. In contrast to DeBakey, he is satisfied by the fact that the interior walls of the pump became coated with a layer of tissue and that the blood showed only the most minor cell damage. On the strength of these facts alone, he proposes using the pump on human beings during open-heart surgery. It is highly significant that he would resort to the pump in cases in which total collapse of the heart occurs on the operating table, so that only a heart transplant might prolong the patient's life. The whole-heart pump would then serve until a donor heart could be obtained.

"In view of the decline of enthusiasm for heart transplantation, this idea sounds somewhat disturbing. For it might seem to warrant short-term experiments on human beings with the available artificial-heart models. The medical technician would argue that, far from imperiling the life of the patient, the temporary implantation of a pump offered the one chance to prolong the patient's life until he could be provided with a living heart. Someone familiar with the situation has assured me that DeBakey would never accept such ideas, let alone permit them to be carried out in practice. It sounded to me like a palace revolution on the part of the impatient clique of technologists."

Domingo Liotta et al. in "Orthotopic Cardiac Prosthesis," January 1969:

"In any case of irreversible cardiac failure, a blood pump must be provided to adequately maintain life pending healing or cardiac transplantation. Thus we have worked at this Center to develop an orthotopic cardiac prosthesis for clinical use. . . . The pump, of impervious Dacron fabric, uses a diaphragm-type design for both right and left ventricles. . . . In ten calves total replacement of both ventricles was carried out for twenty-four to forty-four hours with the animals standing normally. . . . These experiments revealed excellent neo-endocardium formation at the blood pump interface; changes in blood cellular mass were not significant. . . . The first clinical application is envisioned during open-heart surgery in which cardiac function cannot be restored."

Report by Michael E. DeBakey, C. William Hall, J. David Hellums, et al. on trials of biventricular artificial hearts in seven calves from January 30 to March 20, 1969:

TABLE 1. Results of Implantation of Biventricular Artificial Heart Pump in Seven Calves

(Department of Surgery, Baylor College of Medicine)

Calf No.	Date of Implantation	Duration of Experiment	Fate of Calf
4578	1/30/69	59 min	Died on table; technical difficulties.
4576	2/3/69	67 min	Died on table; technical difficulties.
4582	2/13/69	47 min	Died on table; technical difficulties.
4583	2/20/69	50 min	Died on table; rupture of pump diaphragm.
4584	2/24/69	12.5 hrs	Some reflex movement, but calf unable to stand. Rupture of pump diaphragm. Renal failure; no urinary output during last 8 hrs.
4587	3/17/69	8 hrs 25 min	Some reflex movement, but calf unable to stand. Renal failure; no urinary flow. Calf intubated and on resuscitator. Increasing anoxia.
4596	3/20/69	44 hrs	No reflex movement. No urinary output. Calf virtually cadaver from time of implantation. Calf heparinized and given artificial respiration.

April–June, 1969 *Cardiovascular Research Center Bulletin 137*

From these experiments DeBakey concluded that considerable further work would be necessary before any experimentations on man could be undertaken.

3 / Haskell Karp

Los Angeles Herald-Examiner, *April 5, 1969:*

ARTIFICIAL HEART IMPLANT

"Six months ago Dr. Denton A. Cooley said an artificial heart for use in human transplants was three to five years away. Friday night Cooley placed such a device in a 47-year-old Illinois man."

New York Times, *April 5, 1969:*

ARTIFICIAL HEART IMPLANTED IN MAN

"Houston, April 4—The world's first implant of a total artificial heart was performed here today in a three-hour operation by a surgical team under Dr. Denton A. Cooley at St. Luke's Episcopal Hospital. The 47-year-old recipient, Haskell Karp of Skokie, Ill., was reported tonight to be in satisfactory condition."

Thomas Thompson in Life, *April 10, 1970:*

"On the morning of April 5, 1969, DeBakey was in Washington for a meeting of the National Heart Institute. . . . Always a man with a hundred things occupying his mind, he did not read the morning newspaper or listen to the radio. When he walked into the meeting room, he was immediately confronted by colleagues who were hungry for information about the landmark operation that they had heard Denton Cooley had performed the evening before.

" 'What operation?' DeBakey said in effect.

"It was only then that Mike DeBakey learned that Denton Cooley had replaced a critically ill man's heart with a temporary artificial one, the very feat DeBakey had been researching and planning for years."

Haskell Karp, a print shop employee from the small town of Skokie, near Chicago, had read a good deal about Michael E. DeBakey and Denton A. Cooley—their names appeared frequently enough in the newspapers, after all. But he knew little about the medical world of Houston when he set out for Texas in a last effort to save his life.

Haskell Karp was an inconspicuous man of forty-seven with a mustache and horn-rimmed glasses. With his wife, Shirley, forty, and his three sons, Michael, Joel, and Martin, he lived in an apartment on Skokie Boulevard. His father had had a history of what was known as "heart disease" and had died at fifty-seven. He himself had been a traveling salesman until, in 1959, when he was in his late thirties, he was stricken by a first cardiac infarct. He had recovered somewhat, but had been forced to change his occupation and take a less strenuous job. He found one at the Crewdson Printing Company. His new employer was more considerate of Haskell's handicap than is customary in business. But even the relatively easy duties had not spared Haskell a second heart attack in 1966.

Since then he had been in and out of various hospitals half a dozen times for acute heart failure. Finally, in May 1968, a pacemaker had been implanted; by this time the greater part of his heart muscle had been destroyed, as well as the stimulus system that regulates the heartbeat. The pacemaker battery was inserted in the right side of his chest. Night after night Shirley Karp had not been able to sleep for fear that the battery would lose power and Haskell's heart would suddenly stand still. In fact, Haskell had simply grown progressively weaker; the deterioration of his heart muscle apparently could not be checked. Finally his doctor, foreseeing his patient's certain death, got in touch with Denton A. Cooley in Houston and described Karp's case.

Denton A. Cooley to Jerry LeBlanc, 1970:

"Haskell Karp was . . . referred to us by Dr. Albert J. Levine of Skokie, Illinois, a suburb of Chicago. Dr. Levine told me just how sick this man had been. . . . This man was so incapacitated that the mere act of brushing his teeth was enough to give him angina, rapid heart action, make him cold and clammy. . . . Dr. Levine wanted him to come down here and have a heart transplant."

On March 5, 1969, Haskell and Shirley Karp, a small, plumpish, motherly woman, said good-bye to their three sons in Skokie and set out for Houston. Dr. Levine had prepared his patient for the trip as well as he could by giving him a high dosage of digitalis. Nevertheless, Karp suffered considerably on the flight. His pink complexion gave him a deceptive look of health. But anyone who heard his painful breathing would have realized that he was a severely ill person, and the stewardess asked Shirley Karp several times whether she could do anything for her husband.

Haskell Karp was following Dr. Levine's advice and going to Texas because behind him, in Skokie, nothing but death waited. However, he no longer believed that a transplant could make his life more bearable. Whenever some doctor had explained to him, as several had during the past few months, that the effectiveness of the heart drugs and the pacemaker was exhausted and that only a transplant could help him now, Haskell Karp had put up an inward resistance. When he was almost ready to give up any hope, he had read a newspaper article reporting on surgical repair of even acutely ill heart muscles. The article described how surgeons like Cooley had performed such repairs before the rage for transplants swept the world. Cooley had succeeded in excising parts of heart muscles cicatrized by cardiac infarcts and repairing weakened spots in the walls of the ventricles by inserting plastic sections. Since Haskell Karp was only human, with a human craving for hope, he now based new hope on repair to his heart by Cooley.

It was explained to him that heart muscle repair was more difficult and more dangerous than a transplant. No matter—he would be left with his own heart, which was quite another thing from having to live with a foreign heart that one's body was bent on rejecting. All he wanted was to go on a little longer and with less suffering, to live to see his eldest son's wedding in September—Michael was now twenty-two—and beyond that to watch his youngest son, Martin, growing up. And he wanted to believe that if his heart were repaired by Cooley's world-famous hands, he would be granted that little extra time he craved.

After the landing in Houston, the walk through the airport terminal was like going through the antechamber of hell for Haskell Karp. Arrival in St. Luke's Hospital was a relief. He looked up at the mighty scaffolding of the Texas Heart Institute, growing story by story and in Houston already bearing the name "Cooley Tower," and felt a surge of confidence.

Denton A. Cooley to Jerry LeBlanc, 1970:

"When Mr. Karp got here, there had been some bad news about heart transplants at that time. . . . Even Everett Thomas had already died, so this man was aware of some of the bad news and he was disinclined to accept what was necessary for him. . . . He had read some accounts in the newspapers of success in doing tailoring operations on these sick left ventricles, and he wanted to try something like that and keep his own heart."

Denton A. Cooley in the American Journal of Cardiology, *1969:*

"Complete atrioventricular block was identified in the electrocardio-gram recorded on admission, and the ventricle was activated by the pace-maker impulse. . . . Coronary arteriograms revealed severe narrowing of the right coronary artery . . . and complete occlusion of the anterior de-scending and left circumflex arteries, with small collateral arteries supply-ing the myocardium."

Recollections of a Houston newspaper correspondent:

"When Haskell Karp arrived in St. Luke's he had no inkling that Coo-ley was embarking on a new psychological phase and getting ready for a new surgical adventure—even riskier than heart transplantation. After-ward, of course, there were people who considered Karp a poor devil who had fallen into the hands of a totally unscrupulous and ambitious surgical team.

"The wave of heart transplants had carried Cooley out from under the shadow of DeBakey into the world spotlight. But when the wave broke, when hopes turned to disappointments, Cooley looked for new ways to advance into unknown territory. By now the professional journals have more or less filled us in on what happened in and around Cooley between the end of 1968 and March 1969, when Haskell Karp arrived in St. Luke's Hospital. Cooley knew that heart transplants were not living up to their promise. He decided that DeBakey, with his faith in an artificial heart as the more likely solution for the future, might well be on the right track. In November 1968, Cooley, at a congress of surgeons in Chicago, had spoken words that should have made everyone present prick up his ears. In re-sponse to a question about his views on the future of heart transplantation, Cooley had replied that in the future surgeons would have better luck in the struggle against rejection. But then he had added: 'Although at pres-ent I regard heart transplantation as a possible way to save hopelessly sick patients, it seems to me more correct to consider transplantation a step on the way to a more practicable future solution—to an artificial heart.'

"In other words, Cooley was trying to get into the act. However, he had never done any work on the problem of an artificial heart. He was building his Texas Heart Institute, but as yet he had no laboratories, no trained and experienced associates. That is to say, he could not enter this field as quickly as his temperament demanded. On the other hand, De-Bakey at Baylor and Rice universities had a team which had been engaged in this project for nine or ten years. Models of pumps that might sometime in the future take over the work of the entire heart were already in existence.

"Cooley might well tell himself that the team developing artificial hearts was not the private property of DeBakey, but a part of Baylor and Rice universities, and that he himself was likewise a professor at these universities. Consequently, he should have the right to use the team's plastic hearts. But he was aware that this was theoretical. The funds for the team came from the National Heart Institute, whose trust DeBakey had won by his many years of research work. As a latecomer Cooley had little chance of climbing aboard the moving train without submitting to the authority of DeBakey and his more and more cautious scientific program. For a man of Cooley's temperament there could be only one answer: artificial hearts under a program of his own.

"He had about reached this point in his thinking when he learned that some members of DeBakey's team, headed by Liotta, were dissatisfied and impatient with DeBakey's attitude. Around the end of 1968, Cooley got in touch with Liotta. He proposed that Liotta work for him building artificial hearts for clinical tests, and promised that Liotta would have the chance to see more rapid practical application of the artificial heart than would be likely under DeBakey.

"Liotta was aware of Cooley's leaning toward fast, venturesome action. For himself, he saw a chance to escape from DeBakey's restrictions and advance more rapidly toward his goal of early practical tests for the artificial heart. Today it is pointless to discuss who deceived whom. But the allegation has been published, and not denied, that Liotta, lacking suitable laboratories in Cooley's domain, secretly used the laboratories of the DeBakey team and appropriated the preliminary work financed by the National Heart Institute, and developed by several of his former associates, to build three pump models for Cooley. Cooley's contribution consisted of Japanese artificial heart valves, which seemed to him more promising than the valves hitherto used. What was more, Liotta persuaded an engineer of the DeBakey team, William O'Bannon, to copy the compressor and regulator that the team used for its animal experiments. At home, allegedly working in his garage, O'Bannon built the machine at a cost of approximately $20,000. When he delivered it at the beginning of April, he took the precaution of adding an instruction sheet emphasizing that it had been built only for animal experiments."

Washington Star, *August 1969:*

"During March technicians at Baylor put together three of the double-chambered pumps, each consisting of three parts which were made from three hand-cast aluminum molds. . . . Mrs. Susanne Anderson, a plastics technician, . . . was under great pressure from Liotta to complete the job in a hurry. . . . 'The last three pumps I made I knew would not go into animals because Dr. Liotta continued stressing the importance of perfection and continually told me that I would kill someone if the pumps were not perfect.' "

Recollections of a Houston reporter:

"When I consider that, as we now know, the last experiment on a calf in the Baylor laboratories took place on March 20, 1969, and the calf was essentially a cadaver during the entire forty-four hours in which the heart pump was working, the question arises what prompted an audacious but never unfeeling or unscrupulous surgeon like Cooley to implant a pump of the type that had failed in animals in a human being.

"Liotta has been blamed for having given Cooley too optimistic a report—in his own unreserved enthusiasm for the pump. It has been said that after the decline of heart transplantation Cooley wanted to be the first to implant an artificial heart in a human being; that he wanted to push open the door and forestall DeBakey. The story goes that Liotta not only supplied him with the artificial heart, but also suggested that it be used to bridge the gap between a patient's total heart failure on the operating table and the transplant of a donor heart. Liotta is also supposed to have pointed out that such a procedure would avert the charges of unscrupulous experimentation which would otherwise be raised if Cooley removed a patient's heart—even a dying patient's heart—and installed in its place a novel and untested plastic pump in order to study the functioning of the pump until the patient died. I personally cannot judge the issue. Only Liotta and Cooley know what really happened."

Denton A. Cooley's recollections:

"Well, here's the thing. Dr. Domingo Liotta and I had been working with this thing. We'd developed it, put some valves in it, thought it had the best possible function, and had used it in four or five calves. The longest survival we got was forty-four hours. But, nevertheless, we were convinced that it would function longer in a human being. We've had the experience of seeing things which fail in the laboratory being successful in the operating room. That's true of open-heart surgery. It's still no good in dogs or cats, but it's great in patients. We sort of translated those laboratory results into terms of a human being and thought that we could at least keep a man alive for forty-eight hours. That's thirty-six hours in which we ought to be able to get a cardiac donor somewhere. . . .

"Cardiac transplantation was going into disrepute. If it was ever to be tried as a two-stage procedure, this would be it. It seemed to me that this was the justification for doing the operation at that time and on this patient, because we had a backup. We weren't just putting in this mechanical device to see how long the device would work. That would be taking a position that would be difficult to defend. But we had this heart transplant in mind; we knew we could do that; we had patients living nine months on that. . . . Don't think I didn't think a lot about it beforehand, and ponder and deliberate as to what was proper. I came up with the decision that we would go ahead under these circumstances and let the chips fall where they may. . . . We had to try it sometime and here was the ideal patient."

The ideal patient had to be one suffering from irreparable heart disease. If Cooley attempted a conservative heart repair on such a patient and failed, there was only one chance to save the patient's life—even if only for a short time—and that was a heart transplant. But, as experience had shown, a donor could not be had to order. Therefore it could be regarded as an emergency act to implant the artificial heart and preserve the patient's life, meanwhile searching for a donor. Cooley might well have counted on finding such a donor within a short time, for the sensational announcement of the implantation of an artificial heart would help. If this announcement were accompanied by an appeal for a donor heart, a suitable donor would—Cooley assumed—soon turn up and provide him with the opportunity to exchange the artificial heart for a living heart and thus save the patient (surgically, at any rate). If he carried out this program, he would have implanted the artificial heart not for its own sake but to keep a human being alive long enough to receive a heart transplant.

Haskell Karp was that ideal patient. One March day after another passed for him, while Cooley's cardiologists and other specialists put him through the usual tests, taking angiograms and coronary arteriograms. Then one day Cooley appeared at his bedside for the first time. It was like the Day of Judgment for Karp, and he looked up to Cooley as if he were somehow equivalent to the Supreme Judge—who would have the last word, of course, but with whom Karp had to discuss the situation so that the last word would not be "transplant." We do not know what was said on that April 3; but after Denton A. Cooley had spoken in his friendly, open way with Karp, the patient gave up his resistance to a transplant and also consented to a desperate experiment with the artificial heart.

Denton A. Cooley to Jerry LeBlanc, 1970:

"He was a drowning man. A drowning man can't be too particular what he's going to use as a possible life preserver. It was a desperate thing and he knew it."

Henry C. Reinhard, Jr., administrative assistant at
St. Luke's Hospital, 1970:

"I met Karp a day or two before his surgery when it became apparent we were going to operate his condition. . . . I was responsible for making sure he understood what he was about to undergo, and that he sign the consent form. . . . He wanted Dr. Cooley to do it in a more conventional way. Dr. Cooley finally agreed he would attempt it, and explained it to Mr. Karp. In our conversation I'm convinced he understood that if Dr. Cooley attempted the conventional repair and failed, he would die on the table unless some other steps were taken, and in the absence of a human donor it would be necessary to use a mechanical device."

Reinhard spent about twenty minutes with Haskell Karp on April 3. He found him sitting on the edge of his bed and tried joking a little about the rosy color of his face. Karp replied: "Well, I look pretty good on the outside, but I'm sure a mess on the inside." Then he spoke of his firm conviction that Cooley would succeed in repairing his heart. And Reinhard assured him that Cooley would do everything in his power in his attempt at repair. Finally Karp signed his name under the following sentences:
"In the event cardiac function cannot be restored by excision of destroyed heart muscle and plastic reconstruction of the ventricle, and death seems imminent, I authorize Dr. Cooley to remove my diseased heart and insert a mechanical cardiac substitute. I understand that this mechanical device will not be permanent and ultimately will require replacement by heart transplant. I realize that this device has been tested in the laboratory but has not been used to sustain a human being and that no assurance of success can be made. I expect the surgeons to exert every effort to preserve my life through any of these means. No assurance has been given by anyone as to the results that might be obtained."

Denton A. Cooley to Jerry LeBlanc, 1970:

"Here was the ideal patient; it was the ideal time because we could have a backup. Like the space program, they always have a backup—

thank God they do or our boys wouldn't have got back from the moon. Our backup was a heart transplant."

Thus Haskell Karp agreed to the first great adventure in artificial heart implantation. Good Friday, April 4, 1969, was set for the day of the operation. The preparations began at once—and were of an unusual nature.

Not that Cooley modified his ordinary operating program for that day. The operation on Karp was the sixth heart operation of the day. It was scheduled to start at two o'clock in the afternoon. Liotta was ready; three heart pumps of different sizes had been brought from a Baylor laboratory to St. Luke's and readied in Operating Room 1. The compressor and regulating apparatus were set up there. Since he needed an experienced engineer to supervise the installation, he turned to O'Bannon and proposed that he handle this job. The time was favorable. DeBakey was off at a conference of the National Heart Institute in Washington. But O'Bannon refused as soon as he learned that an experiment on a human being was involved. Finally Liotta obtained the help of other engineers—one of them being Sam Calvin, whom he swore to secrecy.

Reinhard, meanwhile, was making further preparations. In order to avoid needless moving of the patient after implantation of the pump, Operating Room 1 was set up as an intensive-care unit. Reinhard hired nine retired policemen to guard the entrances. He also saw to it that thirty-three laboratory assistants, three electrocardiograph assistants, five X-ray technicians, and twenty carefully chosen nurses were available for day and night shifts. To ensure that no electric power failure would stop the heart pump, St. Luke's emergency power supply was placed on alert and three electricians assigned to twenty-four-hour duty. Cooley wanted the operation to be recorded on film. For this purpose two Baylor University photographers were assigned to the operating room. Reinhard also started the search for a heart donor. Six administrative employees and two members of the public relations department were appointed to hold press conferences, to check telephone calls offering donors, and to arrange for the transportation of donors.

Haskell Karp was told nothing about the machinery that had been set in motion all around him. He spent the last hours before the operation with his wife and his son Michael, who flew from Skokie to Houston as soon as the decision was made. Later Karp talked with Nathan Witkin, a St. Luke's rabbi, and told him about the unusual consent form he had signed. But it was clear that he hoped Cooley would be able to preserve his own heart. He asked Witkin to pray for that.

Then he was caught up in the usual preliminaries to surgery, which scarcely gave him time to think until, shortly before two o'clock, he was wheeled into the operating room. A few minutes later he went under, and Cooley, Liotta, and the others began their work, with the cameras clicking. In the first three-quarters of an hour, until the heart was exposed, it was all routine. Only then did the drama begin.

Before Cooley's eyes lay a heart with two-thirds of its muscle hardened by scars and crippled by aneurysmlike changes right into the septum between the ventricles. Cooley did what he had promised Haskell Karp he would do. But from the first incision on it was evidently a hopeless undertaking. Too much of the muscle substance had been destroyed for him to excise it; there was too little healthy muscle to be patched together. Nevertheless, he tried. After an hour he began his attempt to make this remnant of a heart, covered with sutures, begin beating again, as he had done with thousands of hearts in the past. But Karp's heart did not stir, did not even flutter. All that was keeping Karp alive was the heart-lung machine. Here was the hoped-for moment for implanting the artificial heart.

As Cooley severed Karp's aorta and pulmonary arteries and finally the walls of the atria, and lifted the shattered, bleeding heart from the thoracic cavity, excitement gripped everyone present. So far, his procedures scarcely differed from those he had performed on his transplant patients, from Thomas to Willoughby, from Fierro to Everman. But all this was only the prelude to the decisive act.

Liotta handed him the left ventricle section of the plastic device that best matched the size of Karp's heart. Cooley fitted the section in, linked it to the left atrium, took the right artificial ventricle from Liotta's hand, clipped its funnel with his usual deftness, and made the suture. In the "Operative Proceedings" it all sounded like cool routine work:

"The left atrial wall was attached by continuous suture to the Dacron felt atrial component which was trimmed to size. . . . Suture anastomosis —first of the pulmonary artery, then of the aorta—was made to the woven Dacron vascular grafts." Then: "Gas pressure lines were led out from the chest through a subcutaneous tunnel." And finally: "A stable circulation was obtained." Words, without emotion. In reality the suspense mounted steadily throughout the operation, and at the phase described in the last sentence it became almost unbearable. After all, in Calf 4596 the pump had also forcibly established a stable circulation, but there had never been a resumption of real life in the animal or a single reaction from its brain.

Would Haskell Karp return to life? Would his brain indicate by some reflex, by a single movement, that the pump was supplying him with enough blood to live?

Denton A. Cooley to Jerry LeBlanc, 1970:

"Another thrilling moment in my professional career was when Haskell Karp opened his eyes, on the operating table. . . . He opened his eyes and looked around the room. Well, this was just amazing; no one has ever had his heart completely replaced with an artificial device and the circuits have enough normal circulation. The first thing we know when a man opens his eyes is that his brain is functioning. We'd saved his brain, which is the person, after all."

Cooley was not alone in his sense of the uniqueness of this moment.

Henry C. Reinhard, Jr., 1970:

"It was almost incomprehensible to see him lying there and to know that he did not have his own heart in his body, that he was depending on an artificial device. He looked better than many patients postoperatively. The artificial heart had polyethylene tubing that came out of the chest wall and was attached to a pneumatic device at the bedside. . . . If you've ever been in a modern dairy and heard a milking machine, that's what it sounded like, the clicking sound of the pneumatic valves as they open and close."

Recollections of a Houston reporter:

"Cooley came out to a conference, casual as always. Liotta followed. And then Cooley exploded his bombshell—he knew quite well that it was a big bomb. He declared that in the past several months Liotta and he had developed an artificial heart. Whereupon he distributed pictures of it. He added that they had tested it on animals and kept a calf alive on it for forty-four hours. (This sounded strange to me, for I knew Liotta only as an employee subordinate to DeBakey.) Cooley then told us that the whole operation had not been intended as a violent medical shock-troop enterprise to use the artificial heart. Rather, he had entered the operating room intending to perform a heart muscle repair on Haskell Karp. During the operation it had become evident that Karp's heart was so badly damaged that it could not be restarted. Only a transplant could have saved him. But, Cooley continued, we knew what the heart donor situation was. He didn't have any. And so in a desperate attempt to save Karp's life they had resorted to the artificial pump in order to keep him going until a donor could be found.

"The pump was working amazingly well. Karp had awakened like a man with his own heart, and Cooley was hoping that the artificial heart would continue to function for many hours. Of course, no one could predict how long it would go on, and therefore there was now one urgent task: to find a heart donor for Karp. He begged us to do everything we could to publicize his appeal for a heart donor with Karp's blood group, O Rh-positive.

"So that is how the story was published in the newspapers. And on Good Friday and Saturday morning we had the medical sensation of the year: the first human being with a pumping machine inside his chest instead of his own heart. Cooley was leading the pack again, and there was no question about it—we would do everything we could to find a heart donor for Haskell Karp. We were also handed pictures of Karp in his hospital bed."

Meanwhile, Haskell Karp returned to full consciousness. He felt a strange, beating pressure in his chest and tried to make out what his situation was in this room full of machines, doctors, and nurses. The tracheal tube that had been used for anesthesia was still in his windpipe, so that artificial respiration could be swiftly administered if there were any disturbances in his breathing. When Karp tried to talk, he was able to make only indistinct noises. He raised his hand and gestured for paper and pencil. Then he wrote in an unsteady but legible hand: "What kind of operation?"

A doctor explained to him that the planned repair of his heart had proved impossible and that the artificial heart pump had saved his life. With an optimistic smile the doctor added that the pump was working magnificently and that everything was being done to bring a heart donor to Houston.

Karp's color changed and he closed his eyes as if fending off the truth. When he opened his eyes again after an interval, he had composed himself somewhat, with that resignation which had for so long accompanied each stage in his physical decay. He tried to direct his weary eyes, which saw only dimly without his glasses, toward his chest, in which he now felt a strong pulsing pain. That brought home to him the fact that he no longer possessed his own heart, only a machine that was pumping for him and presenting the alarming question of whether it would always cause such pain. If so, he could not hold out long. He had endured an enormous amount of pain, but this was unlike anything he had ever felt. They would have to hurry with that new heart, he thought, so that this harsh, cold, unendurable pain would pass.

At this point he heard a voice asking whether he was in pain. He nodded, felt the prick of a needle, and the pain vanished. So did his thoughts. He awoke again to hear a voice saying to him that his wife could visit him now. Then Shirley was admitted, in sterile clothing, a sterile hood covering her dark hair. Shortly afterward Michael's thin face appeared in the spectators' gallery above the operating room—at least he could see his father from a distance. Since the tube in Karp's throat made him mute, he had to keep to himself what he was feeling. But he pointed to his eyes to signify that he wanted his glasses, in order to see Shirley and Michael better. The glasses were handed to him. Feebly, he waved up to his son. Silently, he extended his hand toward his wife. And now for the first time he saw clearly the tubes, wires, gas bottle, and pumping machinery at the left side of his bed, and the technician—his face half-hidden behind a surgeon's mask—who sat at this machine watching screens and signal lights and moving switches. Later he indicated that he was again feeling pain in his chest. He received another injection and submitted, dozing off once more, to the machine he was now fettered to.

Denton A. Cooley's recollections:

"The word that we needed a donor went out about an hour later to the news media, and we got a call from a little town up here in East Texas, Cleveland, only about seventy-five miles from here. . . . Actually, the donor was dead when they called us. . . . This patient suffered multiple emboli, and probably emboli to the heart as well as to the brain. . . . Anyway, it couldn't be used. It was one of those moments of high expectation and then bitter disappointment."

In order to prepare for the intended heart transplant, Cooley ordered that Karp be given high doses of Imuran. He wanted to start the antirejection treatment as soon as possible, even at the risk that it might be too soon and Haskell Karp would be left without defenses against infection.

The switchboard operators and secretaries who were waiting for word of heart donors kept receiving calls every five or six minutes, some from Canada, Argentina, England, France, and Australia. But these calls were either queries from newspapers and radio and television stations, or offers of donors who couldn't be used. Hysterical and insane persons also telephoned, offering Cooley their living hearts to be implanted in Karp.

The situation grew disturbing when the constant checks on Karp's circulation and blood chemistry began to show creeping and then more and more patently suspicious changes. Whenever Cooley entered the operating room, he could hear the regular, outwardly reassuring sound of the pump; but the technicians running it reported that the pump's performance periodically diminished because resistances to the blood stream were forming in Karp's vascular system. These resistances could not be overcome by forcing larger quantities of carbon dioxide into the chambers of the pump. In some mysterious fashion Karp's blood vessels had narrowed. The narrowing continued until his entire vascular system had been transformed into a network of rigid, hardened pipes.

The cardiologists whom Cooley consulted expressed the fear that the arteries and veins could not endure the harsh mechanical beat of the plastic pump and were fighting it by convulsive contractions. It was also conceivable that other, less mechanical factors lay behind this rigidity of the blood vessels. Perhaps the pump, which had produced so many mysterious changes in the calves, was in man leading to unknown disturbances of the blood which resulted in an abnormal secretion of vessel-contracting hormones.

The cardiologists recommended trying the drug Arfonad, which has dilating effect upon the vascular system. While Haskell Karp lay half awake, immobile, condemned to silence, X-ray technicians with a portable apparatus measured the performance of the pump; X-ray–opaque dyes had been injected into Karp's blood vessels. The vascular rigidity finally yielded to the effects of Arfonad.

Meanwhile, further complications were developing. The hemoglobin content in Karp's blood serum, which indicated the degree of destruction of red blood corpuscles, had been rising steadily from the time the artificial heart took over. Karp was excreting bloody urine. Liotta argued that this condition would improve as soon as the inner walls of the pump became coated with fibrin. He was right about that. But the question of what was happening to Karp's kidneys remained to be answered. Calves, after all, had died of total kidney failure.

On the night of April 4 and in the early hours of the morning of April 5, Karp developed difficulty in breathing. He awoke from his drugged doze and began struggling for breath. The respirator helped this condition. But the laboratory technicians reported that his body was having difficulty diffusing the oxygen it received. Only part of the oxygen was combining with his blood. Perhaps this was similar to what had happened with Calves 6 and 7, which had been artificially respirated toward the end, but whose tissues had nevertheless lost their vitality and died because even the pure oxygen the animals were breathing could no longer make its way to their cells. Shortly afterward the next ghastly symptom appeared: Karp's kidney excretion diminished from hour to hour.

There it was again, the old menace of the deadly effect artificial heart pumps seemed to have upon the renal system—the experience DeBakey had already had with his by-pass pump.

Denton A. Cooley to Jerry LeBlanc, 1970:

"Well, the ensuing three days were rather harrowing for us because we kept hoping, expecting we were going to get a donor and didn't."

On the morning of April 5 the pump itself continued its regular beating. Haskell Karp lay motionless on his back most of the time. He was lethargic or, during his brief waking periods, stared up through his large, dark horn-rimmed glasses at the ceiling. When the respirator and the tube in his windpipe were removed for a while, he said a few words and also drank from a glass his wife handed him. If he was able to put into words the real feelings of a man with a mechanical pump in his chest, either he did not do so because of the effects of the sedatives he received or what he said never penetrated the walls of the operating room to the outside world. The difficulties with oxygen diffusion persisted, and the kidney excretion continued to diminish. When Dr. Robert O. Morgan, the urologist, was consulted, he found almost total anuria, lack of urine production. Intravenous doses of the diuretic drug Mannitol proved ineffective.

Shirley Karp felt that Haskell was somehow suffering inner damage, but she kept her hopes fixed on his good facial color. That seemed to her equivalent to life. She was a devout woman, and although she had also signed the consent form for the use of the artificial heart, she had done so in the hope that it would not be necessary. The longer she listened to the fearfully monotone, soulless noise of the machine, the more she felt how unnatural such a contraption was. When, hour after hour, no donor was found, she asked to be allowed to plead for a heart for Haskell over the radio or through the newspapers. Reinhard's public relations men saw to it that her plea was published in the morning newspapers on April 5.

Plea for a Heart—

Someone—somewhere—please hear my plea. A plea for a heart for my husband. I see him lying there breathing and knowing that within his chest there is a man-made implement where there should be a God-given heart. How long he can survive, one can only guess.

I cry without tears. I wait hopefully. Our children wait hopefully and we pray.

The Lord giveth and the Lord taketh. But the Lord also gave us gifted men —such as Dr. Denton Cooley and Dr. Domingo Liotta, who are instrumental in prolonging life.

Maybe somewhere there is a gift of a heart for my husband. Please—

Millions read or heard this appeal. But more hours passed, and Cooley was no nearer his goal. The heart pump continued to function; there were no signs of technical hitches, no failures of the instruments that measured the pressure in Karp's artificial ventricles, no disturbance of the monitors. Nor was there any rupture of the pump membranes, such as had killed at least one of the calves. It seemed to add up to technological triumph. Yet Haskell Karp's vitality continued to ebb in a manner that escaped all the resources of technology.

Denton A. Cooley to Jerry LeBlanc, 1970:

"Karp didn't know about the difficulties in getting a donor. We assured him we were making every effort . . . and that the next stage of his salvage was on the way."

The public relations staff desperately issued new communications from Cooley and Shirley Karp to the press:

Cooley: "I'm disappointed and somewhat alarmed that we haven't had a donor."

Shirley Karp: "If I myself could give up my heart to my husband I would do it. My husband is a young man. . . . He suffered for ten years already. I think it's time something good happens."

But instead of the hoped-for news of a donor, Reinhard received a telephone call from a hysteric carried away by the idea of a sensational sacrifice for humanity. It came from Atlanta.

"What would you do if I came to Houston, stood over Mr. Karp, and blew my brains out?"

"We'd put you in the morgue."

"You mean you wouldn't use my heart?"

"No, sir. We would not use your heart."

"Well, why not?"

"Because we couldn't do so without the consent of your next of kin."

"Well, they don't give a damn what happens to me. Don't let that bother you. . . . It's my heart. I ought to be able to do as I damn well please with it."

"I'm sorry, sir. I really can't talk to you any longer. . . ."

"That's all right. Don't worry about it. I'm coming to Houston."

Reinhard ordered the guards at the operating room to increase their vigilance. Meanwhile, the day of Sunday, April 6, began. The engineers, doctors, and nurses of the night shift took their places. At the emergency power center technicians spent their second night on alert. Reporters from Chicago were told by a hospital informant that Karp was in a joking mood and had said: "I always was a lousy golfer. But when this is over, I'd like to try golf again." That was the kind of anecdote they needed, as in the transplant era, to eke out their story of a medical miracle and bring a glow of cheer to the credulous millions who followed the case in the papers.

In actuality Haskell Karp was in a limbo between life and death where joking had no place. His kidneys were ceasing to function. Blood tests began to indicate a steady decrease of the blood platelets, which govern the coagulation of the blood. In addition there was a sharp drop in the number of white blood corpuscles, the chief defenders against infection. In X rays dark shadows suddenly showed up in the lower right lobe of the lung.

Recollections of a Houston reporter:

"Cooley must have been blind if he did not realize on Sunday that with every passing hour he was coming closer to a fiasco. If Karp died with the pump in his chest, if Cooley did not at least manage to remove him from the operating table still alive, with a donor heart, the end for which he had implanted the artificial heart—according to his own statement—would not have been attained. He could, of course, argue that no one in the whole country had been willing to offer a dead man's heart for Haskell Karp and that Karp had died on that account. And he might have tried to represent Karp's survival, which had now lasted more than forty hours, as a triumph for his artificial heart.

"On Sunday morning a friend called me from Washington to tell me about the meeting of the National Heart Institute. DeBakey was there and was taken completely by surprise when fellow surgeons told him about Cooley's undertaking. He had already delivered his report to the meeting and evaluated the results achieved by his artificial-heart team. He had not glossed over the fact that all his animal experiments had ended disastrously and that extensive development was still needed before there could be any thought of operating on humans. And then the Karp story had broken.

"Hitherto no one had heard about any research by Cooley in the field of artificial hearts. He was known solely as an advocate of heart transplantation, and his claim that he had developed a plastic heart in the past few months was treated with extreme skepticism. The newspaper pictures of the heart now in Karp's body looked uncannily like pictures of the artificial hearts that DeBakey's team had made, and the mention of Dr. Liotta in the stories raised the suspicion that Cooley had come into possession of an artificial heart in a manner not entirely legal. If that was the case, he had implanted in Karp an artificial heart of the type that had already failed in animals. There was a good deal of talk about a reckless try, solely in the interests of ambition, which would bring discredit on the whole artificial-heart project.

"My friend reported that there were rumors of an official inquiry. If Cooley had actually used a heart developed by DeBakey's team with the aid of funds from the National Heart Institute, he should have abided by the institute's rules, which required successful animal experiments before any trials on human beings could be permitted. Cooley had asked no one for permission, probably because he had known that his request would certainly be rejected. DeBakey himself refused to take any position.

"The whole thing seemed mysterious. But I had no opportunity to ask Cooley for any comment, for events began moving very fast. Early in the afternoon word came that Cooley was extremely depressed. The pump had been functioning now about forty-eight hours, but apparently things were not going well for the patient. Then news trickled out that there was prospect of a donor. Supposedly the donor was in Massachusetts, 1,600 miles distant. It was said that Cooley would charter a jet to bring the donor to Houston."

Barbara Ewan had never heard of Haskell Karp, Denton Cooley, or the artificial heart. Since ten o'clock in the morning on April 6 she had been lying in a coma in General Hospital in the Boston suburb of Lawrence. She was receiving artificial respiration. Her heart was still beating, but it was only a question of time when it would stop.

She was a sturdily built woman of forty whose face, even in unconsciousness, suggested that a hard life had made her stoical; that she had been, as people said, a "tigress." She had had little choice, having been widowed when she was only twenty-two and left to fend for herself and her three daughters, Carol, Gail, and Sharon, with no aid from anyone.

Possibly her responsibilities had been too much for her. In any case, on March 9 she had been brought to Lawrence General Hospital suffering from depression. She was treated with electroshock and after one of the shocks she did not come to. All efforts to bring her out of her coma failed. Dr. Robert Lennon, the chief anesthetist of the hospital, knew that she had suffered cerebral death, although her heart was still beating.

On Saturday, Dr. Lennon had heard Cooley's appeals for a heart donor over the radio, but had not for a moment thought of Barbara Ewan. He took the appeals as just another item in the day's supply of dramatic news. When the appeals were repeated on Saturday night it struck him merely as odd that no donor could be found in the whole country. Not until the early hours of Sunday morning did he relate a radio repeat of Shirley Karp's petition to the dying woman in his intensive-care unit.

Half an hour later he had telephoned St. Luke's Hospital. Cooley himself answered, his voice betraying his nervousness. He listened to Lennon's description of the patient and asked about Barbara Ewan's blood group. Lennon had to look up the blood group in the case history and then call back. Cooley's excitement grew when he learned that Barbara Ewan had the same blood group as Haskell Karp. He begged Lennon to do everything in his power to obtain consent from the relatives and to try to keep his patient's heart going. As soon as he heard that things were in the clear, Cooley said, he would send a jet plane to Lawrence with a team of doctors. Of course Lennon could accompany his patient to Houston. Moreover, there would be room for one of the next of kin in the plane. Lennon must realize, he added, that they were under unusual pressure in Houston; time was running out with fatal rapidity.

It is understandable that this link with Cooley and the prospect of playing a part in what might very well be the outstanding medical event of 1969 acted as a spur to Lennon. He got in touch with Barbara Ewan's family doctors, who knew the situation in her household. Then he talked to Carol, her oldest daughter, who at twenty-two was legally able to act in this matter. Somehow he coaxed her into a quick consent—in any case, toward 5:00 P.M. he telephoned Cooley again and reported that the necessary paper was signed.

That call freed Cooley from a pressure that was becoming almost unbearable. In order to lose no time, Reinhard had already made arrangements with a private VIP airline that commonly undertook charter flights for businessmen. Its chief pilot, Charlie Smith, had frequently transported donors and recipients for Cooley, St. Luke's Hospital, or the Texas Heart Institute—though never before over so great a distance. But the assignment was so urgent that by seven o'clock an eight-seater Lear Jet with Smith and his copilot was ready to start. Because the case was so unusual, the Federal Aviation Agency granted them an air route that ran in almost a straight line from Houston via New York to Lawrence. A few minutes after seven Hudkins Landes and Carol Martinshek, two St. Luke's specialists in intensive care, came on board; they would be able to tend Barbara Ewan during the flight. At 7:12 P.M. a last telephone call reported that Barbara Ewan's heart was still beating. The plane rose from the runway and headed northeast.

Meanwhile Lennon and several other doctors had gathered around Barbara Ewan—not, as had been the case only a few hours before, to wait for her heart to stop beating, but to keep it beating with every means at their disposal. They were informed that the flight time from Houston would be three to four hours. If the same time were needed for the return flight, Barbara Ewan's heart must be kept going for at least nine hours. Carol and her younger sisters, Gail and Sharon, waited in an adjoining room. Carol was shivering, not only because in her state of nerves she had forgotten to wear a coat, but also because she was shaken by doubts concerning her decision. Had she done right in allowing her dying—or, as Dr. Lennon said, her already dead—mother to be flown 1,600 miles so that her heart could be cut out and the life of Haskell Karp saved? She had read about Karp in a newspaper that morning. Outside, the red lights of an ambulance turned steadily; it was waiting to take her mother to the Lawrence airport. And at the airport itself the lights on the runway were waiting for the plane from Texas. Carol had grown up in the technological age. Nevertheless, she felt she was living in some weird and dreamlike world where the dead with still beating hearts were put on board jet planes and flown half across the continent to have their hearts cut out and the bodies returned by air for burial.

At 10:30 P.M. the Federal Aviation Agency reported that the plane from Texas had passed over New York. With favorable tail winds the plane had made some 500 miles per hour and would be landing in Lawrence about eleven o'clock. Barbara Ewan was carried out to the ambulance, only her head emerging from the white swathings. Her rigid face was almost concealed by tubes, bandages, and adhesive tape. Carol followed the ambulance in her car. Later she waited, still shivering and tortured by doubts, near the stretcher, beside which the doctors and technicians kneeled, while the roar of jets from the landing plane grew louder and louder.

Someone called out that Haskell Karp was holding his own and that Barbara Ewan should be transported to Texas as planned. At 12:35 A.M. Carol boarded the plane. The stretcher bearing her mother had been strapped across three seats. Dr. Lennon and the two strangers from Houston were bending over her lifeless form or fussing with unfamiliar apparatus. The plane rolled down the runway—and Carol imagined she could feel her mother's helpless body being shaken. Then they were in the air. Carol was so exhausted that she would have fallen asleep had not excitement kept her wakeful. In front of her the pilot and copilot were talking with Houston. As she picked up scraps of the dialogue she finally realized that they were all engaged on a race with death, and that this flight would become pointless the moment her mother's heart or Haskell Karp's plastic heart in Houston stood still.

She did not know how long they had been flying when the pilot suddenly turned his head. "I'm sorry," he said, "but we have some technical trouble. Our hydraulic has gone out. We are over Louisiana and are going to try to land at an Air Force base."

She was too tired to grasp the full meaning of these words at once. The pilot added: "We need a very long runway because we have to land without brakes. We'll be landing in Barksdale-Shreveport. But we've already ordered another plane from Houston to come to Barksdale. It will take all of you to Houston."

All this was meant to be reassuring. But it reassured neither Lennon nor the specialists from Houston. They were thinking not about the danger to themselves but about whether Barbara Ewan's heart would continue to beat after a hard landing, and how much time would be lost. It was now close to 2:00 A.M.

None of them knew that Barksdale was a base of the Strategic Air Command, where fully fueled B-52 bombers loaded with bombs stood day and night in alertness. As such it was a prime object of military security. But they had little time to think much about the emergency landing; they had to concentrate on maintaining Barbara Ewan's respiration and heartbeat while the pilot headed the machine down. They felt the thump of the wheels on the runway, and then the plane rolled on and on and on. It came to a stop only a few feet from the very end of the long B-52 runway. Instantly it was bathed in the glare of searchlights and surrounded by guards with submachine guns. Wild as it seems, for a moment they all thought they had landed in Cuba. The pilot tried to explain to the guards where they came from and what a strange cargo they had with them. But the guards clambered directly into the plane. Only after they saw Barbara Ewan and the respirator were they willing to believe that the landing was not some fantastic attempt at espionage, but actually a case of transporting a dying woman for Dr. Denton Cooley.

Immediately they all became helpful, though they could do no more than move the plane off the runway. Then a wait that seemed endless began. Lennon could see that his patient's strength was dwindling; in spite of infusions and injections, heart stoppage seemed imminent. It was an enormous relief to hear from the airport control tower that the second plane was already flying toward Barksdale and would land in the next few minutes, and that Haskell Karp, after some sixty hours with the plastic pump in his chest, was still alive.

At last, toward 3:00 A.M., the second Lear Jet appeared in the glare of the searchlights beside their plane. The uniformed guards carried Barbara Ewan to it. The passengers were all so keyed up that they scarcely realized the strangeness of this landing in Barksdale until they were airborne again. Then they once more began counting the minutes until, toward four o'clock, the lights of Houston's Hobby Airport appeared below them, and immediately after the landing three ambulances, sirens howling, drove up to them. Once more they moved the dead woman with her still beating heart, this time into one of the ambulances. Then they raced along the final leg of their journey. But this was still not the last stage. Barbara Ewan's heart began to flutter—then it stopped. Could all this have been for nothing, Landes thought, as he desperately began massaging the heart while the driver stepped on the accelerator. They reached the entrance to St. Luke's.

Denton A. Cooley to Jerry LeBlanc, 1970:

"When they arrived at the hospital door there was a great furor and excitement. We could use the electric defibrillator and restore heart action. We almost lost that donor, after a 3,000-mile journey—with all those harrowing experiences, we almost lost the donor in the last few yards."

As the stretcher with Barbara Ewan on it was carried into the operating wing, the heart pump in Haskell Karp's body completed its sixty-third hour of functioning. If it was to be evaluated only as a mechanical implement, it had justified Cooley and Liotta in their belief that it would work longer in a human being than in an animal. But if Haskell Karp was thought of as a living organism subjected to this great adventure in order to be kept alive, then the pump had hour after hour brought him closer to death. His kidneys were lifeless; his other bodily tissues were bit by bit losing those mysterious biological forces that made them really alive. It no longer mattered that Haskell Karp opened his eyes and nodded when Cooley ran to tell him that a heart donor had just arrived at the hospital and that he could now be given a new natural heart.

Denton A. Cooley to Jerry LeBlanc, 1970:

"When the donor was in the hospital and everything was proceeding along, I told him we're going to get on with the second stage. He nodded his head and seemed quite gratified with that."

Shortly before seven o'clock in the morning Haskell Karp lay on the operating table for the second time within three days, to endure the second exchange of his heart. This was after sixty-three hours of being fettered to the machine, after sixty-three hours with that thrusting pump in his chest, after sixty-three hours during which his body was no more than an immobile shell and his drugged brain could think only hazily. But in waking and half-waking moments he had thought and felt. He had felt fear and resignation, and the pain of awakening after a numbing injection. He had had moments of hopelessness, followed by moments of trust in Cooley, whose pump was keeping him alive, or in a kind of limbo, as he had predicted. Whether or not he had formerly had any faith in a transplant—Cooley had saved him to the extent that this half life was a salvation, and perhaps Cooley would also be right about the transplant and give him back a real life.

At seven o'clock he closed his eyes and dropped into anesthetic oblivion.

Denton A. Cooley in Transactions of the American Society for
Artificial Internal Organs, *1969:*

"On April 7, 1969, when an allograft was available from a donor, general anesthesia was introduced and the sternotomy incision reopened. Adherent thrombus material was removed from the prosthesis, which was well contained in the pericardial space. . . . After initiation of by-pass the energizing system to the prosthesis was stopped. The two units were removed by dividing the suture attachment to the atria and great arteries. The donor heart was . . . attached just as the prosthesis had been. Sinus rhythm was restored by direct current countershock. . . . Respirator assistance was continued while the patient recovered from anesthesia."

The operation lasted until 9:15 A.M. This time an anxious full hour passed before Haskell Karp showed the first signs of returning consciousness. Then he half woke and seemed to be listening as he was informed that it was all over and that he now had a new human heart. When Shirley Karp received the news, she felt a flood of relief. All would be well now, she thought. To the reporters who had been hanging around her for days, waiting for every scrap of information, she declared: "Now he has a human heart again. I feel that he has come back from the dead." She thanked Dr. Lennon, who had watched the operation. She thanked Carol, the donor's daughter, who had waited nearby with tears in her eyes and who was now preparing to fly back north with her mother's heart-less body. She thanked Cooley and Liotta.

Recollections of a Houston reporter:

"Amid all the tumult, people did not realize that the funeral bells were already tolling in the background. Liotta acted as if he had won a great victory. He made statements about the excellent condition of the plastic heart after its removal from Karp's chest. To one of my friends on the *New York Times* he said: 'It looked really wonderful. It had a real fine lining. I believe he could have lived six months with it. I believe it was possible. For longer periods? For two or three years? I don't know if it was that durable.'

"If those words were really his, he was guilty of hubris—the hubris of the medical technologist so concerned with the durability of a piece of plastic that he did not even ask whether Haskell Karp could have endured that piece of plastic for two or three years. Cooley's attitude, as far as I recall, was much more composed. Probably he realized, despite his sanguine temperament, that Haskell Karp was lost and that he himself was lucky to have managed to get the transplant into Karp in the nick of time. Meanwhile, moreover, he had probably heard of the reaction in Washington and among surgeons throughout the country. Fresh reports of sharp criticism were arriving hourly. Word had it that an investigating committee of Baylor University would be looking into the circumstances surrounding the implantation of the artificial heart. Cooley's explanation that use of the pump had been prompted by sheer necessity was more and more being called into question, as well as the value of the whole attempt. Some doctors were asking why Cooley—if he had been convinced that the heart repair in Karp's case would fail and that only a transplant could save him —had not from the first bent all his efforts on finding a donor, without taking the gamble of using the artificial heart.

"The clouds were gathering to a degree that Cooley had never experienced in his hitherto so fortunate career. DeBakey, it was said, was on his way back to Houston. In Methodist Hospital people were talking about Cooley's action as a 'murderous attack on science.' And although Shirley Karp continued to believe all would turn out well, no one else gave Haskell Karp a chance. Rightly so."

Denton A. Cooley to Jerry LeBlanc, 1970:

"He regained consciousness after the operation and talked to us, and then he began to feel the effects of the pneumonia and the blood stream infection."

Denton Cooley and his associates did not know fully what was going on in Haskell Karp's body during the last hours of his life. The tests, X rays, and observations showed only that the pneumonia was spreading with brutal rapidity. They showed that there was no resumption of the destroyed kidney function and that Karp, feverish, dependent on the respirator, finally sank into unconsciousness. It may be that the early doses of Imuran had destroyed his defenses against infection too soon. But that could only have been one factor in a process that—much as one might wish to deny it—was connected with the artificial heart and underlined the bitter lesson that successful technology alone has not yet created life or preserved it.

At two o'clock in the morning on April 8, almost at the same time that the body of Barbara Ewan arrived back in Massachusetts on Eastern Airlines Flight 544, Haskell Karp took his last—artificial—breath.

Recollections of a Houston reporter:

"Shirley Karp brought her husband back to Skokie. He was buried on Thursday, April 10. To the omnipresent reporters she said: 'My husband was already dead when we went to Houston. . . . He would have died at once if they had not used the artificial heart.' She added: 'It was my husband's wish. He had a share in medical progress and made a great contribution to it. Perhaps in the future artificial hearts will be universally used.'

"Possibly such words gave her and her children comfort at this moment. In any case, she knew only part of the truth; she was still under the immediate impact of the drama she had been through, and under the spell of Cooley's personality, arguments, and explanations. Unquestionably she did not understand the harsh comments on Cooley's action by many members of the medical profession. And she surely did not understand De-Bakey's condemnation. For DeBakey asserted that the use of an untested device on a human being was criminal. 'Our aim is to prolong life,' he said. 'What Dr. Cooley did was nothing but a prolongation of dying.'

"Meanwhile, the investigating committee of Baylor University was meeting behind closed doors, for those concerned were anxious not to damage the reputation of the university or reveal anything that would endanger the flow of funds from the National Heart Institute. But enough revelations reached the public to force Cooley into a defensive stance. He said a number of injudicious things—even that he had wanted to forestall a Soviet success with the artificial heart. He resigned from his professorship at Baylor and concentrated on building up his own Texas Heart Institute, which was not subject to outside influences. But Haskell Karp's sad end did not mean the end of his resolve to employ artificial hearts someday. He took Liotta—who was forced to leave the Baylor-Rice team —into the service of the Texas Heart Institute to develop an artificial heart on his own.

"Curiosity, and the struggle to prolong life by means of an artificial heart, proved stronger than the shock of fiasco. In addition to Cooley's new team, DeBakey's group pushed on with other projects. In Salt Lake City, in New York, and in many other cities in the United States and outside it, efforts have not ceased to achieve the dream of an artificial heart. From Salt Lake City, Willem Kolff reported somewhat more than a year after the death of Haskell Karp: 'We have just beaten the world's record of a living being sustained with an artificial heart inside the chest. Ours was a calf which survived sixty-seven hours—three hours more than Cooley's patient, Karp.'"

Postlude

New York Times, *April 17, 1971:*

"The widow of the first man to live with a mechanical heart has filed a Federal court suit asking for $4.5 million in damages in connection with the death of her husband two years ago.

"The defendants include Dr. Denton A. Cooley, the Houston surgeon who has performed 21 human heart transplants. . . . In addition to Dr. Cooley, defendants named in the suit are Dr. Domingo S. Liotta, Sam Calvin, the engineer who operated the mechanical power facilities, and St. Luke's Episcopal Hospital."

Comment by Dr. Wilhelm B. on the reports of Shirley Karp's suit:

"Shirley Karp's lawsuit against Dr. Cooley and Dr. Liotta may surprise Europeans who are not familiar with the bent of many American lawyers to leap at every chance to claim enormous damages. Here a woman who in 1969 countersigned the operation consent form, and who after the unfortunate outcome spoke gratefully of the experiment and of the future of artificial hearts, two years later files a damage suit against the surgeons who implanted the heart. The fickleness of human nature? Grief that has changed to avarice? Surely the answers are not so simple. There can be no doubt that Shirley Karp, too, did not learn of the background to Dr. Cooley's action until some time after her husband's death. And that background, to a simple, medically innocent, and trusting woman, must have seemed totally incomprehensible.

"To those who know the vagaries of the American legal system, the outcome of such a lawsuit remains unpredictable. But in any case a suit of this sort should help prevent more such premature experiments on human beings. It should also have the further effect of helping to guide the development of the artificial heart, still fraught with innumerable problems, into the cautious, long-term track proper for such a novel device."

Index

421